PHARMACOLOGY - RESEARCH, SAFETY TESTING AND REGULATION

AUTHORIZED GENERIC DRUGS

SHORT AND LONG-TERM COMPETITIVE EFFECTS

PHARMACOLOGY - RESEARCH, SAFETY TESTING AND REGULATION

Additional books in this series can be found on Nova's website
under the Series tab.

Additional E-books in this series can be found on Nova's website
under the e-books tab.

PHARMACOLOGY - RESEARCH, SAFETY TESTING AND REGULATION

AUTHORIZED GENERIC DRUGS

SHORT AND LONG-TERM COMPETITIVE EFFECTS

EDWARD R. NELSON
AND
JERRY G. WRIGHT
EDITORS

NOVA BIOMEDICAL
New York

LIBRARY OF CONGRESS CATALOGING-IN-PUBLICATION DATA

ISBN: 978-1-62257-075-1

Published by Nova Science Publishers, Inc. † New York

Contents

PREFACE

Rising health care costs have for many years focused congressional attention upon the development and availability of prescription drugs. Recently, the presence of "authorized generic" pharmaceuticals in the drug marketplace has been the subject of congressional concern. An "authorized generic" is a pharmaceutical that is marketed by or on behalf of a brand-named drug company, but is sold under a generic name. The brand-name firm may distribute the drug under its own auspices or via a license to a generic drug company. The price of this "authorized copy" is ordinarily lower than that of the brand-name drug. Some sources refer to authorized generics as "branded," "flanking," or "pseudo" generics." This book presents an analysis of the innovation and public health issues relating to authorized generic drugs beginning with a review of the procedures through which independent generic drug companies receive government permission to market their products and resolve patent disputes with brand-name firms and consumer welfare.

Chapter 1 - This Report analyzes the competitive effects of authorized generic drugs ("AGs"). AGs are pharmaceutical products that are approved as brand-name drugs but marketed as generic drugs. AGs do not bear the brand-name or trademark of the brand-name drug or manufacturer, but the brand-name and AG products are manufactured to the brand's specifications. In examining competitive effects, the Report looks both at the price and revenue effects of AG competition and at the potential long-term impacts on incentives for generics to challenge patents on brand-name drugs. The Report also assesses the competitive implications of patent litigation settlements in which brand-name companies refrain from offering an AG when the generic company agrees to defer its entry (so-called "pay-for-delay settlements"). For more than a decade, the Commission has expressed concern about brand-name companies paying generics to delay entry. As this Report observes, promises not to compete with generic entrants by marketing an AG are a common form of compensation to generics in such arrangements, and the competitive effects of such promises should therefore be analyzed in the same manner as other forms of consideration paid to generics. Authorized generics have a unique impact during the first six months of generic competition. Under the Hatch-Waxman Amendments, when the first generic (the "first-filer") challenges the brand's patent, the FDA may not approve any additional generic competitors until 180 days after the first-filer launches its product. During that period, because of the absence of competition, both the generic drug price and the first-filer's revenues are significantly higher than they would be when there are additional generic competitors. Congress created this exclusivity as an incentive for generic companies to enter as soon as possible by challenging invalid patents or patents that are not infringed.

Chapter 2 - The practice of "authorized generics" has recently been the subject of considerable attention by the pharmaceutical industry, regulators, and members of Congress alike. An "authorized generic" (sometimes termed a "branded," "flanking," or "pseudo" generic) is a pharmaceutical that is marketed by or on behalf of a brand-name drug company, but is sold under a generic name. Although the availability of an additional competitor in the generic drug market would appear to be favorable to consumers, authorized generics have nonetheless proven controversial. Some observers believe that authorized generics potentially discourage independent generic firms both from challenging drug patents and from selling their own products. These perceived disincentives result from the provisions of the Drug Price Competition and Patent Term Restoration Act of 1984. Better known as the Hatch-Waxman Act, this legislation provides independent generic firms with a reward for challenging patents held by brand-name firms. That "bounty" consists of a 180-day generic drug exclusivity period awarded to the first patent challenger. During the 180-day period, the brand-name company and the first generic applicant are the only firms that receive authorization to sell that pharmaceutical. At the close of this period, other independent generic competitors may obtain marketing approval and enter the market, ordinarily resulting in lower prices for generic medicines.

In: Authorized Generic Drugs
Editors: Edward R. Nelson and Jerry G. Wright
ISBN: 978-1-62257-075-1

Chapter I

AUTHORIZED GENERIC DRUGS: SHORT-TERM EFFECTS & LONG-TERM IMPACT*

Federal Trade Commission

EXECUTIVE SUMMARY

This Report analyzes the competitive effects of authorized generic drugs ("AGs").[1] AGs are pharmaceutical products that are approved as brand-name drugs but marketed as generic drugs. AGs do not bear the brand-name or trademark of the brand-name drug or manufacturer, but the brand-name and AG products are manufactured to the brand's specifications. In examining competitive effects, the Report looks both at the price and revenue effects of AG competition and at the potential long-term impacts on incentives for generics to challenge patents on brand-name drugs. The Report also assesses the competitive implications of patent litigation settlements in which brand-name companies refrain from offering an AG when the generic company agrees to defer its entry (so-called "pay-for-delay settlements"). For more than a decade, the Commission has expressed concern about brand-name companies paying generics to delay entry. As this Report observes, promises not to compete with generic entrants by marketing an AG are a common form of compensation to generics in such arrangements, and the competitive effects of such promises should therefore be analyzed in the same manner as other forms of consideration paid to generics.

Authorized generics have a unique impact during the first six months of generic competition. Under the Hatch-Waxman Amendments, when the first generic (the "first-filer") challenges the brand's patent, the FDA may not approve any additional generic competitors until 180 days after the first-filer launches its product.[2] During that period, because of the absence of competition, both the generic drug price and the first-filer's revenues are significantly higher than they would be when there are additional generic competitors. Congress created this exclusivity as an incentive for generic companies to enter as soon as possible by challenging invalid patents or patents that are not infringed.

* This is an edited, reformatted and augmented version of the Federal Trade Commission, dated August 2011.

Competition from AGs during the 180-day exclusivity period has the potential to reduce both generic drug prices and generic firm revenues. The courts have ruled that 180-day exclusivity does not preclude a brand-name company from entering with its own generic because it already has approval for its product; therefore, it can sell an AG during that exclusivity period.[3] Brand-name companies now frequently launch an AG to compete with the first-filer.

AGs thus have been the subject of controversy. Brand-name companies that offer AGs contend that they are procompetitive – that they make valuable products available to consumers at lower prices than those of brand-name products and provide competition that leads to lower generic prices overall. Some in the generic drug industry, in contrast, contend that AGs harm competition by drawing revenues away from generic firms during the 180-day exclusivity period provided for first-filers that challenge a brand-name company's patents. They caution that this reduces the potential reward available to generics that challenge patents, thereby discouraging patent challenges that facilitate earlier generic competition and reduce prices for consumers. This, the AG critics argue, undermines long-run competition and the goals of the Hatch-Waxman Amendments.

As a first step toward shedding light on this controversy, the Commission in June 2009 issued an interim report that focused on the short-term effects of AGs during the 180-day exclusivity period (the "Interim Report").[4] That report presented an initial analysis suggesting that "consumers benefit and the healthcare system saves money during the 180-day exclusivity period when an AG enters the market, due to the greater discounting that accompanies the added competition provided by the AG."[5] The Interim Report, however, also found that "AG entry significantly decreases the revenues of a first-filer generic company during its 180-day exclusivity period."[6] Apart from a preliminary analysis of the use of AGs in patent litigation settlements, the Commission left most questions of long-term effects – including any possible impact of AG competition on the calculus of generic entry via patent challenges – for exploration in a final report.

This final Report refines the short-term analysis of the Interim Report and expands the analysis to consider long-term effects. It combines information obtained by compulsory process from more than 100 brand-name and generic manufacturers with price and sales data acquired from commercial sources and information gleaned from FDA databases to assess AGs' competitive effects. Moreover, it updates and extends the Interim Report's study of the use of AGs as a form of consideration in patent litigation settlement agreements.

The new analysis finds that, depending on model specifications, competition from an authorized generic during the 180-day exclusivity period is associated with retail generic prices that are 4-8 percent lower and wholesale generic prices that are 7-14 percent lower than prices without authorized generic competition. On average, the retail price of a typical generic drug during the 180-day exclusivity period is 86 percent of the pre-entry brand price without AG competition and 82 percent of the pre-entry brand price when an AG competes. Similarly, the average wholesale price of a typical generic drug during exclusivity, which is 80 percent of the pre-entry brand wholesale price without an AG, falls to 70 percent of the brand price with AG competition. An analysis of authorized generic pricing over the long term provides no evidence that AG prices are higher than prices of other generics, allaying concerns that AGs might be less aggressive competitors.

The new analysis also confirms the Interim Report's finding that authorized generics have a substantial effect on the revenues of competing, generic firms during the 180-day exclusivity period; depending on how the models are specified, they estimate that the presence of authorized generic competition reduces the first-filer generic's revenues by 40 to 52 percent, on average. Moreover, the impact of AG competition on first-filer revenues persists outside of exclusivity. Revenues of the first-filer generic manufacturer in the 30 months following exclusivity are between 53 percent and 62 percent lower when facing an AG.

With regard to long-term incentive effects, the analysis concludes that the reduced revenue stemming from authorized generic competition during 180-day exclusivity has not affected the generic's incentives in a way that has measurably reduced the number of patent challenges by generic firms. Any disincentive effects would likely be experienced in small markets or in situations where the generic had little chance of winning the patent suit anyway. The Report examines a variety of evidence to reach these conclusions.

- Based on economic analysis, revenue lost from authorized generic competition would be most likely to affect decisions to challenge patents on products with small sales.
  - If a challenger anticipates a 50 percent chance of success, an expectation of AG competition could tilt the balance against bringing a patent challenge in markets with brand sales between $12 million and $27 million, a range that accounts for 13 percent of drugs, but given their low sales, approximately one percent of total prescription drug expenditures. AGs, however, are rarely introduced for these small drugs. For the drugs with higher sales that frequently do attract AG competition, AGs may conceivably deter only a narrow range of challenges that the generic believes it will rarely win, meaning that the challenges are unlikely to result in early generic entry even if pursued.[7]
- Considerable evidence suggests that brand-name firms launch authorized generics to preserve their profits following the onset of generic competition. The evidence, however, also reveals that brand-name companies do recognize that authorized generics, when launched, reduce the revenues of generic rivals and could deter future generic entry.
  - Brand-name firm documents frequently note that launching an AG at the time of generic entry increases revenue, but they also recognize that authorized generic competition reduces generic competitors' profits and could discourage future patent challenges. The documents furnish no basis for deeming one rationale more important than the other.
  - Brand-name firm AG marketing practices are consistent with revenue-enhancement following the onset of generic competition and do not suggest a sacrifice of overall profits to discourage generic entry. None of the econometric estimates provided evidence that brand-name firms sacrifice revenues by introducing AGs. Moreover, about two-thirds of the AGs studied were launched after 180-day exclusivity had ended or when no exclusivity had occurred. This does not preclude a disincentive effect for those AGs that *were* marketed during 180-day exclusivity periods, but it does suggest that other explanations for AG marketing should also be considered. Furthermore, almost all AGs marketed during exclusivity continued to be marketed for an extended period. Again, the

pattern suggests that AG marketing provides value to brand-name firms distinct from any potential disincentive effect from devaluing 180-day exclusivity.

- Although none of the generic companies' internal documents expressly discusses authorized generics as a factor in deciding whether to file a particular patent challenge or identifies specific instances when the expectation of an authorized generic dissuaded the company from challenging a patent,[8] some generic companies' internal documents do reflect a general concern that AGs could impact the profitability of patent challenges or suggest that AG competition requires generic firms to better manage their product selection and litigation processes. The document submissions provide no evidence that any firm has substantially abandoned its basic patent-challenge business strategy because of the proliferation of authorized generics. On the contrary, documents submitted by some generic companies question contentions that AGs create significant disincentives to patent challenges. Different generic companies have adopted different business strategies in the face of AG competition, and those strategies appear to reflect how they view AGs and their potential long-term impact.
- Generic companies typically expect authorized generic competition during the 180-day exclusivity period and often build that assumption into their forecasts, which means reducing the expected revenues for the generic challenger.[9] And one company provided an analysis suggesting that this reduction in expected profits had led it to reject or defer filing patent challenges for two products in small markets.
- Finally, despite the presence of AG competition, generic companies have continued to challenge patents, even on brand-name drugs with small markets.
  - From 2003 through 2008, 17 percent of the drugs subject to a first patent challenge had sales below $50 million. The median revenue of drugs subject to a first patent challenge fell during this period, while AGs were becoming common, from $553 million to $131 million.
  - The number of drugs receiving their first Paragraph IV certification approximately doubled between 2003 and 2008.[10]
  - Generic companies' willingness to pursue Paragraph IV challenges when they know that they are likely to share exclusivity with other generic companies indicates that AGs have not deterred generic challenges. The evidence comes from examination of patent challenges for new chemical entities, a category of drugs for which first-filers expect to have to share exclusivity.[11] The percentage of such drugs drawing first-day patent challenges has increased greatly despite the likelihood of shared exclusivity, from 6 percent in 2002 to 73 percent in 2008.

Each category of evidence has its limitations. And each category is consistent with some expected impact on incentives to challenge patents, particularly for drugs in small markets. On the whole, however, whether viewed from the perspective of a break-even analysis drawn from quantitative data, brand-name firm strategic documents and marketing practices, generic firm memoranda and forecasts, or the number of patent challenges observed even for small-market drugs, authorized generics appear not to have substantially altered generic firms' willingness to enter by challenging questionable patents.

While there is little evidence of authorized generic competition affecting the number of patent challenges, there is strong evidence that agreements not to compete with an authorized generic have become a way for brand-name companies to compensate generic competitors for delaying entry. These agreements can be part of "pay-for-delay" patent settlements, which have long concerned the Commission.[12] These agreements involve a brand-name firm compensating a generic and the generic agreeing to delay its entry. One form that compensation can take is the brand's commitment, in exchange for the first-filer's agreement to delay entry, not to sell an AG during the first-filer's 180-day exclusivity period. Because the first-filer's revenue will approximately double absent an authorized generic, its revenues will be much larger by agreeing to delay than if it litigated, won, and faced AG competition. The generic firm benefits from greater profits during its 180-day exclusivity; the brand-name firm benefits from later generic entry; but consumers suffer from delay of generic competition. Because generics often are priced substantially below the price of brand-name drugs,[13] even a few additional months without generic competition can significantly increase overall prescription drug costs.

Settlements in which the brand-name company agrees not to compete with an AG have become commonplace. Between FY 2004 and FY 2010, 39 of 157 patent settlements with first-filer generics (approximately 25 percent) contained such provisions, which have been used with some frequency and have become common in agreements with pay-for-delay provisions.[14] The average delay for the 39 agreements was 37.9 months, and the total market for the drugs involved (an indeterminate amount of which represented consumer harm tied to the practice) exceeded $23 billion. The promise to suppress AG competition – not the AG itself – is responsible for any ensuing consumer harm.

In conclusion, this Report finds that, during the 180-day exclusivity period, competition from authorized generics lowers prices for consumers and lowers revenues for the independent generic competitor. Over the longer term, lower expected profits could affect a generic company's decision to challenge a patent on products with low sales, and one company provided a few examples where it claimed the expectation of an authorized generic led it to reject or delay such a challenge. Overall, however, patent challenges, even on drugs with low sales, remain robust and, by most measures, have increased despite the prevalence of authorized generic competition. Moreover, as a consequence of an authorized generic's significant negative impact on a generic's revenues, some brand-name companies have used agreements not to launch an authorized generic as a way to compensate an independent generic in exchange for the generic's agreement to delay its entry. The frequency of this practice and its profitability may make it an attractive way to structure a pay-for-delay settlement, a practice that causes substantial consumer harm.

1. INTRODUCTION

This Report presents the results of a study undertaken by the Federal Trade Commission on the effects of authorized generic drugs[15] ("AGs") on competition in the prescription drug marketplace. The Commission undertook this study at the request of Senators Grassley, Leahy, and Rockefeller, who asked the Commission to examine "the short term and long term effects on competition of the practice of 'authorized generics,'"[16] as well as Representative

Waxman, one of the co-authors of the Hatch-Waxman Amendments,[17] who requested the FTC to study "the impact of so-called 'authorized generics' on competition in the prescription drug marketplace."[18]

Since their marketing surged beginning in 2003,[19] AGs have been the subject of controversy. Brand-name companies that offer AGs contend that they are procompetitive – that they make valuable products available to consumers at substantially lower prices than those of branded products and provide competition that leads to lower generic prices overall. Some companies in the generic drug industry, in contrast, contend that AGs harm competition by drawing revenues away from generic firms during the 180-day exclusivity period provided by governing statutes for first-filers that challenge a brand-name company's patents, thus discouraging future challenges that would allow earlier generic competition and reduce prices for consumers. Opposition to AG marketing during the 180-day exclusivity period has been voiced in citizen petitions filed with the FDA[20] and raised in litigation.[21] This study seeks to shed light on this controversy by examining the competitive effects of AGs based on substantial data sets obtained from governmental and non-governmental sources and on documentary information produced by brand-name and generic companies in response to compulsory information requests.

This Report substantially extends the analysis presented in an interim report in June 2009.[22] The Interim Report examined two sets of topics: (1) the short-term impacts of AGs on retail prices, wholesale expenditures, and sales quantities; and (2) the use of AGs in patent litigation settlement agreements. Whereas the Interim Report looked at the short-term impacts in terms of weighted and unweighted averages, this Report applies more sophisticated statistical techniques to refine that analysis. This Report then provides a comprehensive look at the long-term impacts of AGs, examining from a variety of perspectives their potential impact on generic firms' incentives to challenge patents. Finally, this Report updates the analysis of patent litigation settlement agreements, highlighting the increasing use of brand-name company commitments not to market an AG as compensation to generic firms for agreeing to defer entry.

I. The Basic Regulatory Framework and the Hatch-Waxman Amendments

The Food and Drug Administration ("FDA") must approve the marketing of all pharmaceutical drugs, both brand-name and generic, in the United States. The Federal Food Drug and Cosmetic Act, as amended by the Hatch-Waxman Amendments, establishes the regulatory framework. Typically, a brand-name drug obtains FDA approval through a New Drug Application ("NDA").[23] A generic drug manufacturer obtains FDA approval through an Abbreviated New Drug Application ("ANDA")[24] in which it is allowed to rely on the clinical data first submitted by the brand-name drug manufacturer to establish the safety and efficacy of the generic drug.

To encourage generic firms to pursue entry as soon as warranted by challenging questionable patents covering brand-name drugs, the Hatch-Waxman Amendments allow generic drug manufacturers, in certain circumstances, to seek FDA approval prior to expiration of claimed patent protection for the corresponding brand-name drug. To do so, a generic drug manufacturer must first submit to the FDA a "Paragraph IV" ANDA[25] in which it certifies that (a) its generic drug will not infringe patents listed in the FDA's "Orange

Book" in regard to the relevant brand-name drug product, and/or (b) that the relevant Orange Book patents are invalid.[26] At that time the applicant must also provide notice of its certification to the NDA filer and any other patent holders, including a detailed statement of why it believes the patent is invalid or will not be infringed.

For ANDAs with Paragraph IV certifications, if the brand-name company files a patent infringement suit within 45 days after receiving the required notice from the generic firm of the Paragraph IV ANDA, the FDA may not approve the generic drug until 30 months after that notice (or until a decision that the patent is invalid or not infringed, if earlier). At that point the FDA may authorize the marketing of the generic drug, and the first-filed Paragraph IV ANDA applicant becomes entitled to 180 days of marketing exclusivity.[27] This exclusivity protects the first FDA-approved Paragraph IV ANDA applicant from competition against other ANDA marketers during the 180-day period, thereby providing an incentive for ANDA applicants to challenge patents on brand-name drugs and to seek generic entry prior to patent expiration.

Some commentators have credited this regulatory framework with helping to foster immense growth of generic drug offerings.[28] In 2009, 74 percent of all U.S. prescriptions reportedly were filled by generics,[29] up from 43 percent in 1996 and only 19 percent in 1984, when the Hatch-Waxman Amendments were enacted.[30] The Generic Pharmaceutical Association ("GPhA"), a trade association comprised of generic drug companies, attributes much of the health of generic marketing to Hatch-Waxman exclusivity, maintaining that "[t]he vast majority of potential profits for a generic drug manufacturer materialize during the 180-day exclusivity period."[31]

The 180-day marketing exclusivity does not, however, preclude competition from an AG. The courts have determined that a brand-name company can market an AG during that exclusivity period because the brand-name company does not need the FDA to approve an ANDA. Instead, the brand-name company can rely on its already-approved NDA.[32] As the practice has become increasingly common, however, it has generated increasing controversy, with some generic companies contending that AGs deprive generic companies of the "true" exclusivity that was contemplated by the Hatch-Waxman Amendments, and brand-name companies defending AGs as procompetitive and consistent with the Amendments. A number of industry and academic studies (discussed below) have reached differing conclusions on the competitive effects of AGs, and various bills have been introduced in Congress to address the practice.[33] It is in this context that the FTC has undertaken this study.[34]

II. The Key Issues Addressed in This Report

Policy discussions surrounding AGs generally focus on opposing short-term and long-term competitive effects: (1) whether, and to what extent, AGs offer consumers a short-term benefit by lowering prices during 180-day exclusivity through competition with the first filer's ANDA-generic drug; and (2) whether, and to what extent, by reducing ANDA-generic revenues during 180-day exclusivity, authorized generics deter future Paragraph IV filings, which then could delay generic entry, diminish generic competition, and reduce consumer benefits from lower-priced generic products.

A number of industry and academic studies have reached varying conclusions. For example, a study conducted by IMS HEALTH on behalf of the Pharmaceutical Research and

Manufacturers of America ("PhRMA"), a trade association composed largely of brand-name firms, concluded that the presence of AGs significantly reduced wholesale prices during the 180day exclusivity period.[35] On the other hand, a study announced by GPhA found that retail price effects of AGs on the same set of drug products were minor, with "the prices faced by most consumers . . . virtually unchanged by the presence or absence of AGs."[36] Another study, funded by PhRMA, concluded that AGs have not deterred patent challenges, citing data showing that the number of Paragraph IV challenges has remained steady.[37] Yet another study, commissioned by PhRMA and submitted to the FTC while this Report was in preparation, concluded that any effects of AGs on patent challenges would be confined to markets with annual sales between $50 million and $110 million.[38]

This Report addresses both the short-term and long-term competitive effects of AGs. With respect to short-term effects, Commission researchers drew upon a considerably larger data set than that analyzed in prior studies in order to enhance reliability of the conclusions and applied a variety of statistical techniques to further refine the results. They took care to isolate the effects of other explanatory variables in addition to AGs. They also broadened the scope of investigation, looking at AGs' effects on wholesale expenditures, as a proxy for the revenues of generic and brand-name manufacturers, as well as prices at both retail and wholesale levels.

With respect to long-term effects, this Report considers whether AGs have deterred patent challenges over time, as their critics have asserted. It examines numerous strains of evidence, including documents from brand-name and generic firms; data regarding the effect of AG marketing on generic firms' revenues and on the sales levels and probabilities of a successful patent challenge needed to break even on, or justify, generic entry via Paragraph IV challenges; and information regarding the frequency and context of Paragraph IV challenges. Each piece of evidence provides insights from a different perspective regarding AGs' potential entry-deterrence effects.

Although discussion generally has been formulated in terms of these short- and long-term competitive effects, the Report presents its analysis within a broader context. Thus, it examines the potential for brand-name firms' AG marketing strategies to serve multiple objectives, preserving a revenue stream following generic entry while reducing the profit opportunities of potential generic rivals. It notes the difficulty of separating these possible objectives when some of the same strategies that create disincentives to patent challenges also yield incremental income without respect to any disincentives. As to the generic companies, the Report describes how firms choose from a package of possible strategies, with some concentrating on pursuing exclusivity periods for their own ANDA-generics and others tending to partner with brand-name firms by marketing AGs. It observes how this choice may affect a generic company's views of AGs.

Finally, the Report examines a different way in which AGs might be used to impair competition. Numerous recent patent litigation settlements combine the brand's agreement not to market an AG in competition with a first-filer generic with the generic's commitment to defer its entry. Such arrangements, though mutually beneficial to the litigating parties, could prolong a brand-name company's monopoly and impose substantial costs on consumers of prescription drugs. The Report examines recent use of these "No AG" agreements, presenting findings regarding their frequency, the duration of periods during which they defer generic entry, and the size of the affected markets.

III. Study Scope and Data Sources

In April 2006 the Commission began the formal process of obtaining authorization for the study. On August 20, 2007, the Commission obtained OMB approval,[39] and in October 2007, under authority of Section 6(b) of the FTC Act,[40] it began service of Special Orders to brand-name, generic, and authorized generic pharmaceutical companies.[41]

Fifty-nine brand-name[42] and 59 generic[43] companies, including all the major firms involved in marketing AG products, were included in the study. Additionally, two AG-only companies – firms that market AGs but do not file ANDAs – also were included. Appendix C lists all companies included in the study. The Commission's Special Orders for the Brand-Name Companies, the Generic Companies, and the Authorized Generic Companies are set out in Appendices D, E, and F, respectively.

Staff identified 119 different oral-solid (tablet/capsule) AG products that were first marketed between January 1, 2001, and December 31, 2008.[44] The Special Orders required the companies to provide detailed data submissions on AGs, as well as the brand-name drugs and ANDA-generics related to the AGs, and information on relevant Paragraph IV filings and 180day exclusivity periods.[45] As described more fully in Chapter 3 and Appendices H and I, staff supplemented this quantitative data with pricing and sales information purchased from commercial sources and also relied heavily on information culled from FDA databases.[46]

Additionally, the Special Orders required the brand-name companies to produce certain categories of preexisting "planning, decisional, or strategy documents" that "evaluated, considered, or analyzed . . . the marketing or possible marketing of an AG or AGs (as a response to current or future generic competition or for other reasons)."[47] The generic companies were subject to a similar request, as well as an additional request for documents reflecting the effects of AGs on the decision to file an ANDA or to make a Paragraph IV certification or on the profitability of ANDA-generic marketing during 180-day exclusivity.[48]

IV. Organization of the Report

The study's detailed findings are presented in the next seven chapters:

- Chapter 2, "An Overview of AG Marketing and Its Relationship to the Exclusivity System," examines trends and industry practices in the marketing of AGs – alternative marketing strategies and key attributes of brand-generic marketing arrangements that may affect the price of an AG and the timing of its presence in the market – and presents basic facts regarding the relationship between AG marketing and exclusivity periods;
- Chapter 3, "Short-Term Impacts of Authorized Generics: Price and Revenue Effects During 180-Day Exclusivity," examines the short-term effects of AGs on retail and wholesale prices and on brand and generic revenues based on quantitative analysis of IMS data;
- Chapter 4, "The Marketing of Authorized Generics: Brand-Name Firms' Objectives and Strategies," describes the brand-name firms' interest in using AGs to maintain an income stream after generic entry has occurred as well as to reduce generic firms'

incentives to enter early via patent challenges and analyzes the brand-name firms' documents and practices for consistency with revenue-enhancement and entry deterrence strategies;

- Chapter 5, "The Marketing of Authorized Generics: Generic Firm Perceptions and Decision-Making," reviews the contemporaneous documents produced by generic companies discussing their concerns with AG competition and the impact of AGs on incentives to challenge brand patents via Paragraph IV certifications;
- Chapter 6, "Long-Term Effects of Authorized Generics: Price, Revenue, and Break-Even Effects," analyzes quantitative data (i) reflecting long-term effects of AGs on retail and wholesale prices and wholesale expenditures and (ii) indicating how AG competition may affect the break-even point – measured, alternatively, in terms of market size and probability of a successful patent challenge – necessary to profitably support generic entry via a patent challenge;
- Chapter 7, "Assessing the Impact of AG Competition from Patent Challenge Data," inquires about the extent to which generic firms have continued to challenge brand-name firms' patents despite the proliferation of AG competition. It presents data on the relationship between patent challenges and sales levels. It also examines generic firms' record of bringing patent challenges under circumstances where they are likely to share exclusivity with other ANDA generics, a setting analogous to sharing exclusivity with an AG; and
- Chapter 8, "The Use of Authorized Generics in Patent Litigation Settlement Agreements," describes the various roles played by AGs in settlement contexts. In particular, the chapter examines the increasingly frequent occurrence of settlements in which a brand-name firm's commitment not to market an AG in competition with an ANDA generic during 180-day exclusivity serves to compensate the generic for deferring entry.

2. An Overview of AG Marketing and Its Relationship to the Exclusivity System

This chapter charts the landscape of AG marketing, describing industry practices and trends that may influence AGs' competitive effects. The overview first considers the extent of brand-name industry marketing of AGs and generic industry participation in their distribution. It then focuses on a central issue regarding AGs: their relationship to the 180-day exclusivity periods granted to ANDA-generic companies.

Consistent with industry reports, the data show that AG marketing surged beginning in 2003, becoming a widespread industry practice around that time. Many brand-name companies distributed AGs, either themselves or through contracts with generic companies. Beginning in 2003, more than half of the 180-day exclusivity periods included an AG. Yet the majority of AGs were not marketed during any portion of a 180-day exclusivity period. Indeed, brand sales level, rather than whether generic entry occurred via exclusivity, appears to have been a key factor in decisions to market AGs. These findings set the stage for analysis of the short- and long-term effects of AGs presented in the chapters that follow.

I. AG Marketing: Trends and Industry Practices

A. The Scope and Time Course of AG Marketing

A total of 119 AGs, each arising from a different capsule or tablet form of a brand-name drug, were launched from 2001–2008.[49] As shown in Figure 2-1, there were few AG launches during the earliest years covered by the study, but, consistent with industry reports, launches surged in 2003 and remained high through 2006. Only seven AGs were launched per year from 2001–2002, but from 2003–2006 the number of launches ranged between 19 and 21 per year. At the same time, the marketing of AGs during 180-day exclusivity periods substantially increased, suggesting the possibility of a new rationale for AG marketing and generating the controversy over AGs.[50]

The increase in 2003 marked a resurgence of interest in AGs arising from several trends in the pharmaceutical marketplace. Although AGs had been marketed during the 1990s, they reportedly were not very profitable, and many companies had abandoned the practice by the end of the decade.[51] One trend that likely contributed to rekindled interest in AGs a few years later was the increase in 180-day exclusivity periods that began at that time.[52]

At the same time, the rate of generic penetration was increasing, with much of the brand share being lost soon after generic entry. This added urgency to the use of AGs as a way for brand-name companies to stem their losses to generic competition and perhaps to reduce incentives for patent challenges by marketing an AG during exclusivity.[53] In addition, rather than incurring the time and expense of buying or developing a generic subsidiary, many brand-name companies began to contract with ANDA-generic companies to market their AGs.[54] The marketing in 2003 of several AGs during 180-day exclusivity, including one with brand sales of more than $2 billion, brought widespread publicity to the practice and the resultant loss to ANDA-generics.[55] Shortly thereafter, both the FDA and the courts affirmed the legality of marketing an AG during 180-day exclusivity,[56] setting the stage for numerous launches from 2004–2006.

Launches fell back to 12–15 per year in 2007 and 2008, however. At least two factors may have contributed. One was a change in the calculation of rebates paid by pharmaceutical manufacturers under the Medicaid Drug Rebate Program, which is intended to ensure that Medicaid pays the lowest price charged by a manufacturer for its drugs. Under Section 6003 of the Deficit Reduction Act of 2005,[57] beginning in 2007 manufacturers were required to include AGs when calculating the "best price" and "average manufacturer price" of brand-name drugs for the purpose of determining rebates. Some public comments submitted in connection with the Commission's study as well as other observers have argued that this requirement will diminish the incentive to market many AGs by reducing the profitability of brand-name drugs with substantial sales through Medicaid.[58]

Another possible cause of the decline could be the increase beginning in 2005 in patent litigation settlements that defer generic entry.[59] Such settlements would also defer the launch of AGs that typically accompanies generic entry.[60] In addition, some settlements that defer generic entry include a promise by the brand-name company not to launch an AG.[61] In 2008, a generic company launched one product that did not face competition from an AG, and the brand was blocked from launching an AG due to a "No AG" provision in a previously negotiated settlement between the brand and the generic.[62]

B. Brand and Generic Industry Involvement in Authorized Generics

The following sections examine industry involvement in two aspects of AGs – the authorization by NDA-holding companies of the marketing of AGs under their NDAs; and the distribution of AGs by companies that may or may not hold the NDAs. Companies that authorize the marketing of AGs under their NDAs are usually, but not always, brand-name companies, as explained below. By contrast, companies that distribute AGs may be subsidiaries or divisions of brand-name companies or external generic marketing partners of brand-name companies. Examination of these marketing patterns provides background for understanding the impact of AGs on industry participants and the differences in companies' views regarding AGs.

In addition, the different marketing patterns might affect brand pricing strategy.[63]

1. Authorization of Generic Drugs by NDA-Holding Companies

The majority of NDA-holding companies included in the study authorized a generic product under their NDAs. As shown in Figure 2-2, 43 companies, about three-fourths of those in the study, distributed or granted rights to distribute AGs pursuant to their NDAs. Most of these companies were brand-name companies, while a few were primarily generic companies or companies with both brand and generic businesses.[64] Most AGs, however, arose from the NDAs of a few large brand-name pharmaceutical companies that have emphasized AG marketing; two companies accounted for 29% of the 119 AGs. Four large companies accounted for 44% of the AGs. Such companies may have developed a reputation for marketing AGs.[65]

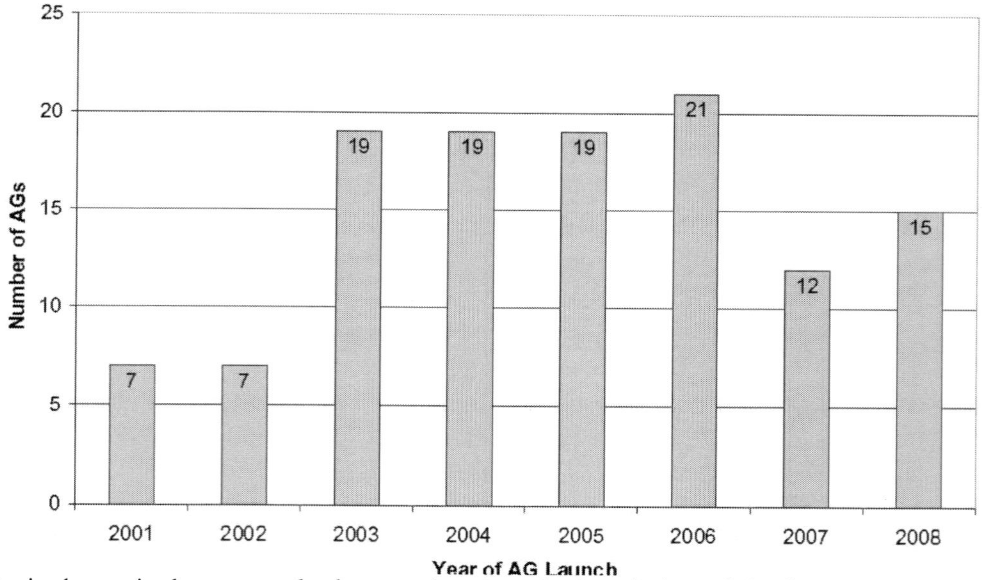

Authorized generic drugs per calendar year, based on the launch date of the first strength that was launched for each drug (NDA). Each NDA is counted only once, even if there were AGs for more than one strength. The figure includes all AGs of "oral solids," including those launched outside of 180-day exclusivity periods as well as those launched during exclusivity.

Figure 2-1. Number of Authorized Generic Drugs Launched.

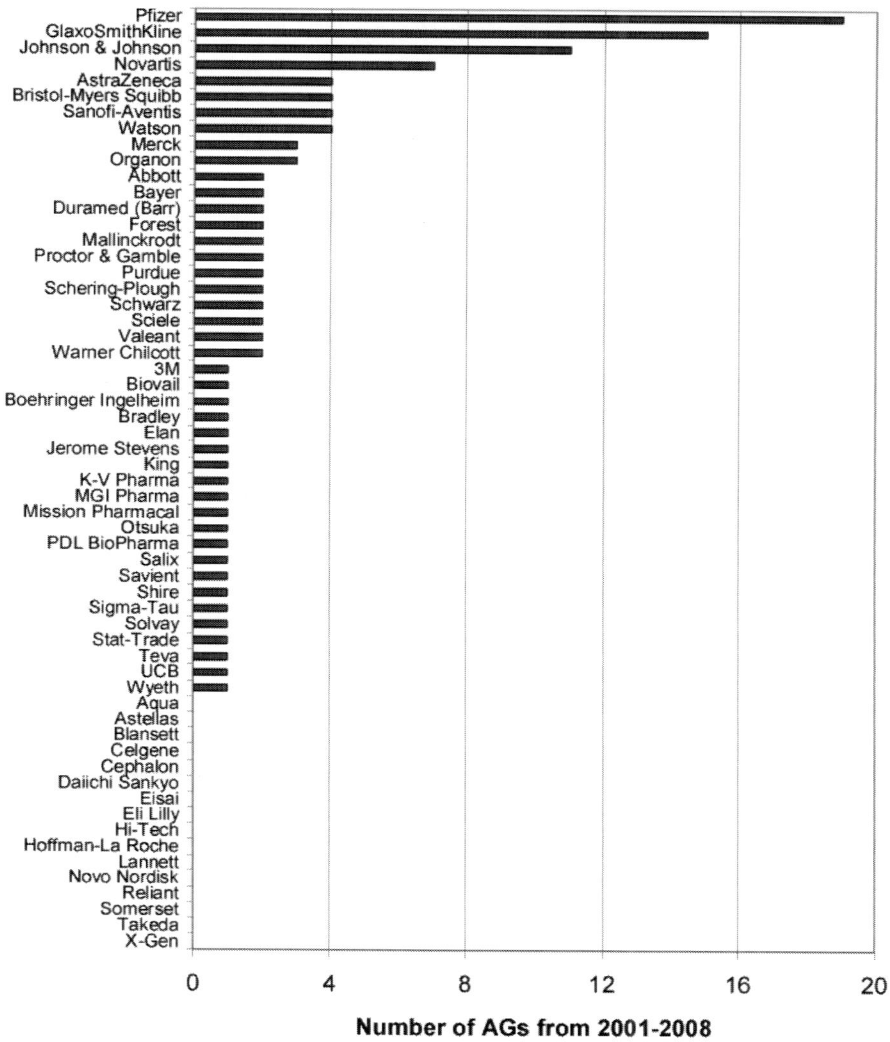

For each company, the graph includes all AGs marketed pursuant to the company's NDAs, whether marketed internally (e.g., by a subsidiary), or through an external generic partner. The figure includes all companies that held an NDA under which an AG shown in Figure 2-1 was marketed, and the other NDA-holding companies included in the study. Most were brand-name companies, but a few were primarily generic or mixed brand/generic companies with rights to market the brand-name drug pursuant to their NDAs. See Appendix H for more information on the categorization of companies.

Figure 2-2. Number of Authorized Generic Drugs per NDA-Holding Company.

Several reasons may explain why about one-fourth of the NDA-holding companies had no AGs. A number of these companies, often small ones, had few or no instances of first generic entry with respect to their brand-name drugs during the period covered by the study. Such companies would have been unlikely to launch an AG.[66] Other companies with no AGs, however, had a number of drugs that experienced generic entry during the study period. Such companies may have relied on strategies other than AGs to address the loss of revenue that occurs with generic entry.[67]

2. Distribution of AGs: In-House Marketing and External Generic Partners

Because brand-name and generic marketing strategies are very different, brand-name companies that authorize generic drugs under their NDAs either enter into distribution and supply agreements with generic companies or develop "in-house" expertise in the strategies and techniques of generic marketing, usually in a subsidiary or division. Brand-name drugs are marketed by emphasizing product differentiation to physicians and consumers and by securing favorable formulary placement with PBMs; such marketing generally drops off following generic entry.[68]

By contrast, generic drugs are commodity products marketed to wholesalers and drugstores primarily on the basis of price.[69] Successful generic marketing may also require consistency of supply and the ability to offer a broad portfolio of drugs.[70]

A breakdown of how the NDA-holding companies distributed AGs is shown below in Figures 2-3 and 2-4. Of the 43 companies listed in Figure 2-2 that had AGs, about a third, listed in Figure 2-3, marketed AGs internally. About two-thirds, shown in Figure 2-4, entered into agreements with outside parties. A few companies marketed AGs both internally and externally, and thus appear in both figures.

a. In-House Marketing

Figure 2-3 shows that a total of fifteen companies marketed in-house 52 AGs arising from the NDAs of their brand-name drugs, approximately 44 percent of the 119 AGs in the study. Ten of these companies were brand-name companies that had generic marketing expertise, usually in a subsidiary or division. These companies marketed 42 AGs arising from the NDAs of their brand-name drugs. Almost half of all AGs marketed in-house were distributed by two brand subsidiaries, Greenstone and Sandoz.[71] Figure 2-3 also includes five primarily generic or mixed brand/generic companies that self-marketed ten AGs for which they held the NDA.[72]

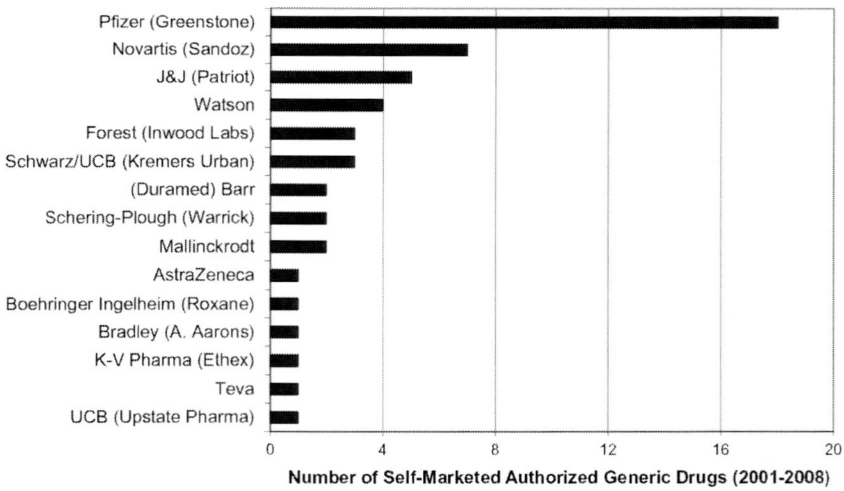

This figure depicts a subset of the NDA-holding companies shown in Figure 2-2, those that distributed AGs in-house. Unlike Figure 2-2, the numbers of AGs shown in this figure include only AGs for which the firm held the NDA and marketed the AG itself, not those marketed pursuant to contract. Subsidiaries are shown in parentheses; the first company listed holds the relevant NDA.

Figure 2-3. NDA-Holding Companies that Distributed Authorized Generic Drugs In-House.

b. Marketing by Contract

i. Brand-Name Companies

While some companies marketed the AGs under their NDAs in-house, about two-thirds, all of which were brand-name companies, imported the necessary generic marketing expertise. As shown in Figure 2-4, twenty-nine brand-name companies marketed a total of 56 percent (67 of 119) of the AGs in the study through arrangements with external generic distributors. Typically, the arrangements transferred only marketing rights, so that the brand-name company retained manufacturing responsibilities.

Although brand-name and generic companies routinely engage in patent litigation, Figure 2-4 shows that most agreements for distribution of an AG by an external marketer did not arise from settlement. Fifty-four of the externally-marketed AGs were distributed pursuant to non-settlement agreements; thirteen were marketed pursuant to distribution agreements that arose from settlements.[73] Of the AGs marketed pursuant to settlements, four were with first-filers of ANDAs with Paragraph IV certifications.[74]

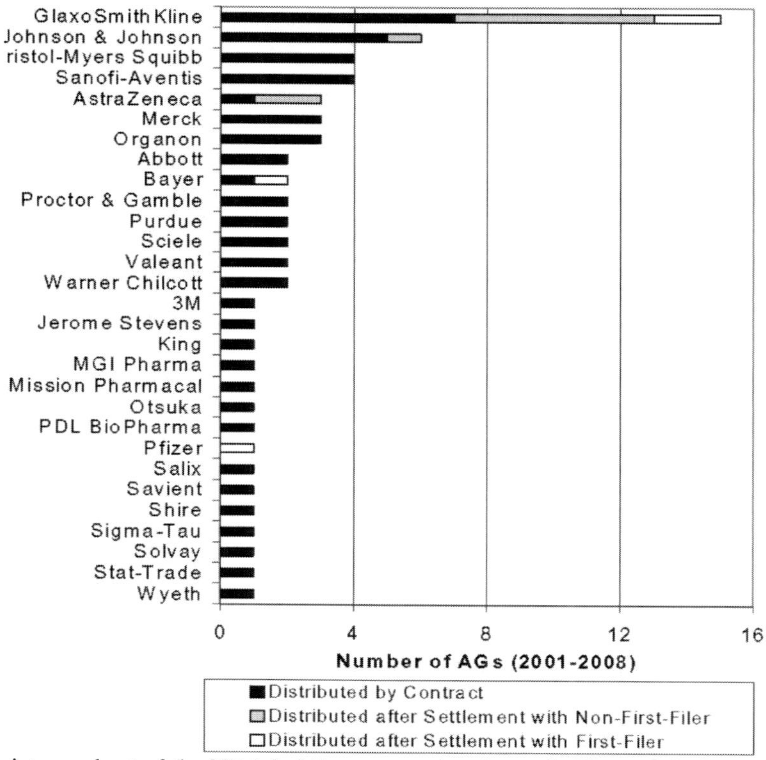

This figure depicts a subset of the NDA-holding companies shown in Figure 2-2, those that distributed AGs by agreement. It counts only AGs for which marketing was by agreement with an external licensee, not those for which marketing was in-house. The categories of agreements are settlements with first filers, settlements with subsequent filers, and non-settlement contracts.

Figure 2-4. Brand-Name Companies that Distributed Authorized Generic Drugs through Agreements with External Generic Companies.

Agreements between a brand-name company and its generic licensee typically are exclusive: the brand agrees that the generic company is the exclusive marketer of the AG. Exclusivity terms may bar competing AG sales by the brand-name firm itself, as well as by other generic marketers.[75] In such cases, the brand may retain the right to market the AG through its subsidiary after the 180-day exclusivity period expires.

The agreements also establish the timing of AG launch. Many agreements provide for launch only after ANDA-generic entry or the date of expected ANDA-generic launch. To ensure that brand sales are not eroded before ANDA-generic competition begins, penalty provisions often apply if the AG marketer launches before generic entry.[76]

ii. External Generic Licensees of Brand-Name Companies

Most ANDA-generic companies do not market AGs. As shown in Figure 2-5, only 21 generic companies, about one-third of the 59 ANDA-generic and two AG companies in the study, entered into agreements with the brand-name companies shown in Figure 2-4 to distribute 67 AGs. Of the 21 companies, three were responsible for more than half of the AGs marketed pursuant to agreement.

Like the 40 generic companies in the study that did not market AGs, the primary business of most external AG marketing partners involves filing ANDAs and marketing ANDA-generic products.[77] Only one of the outside marketers specialized in distributing AGs.[78]

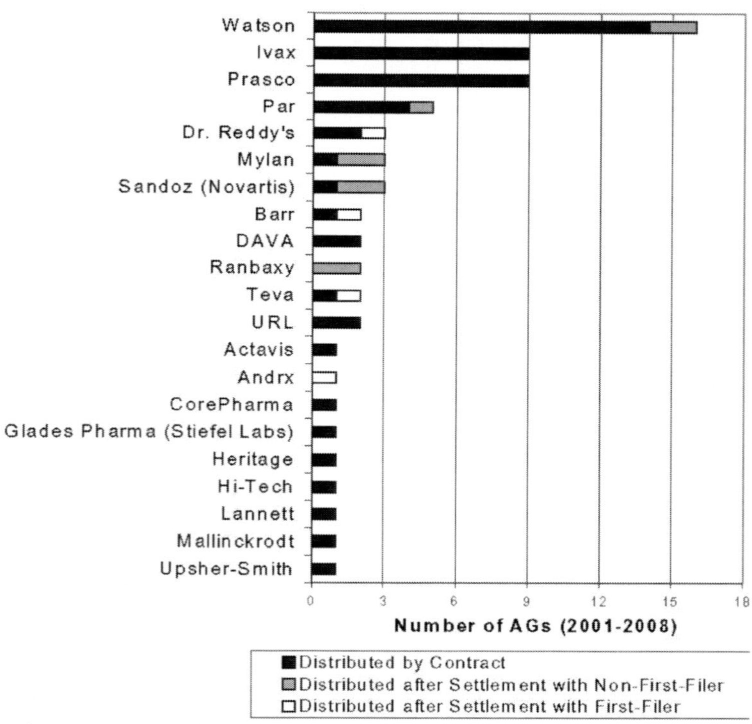

The number of AGs per company includes only AGs distributed pursuant to an agreement with a brand-name company. AGs for which a company held the NDA (e.g., an NDA held by a brand parent) are not included. The categories of agreements are settlements with first-filers, settlements with subsequent filers, and non-settlement contracts.

Figure 2-5. Generic Drug Companies that Distributed Authorized Generic Drugs by Agreement with Brand-Name Companies.

Outside marketing partners that enter into non-settlement agreements for distributing an AG may or may not have filed an ANDA or made a Paragraph IV certification covering the brand-name drug related to the AG. Some brand-name companies will not contract with firms that have filed an ANDA or made a Paragraph IV certification for a bioequivalent product,[79] and some non-settlement agreements prohibit the generic firm from filing or marketing an ANDA product bioequivalent to the relevant brand-name drug.[80] Other non-settlement agreements allow the marketing of an ANDA-generic but require the generic to pay the brand a percentage of the profits, usually similar to the profit split on the AG.[81]

A number of terms affect potential profitability:

- Pricing: Neither settlement nor non-settlement agreements restrict the generic company's authority in setting the price of AGs. Indeed, they frequently affirm that authority.[82]
- Transfer Price: The transfer or supply price establishes the amount the generic company pays the brand-name company for the AG. In some agreements, this price is related by express terms to the cost of manufacturing the AG.[83]
- Profit-Splits: Most agreements provide a profit-split, which governs the distribution of profits between the brand and generic companies from sales of the AG. Many non-settlement agreements require the AG marketer to pay the brand a large percentage of profits on the AG.[84] Profit-splits have implications for generic firms' incentives: although AG distribution agreements can give a generic company that was not the first filer the benefit of being able to market during the 180-day exclusivity period, first-filing status provides the possibility of exclusivity unburdened by a profit-split, albeit with the likely expense of patent litigation.

Generic companies generally appear to choose between strategies that focus either on (i) entering agreements to market AGs or (ii) obtaining first-filing status providing 180-day exclusivity. Figure 2-6 shows that from 2001 through 2008, companies that marketed the most AGs by non-settlement agreement tended to have few 180-day exclusivities.[85] These companies, including one that specializes in AGs and does not file ANDAs (Prasco), appear to have focused on AG marketing, rather than first-to-file status, as a way of enhancing their profitability.[86]

Conversely, Figure 2-6 shows that those companies with the most 180-day exclusivity periods tend to market few AGs. This difference in strategies, where some companies focus on marketing an ANDA-generic during 180-day exclusivity while others seek to market AGs, may contribute to differences in generic company views on AGs, as discussed in Chapter 5.

II. AG Marketing: Relationship to 180-Day Exclusivity Periods and Patent Challenges

By challenging patents, generic companies can bring lower cost drugs to consumers before the expiration of a drug's last-to-expire patent.[87] Some have argued that brand-name companies seek to discourage such challenges by launching AGs during 180-day exclusivity periods, thus reducing ANDA-generics' incentives to bear the cost of patent litigation.[88] To assess the linkage between AGs and ANDA-generics' 180-day exclusivity periods, this section examines the prevalence of AG marketing during, and apart from, exclusivity. Similarly, the section explores the extent to which AGs have been marketed for drugs subject to Paragraph IV patent challenges, as opposed to other certifications. Although AGs have been present during most 180-day exclusivity periods, brand-name companies frequently launched AGs in situations without an exclusivity period or where there was not a patent challenge. The rate of AG launch was similar for ANDA-generic entry with and without exclusivity and was much more closely associated with sales levels than with the presence or absence of exclusivity.

A. AG Marketing During 180-Day Exclusivity Periods

Since 2003, drug companies have marketed AGs during many 180-day exclusivity periods. Prior to that time, most such exclusivity periods featured only ANDA-generic products.[89] Thus, as shown in Figure 2-7, only two of the twelve (17%) exclusivity periods that began in 2001–2002 included an AG. Thereafter, the number of exclusivity periods with AGs increased, and in five of the six years from 2003 through 2008, an AG was marketed during at least half of the exclusivity periods. From 2003–2008, the percentage of exclusivities with AGs was 61%, ranging from 43–71% per year.[90]

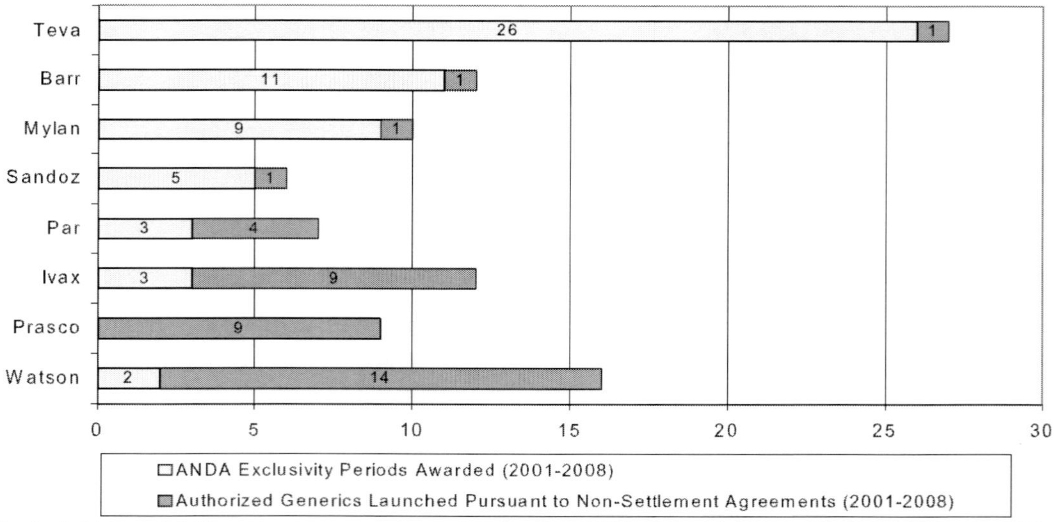

Exclusivities and AGs pursuant to agreement for the four ANDA-generic companies with the most 180-day exclusivity periods, and the four generic companies with the most AGs pursuant to non-settlement agreements. In order to make the figure most useful for examining the extent to which some generic companies seek opportunities to market AGs rather than to pursue patent challenges, AG counts do not include AGs pursuant to settlement agreements (which arise from patent challenges). Similarly, the figure does not include AGs for which the company or a parent or subsidiary company holds the NDA, because that is a reflection of a company's brand-name business.

Figure 2-6. Top Companies for 180-Day Exclusivity Periods and Authorized Generic Drugs by Contract.

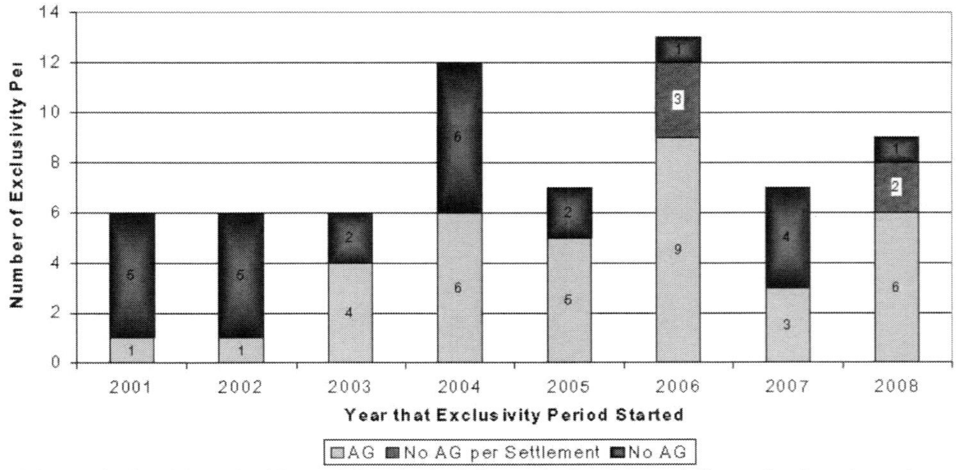

Exclusivity periods with and without AGs. Exclusivity periods without AGs are broken down into those for which a "No AG" agreement prohibited the marketing of an AG and those for which there was no such prohibition. Exclusivity periods are shown by brand-name drug (not by strength). Because the graph focuses on the competitive conditions of exclusivities, the x-axis shows the year during which the first 180-day exclusivity period began for any of the strengths of the drug.. This is not necessarily the year of AG launch. Similar results are obtained when exclusivities and AGs are plotted by strength. For more information, see Appendix H.

Figure 2-7. Number of 180-Day Exclusivity Periods with and without Authorized Generic Drugs.

Moreover, the percentage of exclusivity periods with AGs likely would have been higher had it not been for "No AG" settlement agreements. As explained in Chapter 8, "No AG" agreements, which became common around 2006, are settlements in which a brand promises the first-filer generic that it will refrain from marketing a competing AG during 180-day exclusivity. Such a promise can provide value to persuade a generic to defer entry of its litigated product. As shown in Figure 2-7, three of the exclusivity periods without AGs in 2006, and two in 2008, were subject to a "No AG" agreement.[91] Without these "no AG" agreements, AGs might have been marketed during 92% of the exclusivity periods in 2006, and 89% in 2008. Indeed, without "no AG" agreements, 70% of exclusivity periods from 2003–2008 might have had AGs.

B. AG Marketing Apart from 180-Day Exclusivity Periods and Patent Challenges

Although drug companies marketed many AGs during 180-day exclusivity, they marketed more during non-exclusive periods, and often for drugs that had not been subject to a patent challenge. As shown in Figure 2-8, approximately two-thirds of the 119 AGs launched from 2001 through 2008 were *not* marketed during an exclusivity period.[92] In every year during the study period except 2008, the number of AGs marketed outside or without an exclusivity period was considerably higher than the number marketed during exclusivity. In 2008 a little more than half of the AGs launched were marketed during a 180-day exclusivity period. It remains to be seen whether this shift, which followed a year in which almost all AGs were marketed apart from 180-day exclusivity, has continued.

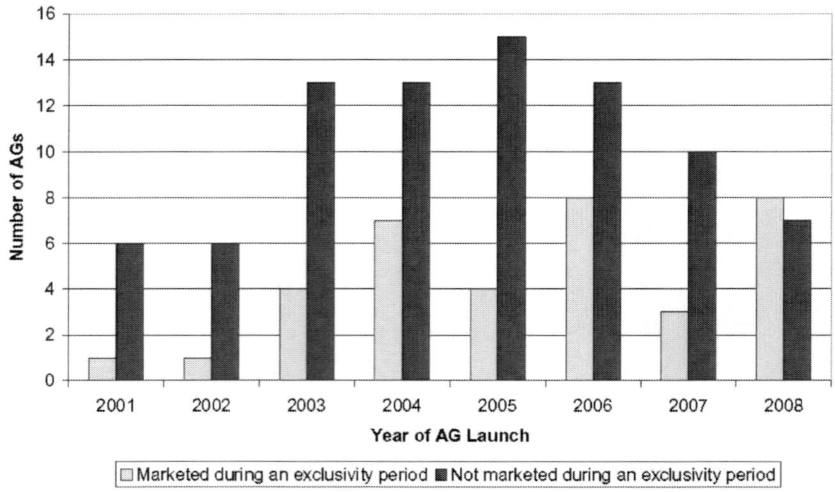

The figure shows the numbers of AGs marketed during and apart from 180-day exclusivity.[93] Because the graph focuses on AGs and the conditions under which they were launched, the number of AGs per year was graphed by the year of launch for each AG. The year of AG launch may not be the same as the year when a 180-day exclusivity period for that drug began. Thus, the number of AGs marketed during exclusivity in this graph is not always the same as in Figure 2-7, which shows the number of AGs marketed during exclusivity by the year the exclusivity began. For more information, see Appendix H.

Figure 2-8. Number of Authorized Generic Drugs Marketed During and Apart from Exclusivity.

Although the overall number of AGs that were not marketed during a 180-day exclusivity period was greater than the number marketed during exclusivity, it does not necessarily follow that the *rate* of AG launch – the percentage of first generic entries for which an AG was launched[94] – was higher when generic entry occurred without exclusivity than with exclusivity.[95] Indeed, because of the high revenues potentially available to an AG during exclusivity,[96] and the potential disincentive to future patent challenges, brands might prefer to market AGs during exclusivity.

As shown in Figure 2-9, however, the rate of AG entry is correlated with pre-entry brand sales, rather than with the nature of generic entry. While the rate of AG entry increases with pre-entry brand sales, there was no consistent pattern as to the relative magnitude of the rates of AG entry for generic entry with and without exclusivity. And within most sales levels, the percentage of drugs with AGs was similar for ANDA-generic entry with and without exclusivity. These data suggest that during the period when AGs have been common, the anticipated sales level, on average, has had greater bearing on brands' decisions to launch AGs than whether generic entry occurred via 180-day exclusivity.

Data examining the patent certification of ANDAs for brand-name drugs for which an AG was marketed are consistent with the data showing that the majority of AGs were not marketed during 180-day exclusivity periods. As shown in Figure 2-10, from 2001 through 2006, more than half of the AGs were versions of drugs that had not been subject to a patent challenge, *i.e.*, no ANDA included a Paragraph IV certification. During 2001–2006, only 41 AG launches involved drugs for which an ANDA with a Paragraph IV certification had been filed, whereas 51 involved drugs for which the highest certifications fell under Paragraphs I, II, or III.[97]

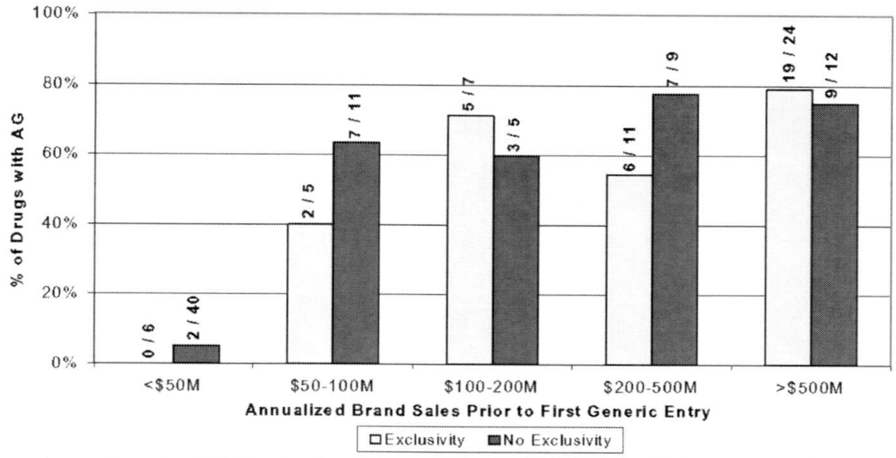

The figure shows the rate of AG entry by pre-entry sales of drugs for which first generic entry occurred between April 1, 2003 and December 31, 2008, which is the largest time window possible using the available IMS data. In each fraction above the bar for a particular sales range and condition (drug with or without exclusivity), the numerator is the number of AGs marketed, and the denominator is the total number of drugs for which first generic entry occurred. Sales levels are annualized based on the three months prior to generic entry, adjusted for inflation as described in Chapter 3, and include all strengths of a drug (NDA). If a 180-day exclusivity period was granted for any strength, the drug was counted as having an exclusivity. Similarly, if an AG was marketed for any strength, the drug was counted as having an AG.

Figure 2-9. Rate of AG Entry by Pre-Entry Brand Sales.

Nonetheless, beginning in 2003 there was a substantial increase in the number of AG launches for drugs that were subject to a Paragraph IV certification, and by 2007–2008 most AGs were versions of drugs for which there had been a Paragraph IV certification. The predominance of AG launches associated with a Paragraph IV certification in 2007–2008 appears to arise more from a decrease in AGs for drugs subject to ANDAs with Paragraph I, II, or III certifications, than from an increase in those subject to PIV. Figure 2-8 similarly shows a decrease in 2007 and 2008 of the number of AGs that were not marketed during a 180-day exclusivity period. Various factors could have contributed to the decreases.[98] In any event, it does not appear that the more controversial aspect of AGs, their launch during exclusivity, is undergoing a similar decline.

Taken together, the exclusivity and patent certification data in Figures 2-8 and 2-10 indicate that during the period when AGs became common, undermining 180-day exclusivity was unlikely to have been the primary rationale for many AG drugs. This does not preclude a disincentive effect or rationale for those AGs that *were* marketed during 180-day exclusivity periods, but it suggests that different or additional explanations for AG marketing also should be considered.

III. Conclusion

AG marketing became commonplace around 2003, with many brand name companies marketing AG versions of their drugs either through subsidiaries or via partnerships with generic companies. AGs frequently were marketed during the 180-day exclusivity periods granted to the first ANDA-filer for a particular drug. Indeed, from 2003–2008, the percentage of exclusivities with AGs was 61%, and might have been 70% without "No AG" agreements.

Nonetheless, AGs marketed during exclusivity were in the minority. More AGs were marketed after exclusivity or when no exclusivity had occurred; many of the latter drugs had not been subject to a patent challenge. The rate of AG launch increased as pre-entry brand sales increased, and within most sales levels was similar for ANDA-generic entry with and without exclusivity; there was no consistent pattern in the relative magnitude of rates of AG entry for generic entry with and without exclusivity. These findings suggest that, on average, the anticipated sales level of the brand-name drug has had greater bearing on decisions to launch AGs than whether ANDA-generic entry occurred via exclusivity. The findings, however, do not preclude a disincentive rationale or effect for AGs that *were* marketed during exclusivity.

The widespread marketing of AGs, especially during exclusivity periods, suggests that AGs could have a number of important short-term effects. They could spur competition that might reduce prices during exclusivity, perhaps generating savings for consumers. Similarly, marketing of AGs during exclusivity periods could have an impact on the revenues of both ANDA-generic and brand-name firms. Chapter 3 addresses these issues based on quantitative economic data.

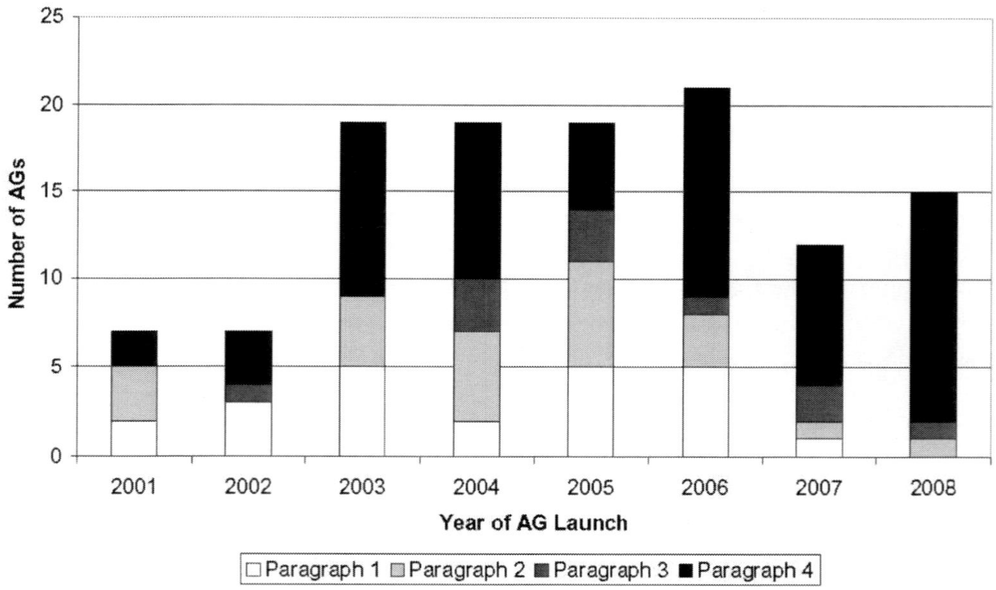

The graph shows the highest patent certification by ANDAs filed with respect to the NDA pursuant to which the AG was marketed, i.e., the NDA for the reference-listed brand-name drug. The number of AGs for which the brand-name drug was subject to an ANDA with a PIV certification is higher than the number shown in Figure 2-8 of AGs marketed during an exclusivity period because not all patent challenges result in an exclusivity period. This figure includes Paragraph IV certifications for five drugs, the same as those discussed in footnote 45, for which an AG was marketed by the first-filer.

Figure 2-10. Number of Authorized Generic Drugs Launched, by Highest Patent Certification in ANDAs.

3. Short-Term Impacts of Authorized Generics: Price and Revenue Effects during 180-Day Exclusivity

This chapter analyzes the effects of AG drug competition on several market outcomes during FDA-granted 180-day exclusivity periods. The market outcomes that are the focus of the analysis are prices and revenues. Preliminary analysis of these data appeared in the Interim Report.[99] This chapter employs more sophisticated tools to account for market characteristics that may systematically differ between AG and non-AG markets, in order to better isolate the effect of the AG.

As discussed in Chapter 1, an important consequence of competition from AGs may be that purchasers face lower prices. This chapter confirms the Interim Report's finding that the presence of an AG during a 180-day exclusivity period is associated with lower retail and wholesale prices. The analysis in this chapter finds that the presence of an AG during an exclusivity period was associated with lower generic prices – ranging from slightly, but not significantly,[100] lower to as much as 14% lower. The estimated impact generally was smaller for retail prices than for wholesale prices.

Another key finding of the Interim Report was that revenues of first-filer generic manufacturers were substantially lower in the presence of AG competition. Again, the more sophisticated analysis in this chapter confirms the findings of the Interim Report, that AG introduction significantly diminishes first-filer revenues during the exclusivity period. This chapter finds that the wholesale expenditures on the first-filer's generic drug – a proxy for revenues – were 40 to 52 percent lower, on average, when an AG was present. AGs could have material long-term effects if their impact on first-filer revenues is large enough to substantially alter the incentives to file Paragraph IV challenges or even to file an ANDA at all. Discussion of the impact on incentives to pursue Paragraph IV challenges is a topic of Chapter 6, where the effects of AGs beyond the exclusivity period are estimated.

A related question about incentives is whether the AG's direct revenue impact alone makes the decision to launch a rational choice, or whether indirect effects, such as potential deterrence of Paragraph IV challenges, must also be present to make the strategy profitable. There is some evidence that brand-name drug manufacturers have higher revenues during the exclusivity period when they introduce an AG than when they do not.

This chapter begins with a review of some prior studies that investigated related topics. That is followed by a description of the data compiled for this study and a discussion of the basic methodology used in the analysis. Finally, the chapter presents new analysis of the impact of AGs on prices and revenues of generics and brands during exclusivity periods.

I. Prior Studies

The short-term price effects of AGs have been examined in a series of prior studies that have not completely resolved the questions raised above. In 2006, IMS Consulting conducted a study commissioned by the Pharmaceutical Research and Manufacturers of America ("PhRMA") to measure the impact of AGs upon costs to the health care system through their influence on generic pricing, both during and after periods of 180-day exclusivity.[101] It compared two groups of generic drugs. The first group included nine drugs for which an AG competed against a single generic firm during the 180-day exclusivity period. The second group included nine drugs for which a generic drug company with 180-day exclusivity did not face AG competition. The study concluded that, relative to the brand price, wholesale generic prices were about 16 percent lower when the first generic faced competition from an AG. (The generic price was 38.8% lower than the brand price with AG competition but only 23% lower when there was no AG.)[102] The statistical properties of these estimates were not discussed, which could be important given the small number of drugs used in the analysis.

The IMS Study was critiqued on numerous fronts by Aidan Hollis and Bryan Liang[103] in a study released by the Generic Pharmaceutical Association ("GPhA"). First, the authors suggest that retail prices, rather than wholesale prices, should have been used. Second, the authors point out that "the PhRMA study appears to examine the average generic price discount off the brand price at any point in time."[104] They argue that this approach is erroneous because brand prices may change over time and instead recommend that generic prices be compared to the brand price that prevailed prior to entry. This issue is especially pertinent because, according to the authors, brand prices tend to increase more following introduction of an AG than they do following introduction of an ANDA-generic. After adopting these two changes, Hollis and Liang conclude that, for the same set of drugs analyzed by IMS, the average generic discount off the pre-entry brand price was 15% without an AG and 20% with an AG.[105] Again, the statistical properties of these estimates are not reported.

Hollis and Liang go further however, and argue that even the 5% difference overstates the immediate benefits from AGs. In particular, the authors argue that each of 18 drugs used in the IMS Study should be weighted by sales. When this is done, Hollis and Liang conclude that the average generic discount off pre-entry brand price is virtually identical with and without AGs (17.1% with an AG and 17.7% without an AG).[106]

The controversy over whether retail or wholesale price is the more appropriate measure of the impact of AGs received further attention in a white paper produced for PhRMA by Howrey and CapAnalysis.[107] It argues that the retail pricing data used by Hollis and Liang do not accurately portray the impact on consumers: many of the reported transactions are for individuals covered by health insurance, so that the data include payments from the pharmacy benefit manager to the pharmacy plus a dispensing fee, in addition to a co-payment paid by the consumer. Furthermore, the white paper argues that retail pharmacies set prices based on many factors that are unrelated to the AG question, making reliance on wholesale prices more appropriate when investigating the effect of a change in the level of competition between rival manufacturers.[108] Howrey also responded to the findings from the FTC Interim Report in a separate white paper produced in 2009. Combining the findings from the Interim Report and their own analysis, they construct a metric of aggregate consumer benefit from the introduction of an AG using the short-term price effect estimates from the sales-weighted wholesale data presented in the Interim Report.[109]

Neither wholesale nor retail data are direct measures of consumer outcomes in these markets, but both can shed light on the impact of AGs on consumers provided that care is taken in their use and interpretation. While the linkage between consumer benefit from a lower retail price is undeniably less direct in pharmaceutical markets than in most other markets,[110] consumers nonetheless benefit from lower retail prices, whether through reduced out-of-pocket payments, lower health insurance premiums, or a diminished tax burden. Furthermore, some portion of the cost savings from lower wholesale prices will get passed on to the consumer, depending on market conditions in the health insurance and retail pharmacy markets, so wholesale prices could be used as a measure of the impact on consumers, or at least as a measure of cost savings to the health-care system.

The second main point of the CapAnalysis paper, that wholesale data more directly reflect changes in competition between manufacturers, seems valid. To the extent that this Report's analysis seeks to quantify measures of competition between manufacturers, it will rely primarily on wholesale data, though analysis of the retail data will also typically be reported for completeness.

II. Description of the Data

The empirical analysis performed for this study relies on information drawn from several different data sources.[111] The FTC acquired a license for both retail and wholesale sales data from IMS Health Services (IMS). It obtained monthly wholesale and retail dollar and quantity sales data for oral solid prescription drugs from January 2003 through December 2008.[112] The licensed sales data have been combined with drug information from the Food and Drug Administration (FDA) and firm submissions. All retail and wholesale expenditures and prices are deflated to December 2008 dollars using the monthly producer price index (PPI) series for finished goods.[113] Whether a product[114] faced a Paragraph IV challenge and the dates of any exclusivity period arising from the challenge were determined using information obtained from the FDA.[115] AGs were identified based on information from the FDA, supplemented and verified using information subpoenaed from the pharmaceutical firms. Among other things, the subpoenaed information reports on whether the brand issued an AG and, if so, the identity of the AG distributor. The study thus builds upon and supplements the data used in prior research regarding the impact of AGs, including the IMS Study sponsored by brand-name manufacturers and the Hollis and Liang study released by the generic manufacturers. Using the combined data, the sample covers 312 products that first faced generic competition during the period between April 2003 and December 2008.[116]

The relationships depicted in Figure 2-9 and Figure I-1 in Appendix I show that AGs tend to be introduced on relatively higher sales products[117] and suggest that market size may influence decisions about both whether to attempt generic entry through a Paragraph IV challenge and whether to launch an AG. One concern is that market size also may be correlated with the amount of discounting that happens following generic entry, which may make it difficult to separate the price effect of AG presence from the hypothesized price effect of market size. Furthermore, market size may not be the only variable that helps explain the competitive environment.

The regressions in this chapter attempt to control for many of these issues by including product-characteristic controls in the analysis of the effect of AG competition on market outcomes. Therapeutic class indicator variables represent an important subset of these product-characteristic controls. Therapeutic class indicators, as defined by the data vendor, IMS, are used to group together similar products that treat similar conditions. The condition treated by the product is the single most important characteristic relating the products in a category together. Therefore, the regression analysis of this chapter uses the therapeutic class indicators to help control for potential differences between products that have an AG and products that do not.[118] The use of these controls is discussed further in Appendix I.

III. The Effect of Authorized Generic Competition during the Exclusivity Period

The introduction of an AG can affect consumers in several ways. Some of these effects may be beneficial, but others could be harmful. For example, in the short-run, consumers may benefit from lower prices associated with additional competition from an AG. However, in the long-run, the expectation of an AG may deter ANDA-generic firms from challenging questionable patents using a Paragraph IV certification. If there were deterrence, consumers would not have the opportunity to choose the generic alternative until the (potentially invalid or not-infringed) patent of the brand had expired.[119] Furthermore, the anticipation of revenues from an AG version of a drug in addition to the brand sales of the drug could potentially provide added incentive for the brand-name company to develop the drugs in the first place, which could also benefit consumers. Whether an AG is, on net, beneficial to consumers depends on the relative size of the beneficial and harmful effects.

Although the analysis will not be able to address the full welfare implications of the introduction of an AG, the empirical analysis attempts to estimate many of the effects that AG competition may have on market outcomes that are relevant in both the short- and long-run. We begin by considering how AG competition affects generic and brand prices and revenues during the exclusivity period.

The price analysis addresses several issues important to consumers. Introducing an AG during exclusivity might be expected to add a competitor to the lone ANDA-generic and, consequently, to reduce generic prices in the short-run. The analysis estimates this effect using both retail and wholesale data. The prices of AGs and rival ANDA-generics are also compared to investigate whether one type of generic tends to be a relatively more or less aggressive price competitor than the other. Because the effect of AGs on generic prices may be somewhat offset or exacerbated by brand-name firm pricing decisions, the analysis also considers the effect of an AG on brand prices. Furthermore, we investigate the extent to which both generic and brand prices depend on the nature of the relationship between the AG marketer and the brand-name firm. For instance, one analysis looks at differences in brand pricing depending on whether the AG marketer is a subsidiary of the brand or an independent licensee.

Firm revenues are also studied. The revenues available during the 180-day exclusivity period may be an important consideration in a generic firm's decision to challenge a patent. This chapter provides estimates of the impact of AG competition on first-filer revenues during exclusivity. In Chapter 6, this information is combined with other findings to assess how the presence of an AG is likely to affect a generic firm's incentives to challenge a patent.

The revenues of the brand-name firm during exclusivity are analyzed to provide insight into its motivation for issuing an AG. Assuming that the brand-name firm is profit-maximizing, a strategy that reduces revenues in the short-run must either decrease short-run costs at least as much, or be motivated by a long-term objective. If the AG diminishes brand-name firm revenues in the short-run, the profitability of offering an AG most likely would be attributable to longer-term effects, perhaps entry deterrence. However, if the brand-name firm earns higher revenues in the short-run by issuing an AG, then the decision to issue an AG may be either a long-run or a short-run strategy.

The analyses compare these market outcomes across groups of products that are distinguished by whether an AG was marketed. They control for product attributes that could potentially confound the effects of an AG with the impacts of other product characteristics in order to estimate the effect of AG entry. Limitations on generic entry during the exclusivity period create a relatively homogenous set of market conditions that do not change very much over time. Approximately 74% of products observed during exclusivity fall into one of two categories: a single ANDA-generic competitor (ANDA-Only); or an ANDA-generic and an AG competitor (ANDA+AG).[120] The competitive environment for individual products tends to be stable during exclusivity. Over 85% of products observed during exclusivity begin and end the period with the same competitive environment (for example, they begin and end exclusivity as an "ANDA-Only" product). Similarly, products with the same molecule typically face identical competitive environments.[121]

A. Market Prices of Generic Drugs

Nearly all of the previous studies of AGs' short-run effects have found that generic prices during exclusivity are lower in markets with an AG than in markets without an AG. However, these studies find effects of different magnitudes because they apply different methodologies to analyze two different data sets, retail and wholesale sales data. The original price analysis in this Report considers the effect of an AG on generic prices using both wholesale and retail data and employing several methodologies as robustness checks.

The measure of quantity used in this analysis is an extended unit. For example, if a pharmacy buys a bottle of 1000 10mg tablets of Alendronate, the extended unit is a tablet, so the quantity associated with that purchase would be 1000. The unit of observation is a product, which as described above, refers to active ingredient(s)-strength-dosage-form combinations.[122] Using measures derived from IMS Health's retail and wholesale data, price is calculated as the total dollars spent on the product during the month divided by the number of extended units of the product sold within the month.

Generic prices are normalized across products by dividing the generic price by the average price of an extended unit of the brand-name version of that product in the three months preceding generic entry. This calculation provides the standard measure of price used throughout this Report, referred to as the "relative price."[123] Normalization is necessary to allow comparisons and aggregation across products that may have very different nominal prices. Normalizing generic prices by the pre-entry brand price accords with recent literature that reports relative prices in terms of the percentage discounts off the pre-entry brand price.[124]

1. Generic Retail Market Prices

This section reports on estimated percent changes in average retail relative prices of generic products due to AG entry. These prices are referred to as market prices because they are averages of ANDA and AG prices, to distinguish them from firm level prices. The estimates are predictions made using the results from a linear regression model relating generic prices to characteristics of the competitive environment.[125]

The empirical analysis in the Interim Report focused on two subsets of products. In the first subset, only an ANDA competitor provided a generic product during exclusivity. In the second, an ANDA competitor was joined by an AG. The Interim Report noted potential problems with comparing summary statistics between these two sets of markets to determine the impact of AG competition because the decision to launch an AG may depend on characteristics of those markets that also affect the summary statistics independent of the AG effect. The regressions in this chapter employ econometric methods to address that concern.

Before turning to the regression analysis, first consider Figure 3-1, which provides graphical evidence consistent with the regression results that follow. Figure I-1 in Appendix I shows that introduction of an AG was substantially more frequent on products with higher pre-entry brand sales. One might be concerned that relative prices may also be correlated with the market size, so Figure 3-1 plots the relative market price for each product in the two subsets (ANDA-Only and ANDA+AG) against the market size for that product in the fourth month of exclusivity.[126] On average, relative market prices in ANDA-Only markets are 0.85, and they are 0.81 in ANDA+AG markets. It is clear from the graph that all of the smaller markets are ANDA-Only markets, but that some of the larger markets are also ANDA-Only. As suggested by the averages, the ANDA-Only products tend to have higher relative prices, and this appears to be true regardless of the market size, though there are exceptions.

In order to more carefully investigate the effect of an AG, several linear regression models are estimated with different types of controls to take account of the possibility that markets with an AG may be inherently different from non-AG markets. All of the models explore the effects on relative generic market prices associated with the number and type of generic marketers.[127] Some of the models also control for the effects of additional factors, other than the presence of an AG, that might also affect price. These models introduce product characteristic controls (or "Full Controls") that include dosage form, the number of months since generic entry, and therapeutic class indicators.

Whether the appropriate model should include such product characteristic controls depends on the nature of AG competition. The decision to market an AG is non-random. The presence of an AG reflects a deliberate choice made by a brand-name manufacturer with a good understanding of the market for that product. Consequently, products that have AG competitors may be systematically different from products without AG competitors. A brand-name firm may choose not to issue an AG when consumers are likely to be reluctant to switch to generic products. Furthermore, an ANDA-generic firm may find it necessary to offer deeper than average discounts for the product in order to entice consumers to switch. In this circumstance, it would be errant to conclude that the lack of an AG *caused* the deep discount.

Controlling for product characteristics may allow the AG effect to be estimated in a way that accounts for unobserved factors, such as a consumer's reluctance to switch from brand-name products to generic products. For example, if consumers are equally as reluctant to switch to generic alternatives for all products within the same therapeutic class, then the inclusion of product characteristic indicators that reflect the therapeutic class would absorb the causes of their reluctance to switch in the product characteristic estimates. In that case, an estimate of the effect of an AG would not include the consumer-reluctance effects, and it would therefore be closer to the true effect of the AG.[128] This is the argument for including therapeutic class controls.

When unobserved factors (e.g., consumers' reluctance to switch to generic products) are not constant within a therapeutic class (because, for example, the reluctance to switch is product-specific), including the product characteristics would not fully separate the causal effect of the AG from these other factors. In addition, the inclusion of therapeutic class controls might distort coefficient estimates if the variables of interest are measured with error. These arguments would caution against adding therapeutic class controls. For these reasons, estimates with and without these controls are reported. With these caveats in mind, however, given the great diversity of drugs included in the analysis, controlling for unobserved characteristics is especially important, so we generally focus on the estimates based on models with the full set of controls.

Table 3-1 presents estimates of the effect of introducing an AG on retail market prices under four model specifications. To interpret the results, consider the "Effect of Adding an AG to ANDA-Only" figure reported in column (i), which is -3.8%. An interpretation of this number is that adding an AG to a market that otherwise would have only one ANDA-generic competitor would lower the retail relative price by 3.8%, compared to the price that would have been realized with only an ANDA competitor, on average.[129] In the simplest model, reported in columns (i) and (iii), the regression includes controls for both the number and the type (ANDA or AG) of competitors in the market, but does not control for any other product characteristics. The more complex model, presented in columns (ii) and (iv), controls for the number and the type of competitors as well, but also includes controls for product characteristics such as the dosage form (e.g., whether the product is an extended-release capsule or a tablet), the therapeutic class (e.g., "Gastrointestinal Medications" and "Analgesics"), the survey year, and the months since generic entry began.

The difference between columns (i) and (iii) is essentially like the difference between a simple average and a weighted average. The unweighted analysis, in columns (i) and (ii), treats each observation of each product equally. The sales-weighted models, in (iii) and (iv), allow contributions to the estimates to be proportional to the pre-entry brand-name product sales, such that products with larger pre-entry brand sales contribute more to the estimation than products with smaller pre-entry brand sales. Because products with identical molecules may not price independently from each other the models cluster standard errors by molecule.[130]

Table 3-1. Effect of AG Introduction on Generic Retail Market Prices

	Unweighted		**Sales Weighted**	
	(i) No Controls	**(ii) Full Controls+**	**(iii) No Controls**	**(iv) Full Controls+**
Effect of Adding an AG to ANDA-Only (Standard Error)	-3.8% (2.8%)	-4.9%** (2.3%)	-4.2% (4.0%)	-7.6%** (2.7%)
ANDA-Only Mean Relative Price		0.86		0.90
Sample Size	666	666	666	666

**Statistically different from zero at the 5% level.

(Note: The statistical test on the AG effect in this and all tables that follow is a two-sided test; testing whether the effect is different from zero.)

+The Full Controls include dosage form, months since generic entry, and therapeutic class indicators.

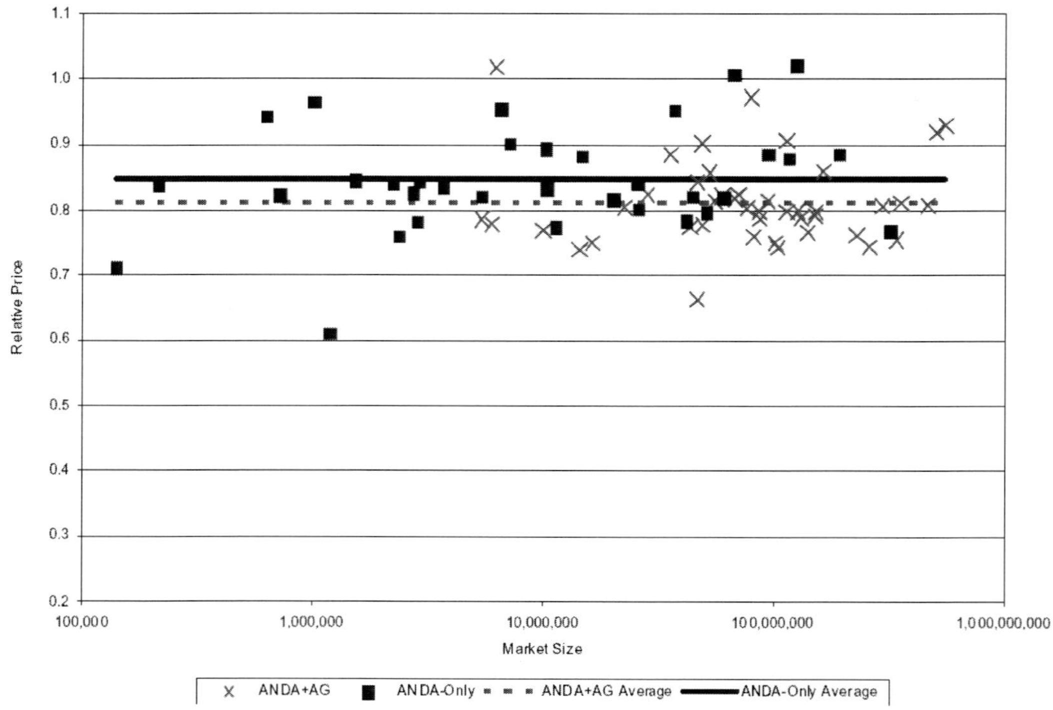

Figure 3-1. Generic Retail Relative Market Prices in Month Four of Exclusivity.

Although all of the estimated AG effects reported in Table 3-1 suggest that changing from a market structure with a single ANDA to one with an ANDA and an AG lowers the average relative price (or, equivalently, increases the price discount), the data do not provide strong, consistent evidence that the true effect of an AG is different from zero. The magnitude of the estimated change ranges from -3.8% to -7.6% of the original "ANDA-Only" price, depending on whether the model sales-weights the observations and controls for product characteristics.

In the unweighted models, the effects appear robust to the inclusion of full controls: the estimates are very similar between the two models and only range from -3.8% to -4.9%. For both weighted and unweighted models, the price decreases are statistically significant at the 5% level only when the full controls are included. The AG effect in the model without controls is insignificant (i.e. not different from zero) at all standard confidence levels, suggesting that the hypothesis that AG competition had no effect during the exclusivity period cannot be rejected. Another way to characterize the statistical properties of this analysis is with a confidence interval.[131] For the unweighted regression without controls in column (i) of Table 3-1, the 95% confidence interval of the AG Effect is [-9.3%, 1.7%].[132]

The sales-weighted model finds somewhat more pronounced effects than the unweighted models. The sales-weighted model without full controls yields an estimate similar to both of the unweighted estimates and is statistically insignificant at all standard confidence intervals. However, including full controls in the sales-weighted models results in larger estimates of effects from the AG. The estimate in column (iv) is roughly twice the size of the unweighted estimates and is statistically significant at the 5% level.

Table 3-1 also reports estimated mean relative prices for ANDA-Only markets. Since a fundamental goal of this analysis is to determine how the presence of AGs impacts markets in which AGs are launched, these mean relative prices are calculated to represent the counterfactual price that would have prevailed in those markets if an AG had not launched. Consequently, the average generic relative prices for drugs in AG markets are calculated, then the estimated AG effect is used to pull out the impact of having an AG in that market. These predicted prices are 0.86 and 0.90 in the unweighted and weighted analysis, respectively. Although these represent fairly substantial discounts off the pre-entry brand price, the prices are much closer to the pre-entry brand price than is typically observed for a generic product outside exclusivity. Results presented in Chapter 6 will show that once further generic entry is allowed outside of exclusivity, the discounts increase.

2. Generic Wholesale Market Prices

This section presents analysis parallel to that of the previous section, except using wholesale data rather than retail data. Figure 3-2 shows the relationship between wholesale relative prices and market sizes for ANDA-Only and ANDA+AG products in the fourth month of the exclusivity period. Here, market size is defined as the annualized wholesale expenditures on the brand-name product just prior to generic entry. The wholesale data show quite a bit more dispersion than the retail data, though qualitatively they are quite similar in many respects. Again, the smallest products are all ANDA-Only products. Controlling for market size, the products with lower relative prices tend to be the ANDA+AG products. The average ANDA-Only price is 0.75, while the average ANDA+AG price is 0.67. Again, relative prices do not appear to vary systematically with market size, though the smaller ANDA-Only products tend to have below average relative prices.

Table 3-2 presents estimates of the effect of introducing an AG on wholesale prices from four model specifications that control for different sets of variables. The model specifications are identical to those in Table 3-1 and the reported results are exactly analogous, except that the sales information used to calculate the results represents wholesale-level sales (sales from manufacturers or wholesalers to pharmacies) rather than retail-level sales. For example, the -6.9% estimate of the "Effect of Adding an AG to ANDA-Only" reported in column (i) means that adding an AG competitor to a market with only an ANDA-generic competitor would lower the wholesale relative price by 6.9% compared to the price that would have been realized had there been only an ANDA competitor, which is reported to average 0.80 two rows down in the table. As with the retail data, AG entry lowers market prices in every model specification. However, the magnitude of the effects is generally larger than suggested by the retail data; the estimates range from -6.9% to -13.5%, depending on whether the model controls for product characteristics and weights the observations by pre-entry brand sales.[133] Moreover, the effects are statistically significant at the 1% level for the models that include the full set of controls.

Controlling for product characteristics in the wholesale data has larger effects in both the sales-weighted and unweighted models than in the analogous retail data. For unweighted models, the AG effect, measured as the percentage change in relative price, increases from -6.9% to -12.8% when full controls are included. Although the two effects are not statistically different from each other, inclusion of product characteristics increases the precision of the AG effect, and allows the hypothesis that the AG effect is zero to be rejected with greater confidence. In the sales-weighted models, the inclusion of the product characteristics also increases the magnitude of the AG effect from -6.6% to -13.5%. Again, the estimate from the model with controls is more precise and significantly different from zero with greater confidence. Weighting the data by pre-entry brand sales had very little impact on the magnitude of the AG effect estimates.

3. Generic Firm Level Pricing Analysis

The analysis above considered the impact of AG entry on the average price paid for a generic version of a product, regardless of whether the product was an AG or an ANDA-generic. This section looks more deeply at pricing within markets for products that have experienced AG entry by comparing the prices for the ANDA products to the AG prices. This sheds light on the possibility that the relationship between the AG and the brand could make the AG a less aggressive price competitor than an ANDA-generic. In addition, understanding the relationship between ANDA-generic and AG prices may provide insight into the mechanism by which the presence of an AG affects market prices.

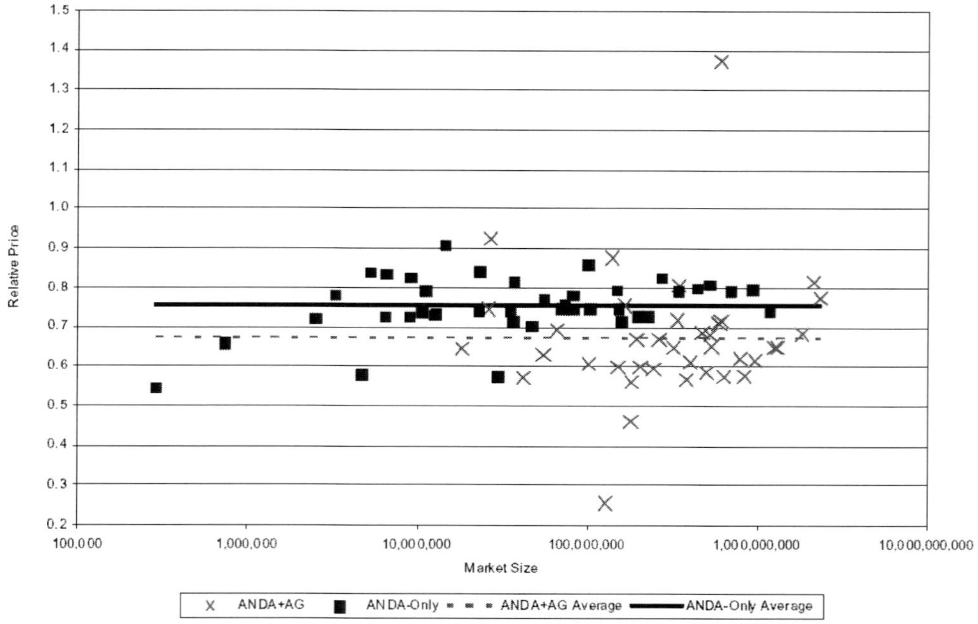

Figure 3-2. Generic Wholesale Relative Market Prices in Month Four of Exclusivity.

Table 3-2. Effect of AG Introduction on Generic Wholesale Market Prices

	Unweighted		Sales Weighted	
	(i) No Controls	(ii) Full Controls	(iii) No Controls	(iv) Full Controls
Effect of Adding an AG to ANDA-Only (Standard Error)	-6.9% (4.8%)	-12.8%*** (2.8%)	-6.6% (5.7%)	-13.5%*** (2.4%)
ANDA-Only Mean Relative Price		0.80		0.83
Sample Size	673	673	673	673

***Statistically different from zero at the 1% level

Table 3-3. Unweighted Price Differences Between AG and ANDA Firms

	(i) Retail	(ii) Wholesale
AG Firm Effect (Standard Error)	-11.4%*** (2.7%)	0.3% (1.0%)
ANDA Firm Mean Relative Price	0.86	0.70
Sample Size	711	715

***Statistically different from zero at the 1% level.

Table 3-3 presents estimates, at both retail and wholesale levels, of the differences in prices charged for an AG relative to the prices charged for a competing ANDA product. Both model specifications include the full set of controls that were included in columns (ii) and (iv) of Tables 3-1 and 3-2.[134]

This analysis shows that retail prices for the AG tend to be lower than the retail prices for corresponding ANDA-generics, and this difference is statistically significant at the 1% level. The value of -11.4% reported as the "AG Firm Effect" estimate in column (i) implies that retail prices for the AG product are 11.4% lower, on average, than retail prices of competing ANDA-generic products, which average 0.86 in the retail data.[135] The analysis of wholesale prices discussed below suggests that this effect is a result of pricing decisions made by pharmacies, which are not a focus of this study, so this difference is not explored further here, though it could be an interesting topic for further research.

The wholesale data tell a different story. This evidence suggests the AG does not price very differently from the ANDA, and that the estimated difference is not statistically significant. The estimated AG firm effect – implying that prices for AG products are 0.3% higher, on average, than prices for competing ANDA-generic products – is positive, small in magnitude, and statistically insignificant. In short, the wholesale data suggest that the AG firm and the ANDA firm price very similarly.

More detailed analysis of these generic prices investigated whether the vertical relationship between the brand-name firm and its AG marketer affects the pricing decisions of either the AG or ANDA generic firms. Although economic theory predicts that the pricing decision of the generic firms need not be affected by whether the AG was marketed by a subsidiary of the brand-name firm or by an independent licensee, depending on the nature of the contracts, one might believe that future potential competitors of the brand (licensees) on other products have different long-run incentives than the brand-name firms' own subsidiaries. However, the estimated impacts of the vertical relationship underlying AG marketing on both AG and ANDA pricing were both economically and statistically insignificant. Put simply, the prices of AGs were similar regardless of whether they were being marketed by a subsidiary of the brand or by an independent licensee, so these results are omitted. The impact of this vertical relationship on brand pricing will be considered below.

B. Market Prices of Brand-Name Products

The pricing analysis, thus far, has focused on the effect that an AG has on the prices of generic products. However, whether a brand-name firm issues an AG may also affect the optimal pricing strategy for its brand-name product. This section considers the impact of an

AG on brand-name product prices using both wholesale and retail data. Brand prices directly affect purchasers of the brand-name product, and they influence the long-run incentives of brand-name firms. How the decision to market an AG affects brand prices is therefore both directly relevant to current consumers and useful for understanding the long-run incentives of the brand-name firm.

Much of the analysis of brand prices is analogous to that of generic prices.[136] It covers the same set of products, employs the same data, and continues to use extended units of the product as the analytical unit. It derives estimates from linear regressions relating brand prices to the competitive environment. The models that examine the impact of an AG on brand prices during exclusivity are nearly identical to those that considered generic prices. These models include the same set of controls and normalize contemporaneous brand prices by pre-entry brand prices. However, because brand prices are also observed prior to generic entry, the analysis can be extended to look at pricing strategies prior to exclusivity.

1. Brand Retail Prices

The regression estimates of the change in relative retail prices for brand-name products due to AG entry can be foreshadowed by consideration of a graph of a time series of retail real price changes over the 18 months prior to generic entry and the six months after generic entry.[137] Figure 3-3 plots these series separately for products with and without an AG.[138]

For most of the period prior to generic entry the two series track each other closely. Prices for products that eventually experience AG entry increase at a rate that appears linear over time, and is very similar to that for products that never experience AG entry. This real rate of price increase is consistent with price increases observed across all brand-name products over this time. Beginning roughly five months before generic entry, the time path for products that never face an AG becomes steeper relative to brand drug prices in AG markets, but any apparent differences in the rates (or the levels) are not statistically different from each other. Finally, during exclusivity, the prices of products with an AG change course and begin to fall, while prices for products without an AG continue to rise at roughly the same rate as prior to generic entry. Although the graph shows an abrupt change of course in the direction of prices, the differences are not statistically different from each other.

Table 3-4 reports the results of regression analysis estimating the impact of introducing an AG on brand prices during the exclusivity period. It does not show statistically significant evidence of an effect. These results are consistent with what is observed in Figure 3-3. During exclusivity, the presence of an AG lowers estimated relative brand retail prices by between 4.2% and 7.2% relative to pre-entry brand prices depending on the controls that are included in the regression model, but these estimates are generally not statistically different from zero at any reasonable significance level. The magnitude of these estimated effects is similar across all four models.

2. Brand Wholesale Prices

This section presents analysis parallel to that of the brand retail prices, except that wholesale data rather than the retail data are employed. Figure 3-4 shows the time series of wholesale relative prices for products that will eventually face an AG and products that will not. The figure is exactly analogous to Figure 3-3 except that it uses wholesale prices rather than retail.

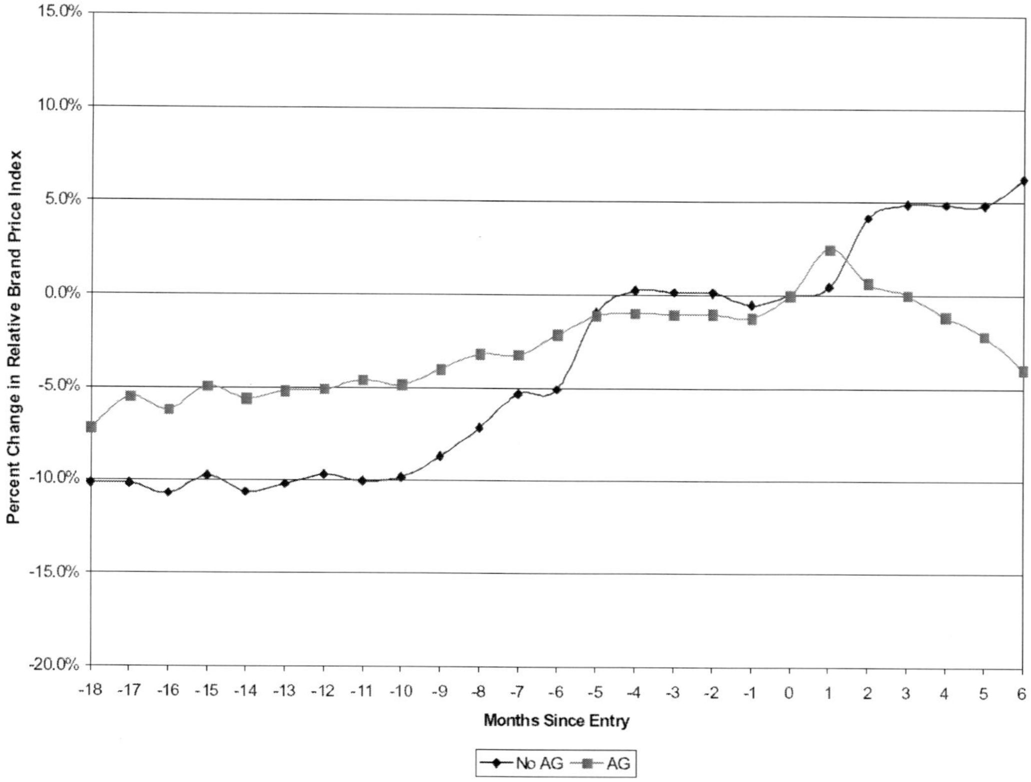

Figure 3-3. Average Brand Retail Price Changes Over Time.

The wholesale data reveal price patterns nearly identical to those shown by the retail data. Prior to generic entry, the two time series of prices are very similar. As in the retail data, the slopes of the two price series are not statistically significantly different from each other. Also similar to the retail analysis, wholesale prices for brand-name products that experience AG entry decrease during exclusivity. The magnitude of this decrease, however, is much larger for wholesale prices than for retail prices. Unlike the retail pattern, brand wholesale prices in markets without an AG also decline during exclusivity, but to a lesser extent than for products associated with an AG.

The relationship between AGs and wholesale prices is investigated further using regression models. Table 3-5 presents estimates of the impact of an AG on relative brand wholesale prices. These results are exactly analogous to those presented in Table 3-4, except that the relationships are estimated using wholesale data rather than retail data.

The average ANDA-Only contemporaneous brand price is 4% lower than the pre-entry brand prices in the unweighted sample and 11% lower than pre-entry brand prices in the sales-weighted sample.[139] During exclusivity, the presence of an AG lowers relative brand wholesale prices by between 7.7% and 12.2%, depending on the controls that are included in the regression model. These estimates are qualitatively similar to those from the retail data, but they are nearly twice as large in magnitude. Moreover, the estimates from all four models are statistically significant at the 5% confidence level.[140] These results are explored further below.

3. Investigating Lower Brand Prices During Exclusivity

One might believe that part of the strategic value of issuing an AG is to allow the brand-name firm to segment the market into groups of consumers, some of whom are price elastic (i.e., sensitive to price reductions) and others who are price inelastic. In this scenario, the lower-priced AG would capture the demand of price elastic consumers, while the price inelastic consumers would remain with the brand. This segmentation in other contexts often results in a higher price for the brand-name product.

Table 3-4. Effect of AG Introduction on Brand Retail Prices During Exclusivity

	Unweighted		Sales Weighted	
	(i) No Controls	(ii) Full Controls	(iii) No Controls	(iv) Full Controls
Effect of Adding an AG to ANDA-Only (Standard Error)	-4.2% (4.1%)	-4.8%* (2.4%)	-7.2% (6.8%)	-6.5% (4.1%)
ANDA-Only Mean Relative Price	1.05		1.01	
Sample Size	666	666	666	666

*Statistically different from zero at the 10% level.

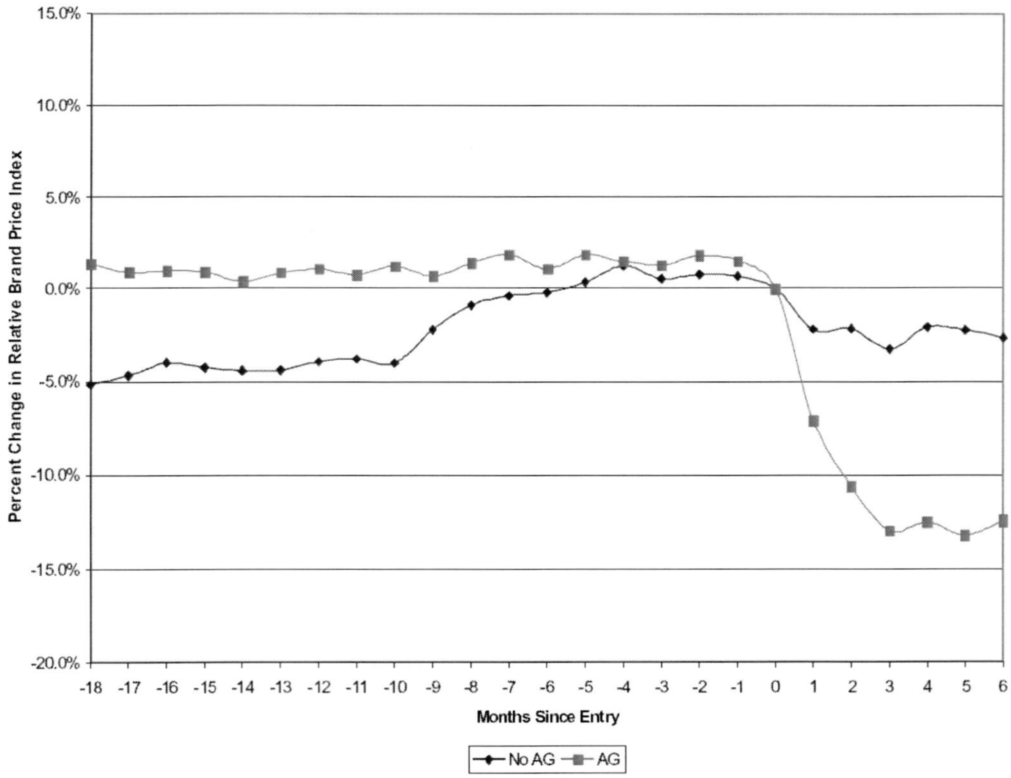

Figure 3-4. Average Wholesale Brand Price Changes Over Time.

Table 3-5. Effect of AG Introduction on Brand Wholesale Prices during Exclusivity

	Unweighted		Sales Weighted	
	(i) No Controls	(ii) Full Controls	(iii) No Controls	(iv) Full Controls
Effect of Adding AG to ANDA-Only (Standard Error)	-9.5%** (3.1%)	-10.6%*** (2.4%)	-12.2%** (5.6%)	-7.7%** (2.5%)
ANDA-Only Mean Relative Brand Price		0.96		0.89
Sample Size	673	673	673	673

**Statistically different from zero at the 5% level; ***at the 1% level.

The circumstances surrounding the decision to issue an AG may help explain the lower brand-name product prices of drugs with an AG during exclusivity. Although some brand-name firms may issue an AG in order to segment the market, in other cases the presence (or more often, absence) of an AG is determined by the terms of a settlement of a patent dispute.[141] For example, some settlement terms specify that the brand-name firm may not issue an AG or that the ANDA-generic firm can become the AG marketer. In these scenarios, the brand-name firm has forgone the ability to segment the market using an AG for some other advantage, such as deferred entry by the ANDA-generic firm. Consequently, the brand-name firm's strategy may differ in these settings from the standard scenario described in the previous paragraph.

This relationship is investigated further by considering how different competitive environments affect brand pricing strategy. Table 3-6 provides the pricing results for two market scenarios chosen to describe the nature of competition in the market.[142]

One factor to consider is whether the AG is distributed by a subsidiary or by an independent licensee. Depending on specific licensing terms, the brand-name firm may retain more of the profits from customers who switch from the brand to the AG following a brand price increase when a subsidiary, rather than a licensee sells the AG. If so, this would make a brand price increase more attractive (or a brand price decrease less attractive). Consequently, one might expect that brand prices would be higher in markets where the AG is distributed by a subsidiary than in markets where the AG is distributed by a licensee.

Table 3-6 reports evidence supporting this hypothesis. Analysis of both the retail and the wholesale data suggests that the brand price is higher in markets where the AG is distributed by the subsidiary. The wholesale data show that brand prices are almost 22% higher when the AG is distributed by a subsidiary than when it is distributed through an independent licensee. This result is statistically significant at the 1% level. The retail data reveal a similar positive subsidiary effect, but the effect is smaller in magnitude.

Another factor that could influence brand pricing is whether the brand-name and generic companies have resolved a patent dispute with an agreement that includes provisions relating to the launch of an AG. These settlements often stipulate either that an AG will not be issued or designate the generic party as the AG distributor. In either case, the brand-name firm's ability to segment the market via an AG is constrained by the settlement, which may induce the brand to try to retain market share by lowering the brand price. The analysis of wholesale prices presented in Table 3-6 finds evidence that brand prices indeed were 6.8% lower when the brand-name firm was party to a settlement that involved the AG, and this effect is statistically significant at the 5% level. No such effect is found in the retail data.

Table 3-6. Effect of AG Competition Type on Brand Prices

	Subsidiary instead of Licensee		AG Involved in Settlement?	
	Wholesale	**Retail**	**Wholesale**	**Retail**
Percent Change in Relative Brand Price (Standard Error)	21.6%*** (5.0%)	12.7%** (5.1%)	-6.8%** (3.2%)	3.2% (2.9%)
Sample Size	382	405	673	666
Sample	Only AG Products		All Products in Exclusivity	

Statistically different from zero at the 5% level; * at the 1% level.

C. Wholesale Expenditures

This section presents an analysis of total wholesale expenditures using the same set of products considered above with regard to prices. Wholesale expenditures are employed as a proxy for revenues of the relevant firm. As explained above, a generic firm will decide whether to challenge a patent based, in part, on the revenues it expects to earn during exclusivity, which, in turn, could depend on whether it expects to face AG competition. In this way, the presence or absence of AG competition could affect long-run outcomes, such as patent challenges.

The brand-name firm's revenues also could provide insight into whether the AG affects long-run outcomes. If brand-name firms that offer AGs earn less revenue during the exclusivity period than brand-name firms that do not, then issuing an AG cannot be profit-maximizing in the short-run.[143] If issuing an AG is not profitable in the short-run and the brand-name firm is maximizing profits, the introduction of an AG must be part of a long-run strategy. This chapter focuses only on market outcomes during exclusivity periods. However, AG introduction may also impact brand-name firm revenues beyond the exclusivity period. The combined short-run and long-run effects ultimately measure the total impact on brand-name firm incentives. Longer term effects will be addressed in Chapter 6.

The following analysis uses wholesale expenditures by pharmacies rather than retail sales to approximate the revenues of generic and brand-name manufacturers. Wholesale expenditures represent purchases by pharmacies from manufacturers and wholesalers.[144] They are a better reflection of the revenues received by manufacturers than are retail sales dollars, which likely include both wholesale and retail mark-ups. Retail margins likely differ across retailers, geographic location and time and, consequently, might mask the effects of an AG on revenues received by the product producer. The wholesale data are closer in the supply chain to the producing firm, do not include retailer margins, and should therefore better represent the firm's revenues. For ease of exposition, wholesale expenditures on particular drug products will often be referred to as the revenues created by those products, with the understanding that wholesale expenditures are an imperfect measure of revenue.[145]

Just as with prices, expenditures have been normalized in terms of corresponding data from the brand-name product prior to generic entry. Monthly wholesale expenditures are divided by average monthly expenditures on the brand for the three months prior to generic entry, and are referred to as "relative expenditures." Again, the normalization facilitates aggregation across products.

1. Wholesale Revenues of ANDA-Generic Firms

The primary reason for considering the wholesale expenditures on products of ANDA-generic firms during exclusivity is to approximate how the revenues of a first-filer generic manufacturer are affected by competition from an AG.[146] Consider first a simple comparison of first-filer contemporaneous revenue shares across markets with only an ANDA competitor (ANDA-Only) and markets with both an ANDA and an AG. As noted in the previous sub-sections, ANDA-Only products and ANDA+AG products represent the largest fraction of products in the sample during exclusivity and were the focus of the empirical analysis in the Interim Report.

Figure 3-5 compares the contemporaneous revenue share of ANDA products in ANDA-Only markets and in markets with both an AG and an ANDA competitor in the fourth month following first generic entry. Clearly, even when controlling for market size, the ANDA-generic product usually takes a larger share of the market when it does not face an AG competitor. The difference between average generic revenue shares across these two groups of markets is 25 percentage points.

Table 3-7 reports the results of a linear regression analysis of the impact of AG introduction on the revenue of the ANDA-generic firm during exclusivity as a percentage of what the firm would have earned had the AG not been introduced.[147] For example, the "Effect of Adding an AG to ANDA-Only" figure reported in column (i) is -45.1%, which means that adding an AG to a market with only an ANDA generic competitor would reduce the ANDA competitor's revenues by about 45% relative to what it would have earned without AG competition.[148]

As shown in Table 3-7, introducing an AG has a large and negative effect on ANDA revenues in every model specification. All of the models predict effects that are statistically significant at the 1% confidence level. The magnitude of the AG entry effect is between -39.6% and -52.0%, depending on whether the model sales-weights observations and includes full controls. However, the differences across model specifications are small relative to the estimated AG effects, and none of the estimates is statistically different from the others.

Regardless of which of the four models one favors, the estimated impact of AG entry on wholesale expenditures on the first filer's product is quite a bit larger than the estimated price effects reported in Table 3-2. Revenue impacts depend on both prices and quantities. The evidence so far suggests that increased pricing pressure from AGs only partially explains the impact on first-filer revenues. By construction, the remainder of the revenue effect must be due to AG impact on first-filer quantities.

Table 3-7 also reports that expenditures on ANDA-generics operating in markets without an AG average between 51% and 70% of the pre-generic entry brand expenditures in the 180-day exclusivity period. This not only indicates that they have much to gain by obtaining the exclusivity, but also likely indicates that generic entry can have substantial impact on brand revenues, which is the focus of the next section.

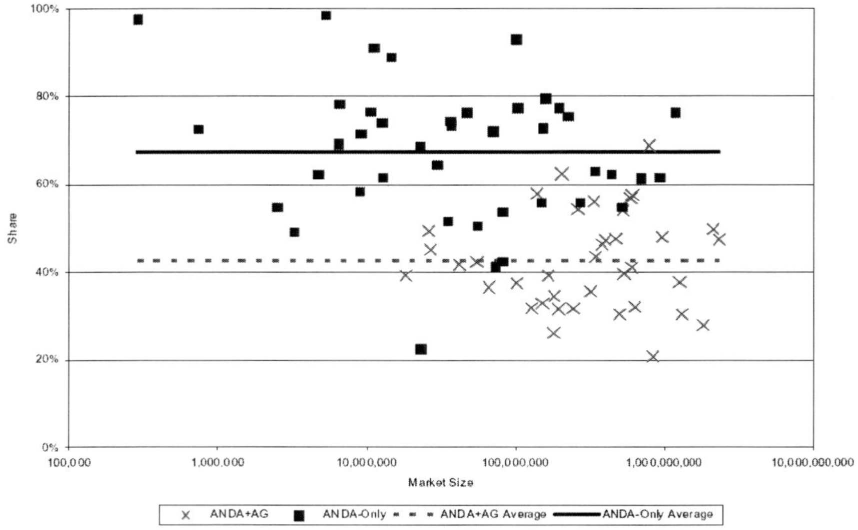

Figure 3-5. Revenue Share of ANDA Generic in Month Four of Exclusivity.

Table 3-7. Effect of AG Entry on ANDA-Generic Product Revenues

	Unweighted		Sales Weighted	
	(i) No Controls	(ii) Full Controls	(iii) No Controls	(iv) Full Controls
Effect of Adding AG to ANDA-Only (Standard Error)	-45.1%*** (7.2%)	-52.0%*** (10.6%)	-40.1%*** (5.9%)	-39.6%*** (10.8%)
ANDA-Only Mean Relative Expenditures	0.70		0.51	
Sample Size	630	630	630	630

***Statistically different from zero at the 1% level

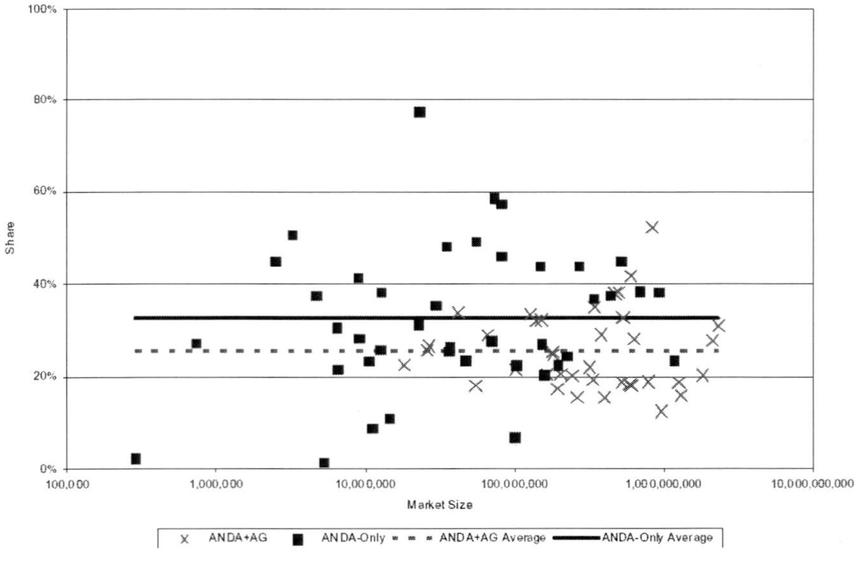

Figure 3-6. Revenue Share of Brand-Name Product in Month Four of Exclusivity.

Table 3-8. Effect of AG Entry on Brand-Name Product Revenues

	Unweighted		Sales Weighted	
	(i) No Controls	(ii) Full Controls	(iii) No Controls	(iv) Full Controls
Effect of Adding an AG to ANDA-Only (Standard Error)	-26.8%*** (6.8%)	-49.0%*** (7.9%)	-27.8%*** (9.2%)	-47.2%*** (9.6%)
ANDA-Only Mean Relative Expenditures	0.49		0.44	
Sample Size	673	673	673	673

***Statistically different from zero at the 1% level

2. Wholesale Revenues of the Brand-Name Product

A potential cost of AG introduction is the cannibalization of brand-name product sales by the AG. This section directly addresses this issue by considering the extent to which an AG affects the revenues of the brand-name product. Figure 3-6 shows that even when controlling for market size, the brand-name product captures a smaller share of revenues in markets with an AG than in markets where it faces the ANDA-generic alone. In the fourth month following generic entry in markets with an AG, the brand-name product's share of revenues is approximately seven percentage points lower than in markets without an AG.

Table 3-8 presents results from four regressions that estimate the effect of introducing an AG on the brand-name products' revenues during the exclusivity period. The model specifications are very similar to those in Table 3-7. The regressions are used to control for how the number of manufacturers and their type affect relative expenditures on the brand-name product.

Table 3-8 examines how introducing an AG affects the revenues of the brand-name product as a percentage of what it would have earned if no AG had been introduced. For example, the "Effect of Adding an AG to ANDA-Only" figure reported in column (i), -26.8%, means that introducing an AG into a market with only an ANDA-generic competitor decreases the revenues of the brand-name product by about 27%, compared to what it would have earned if no AG had been marketed. As shown in Table 3-8, the revenues of brand-name products in AG markets are lower on average than the revenues of brand-name products in No-AG markets. The AG effect estimates range from between -26.8% and -49.0%, and are all statistically significant at the 1% level. Although the differences between the various models can be relatively large in absolute terms, the estimates are not statistically different from each other.[149]

Reduced revenues for the brand-name product, however, do not equate to reduced revenues for the brand-name firm. As discussed in the next section, the brand-name firm receives revenue from the AG as well as from the brand-name product, and both revenue streams contribute to the firm's overall revenues.

3. Wholesale Revenues of Brand-Name Firms

Brand-name companies earn revenues not only from the sale of the brand-name product, but also from the AG, when one is launched.[150] The effect of AG marketing on brand-name company revenues provides some insight into the strategy of the brand-name firm. Because brand-name product sales during exclusivity are more heavily cannibalized in markets with

AGs, as shown in Table 3-8, an important question is whether the brand-name company is able to recoup those lost sales with AG sales. If so, the launch of an AG is in the short-term interest of the brand-name company. If not, perhaps the introduction of an AG is part of a long-term strategy. Long-term strategies might include settlements that designate an ANDA-generic firm as the AG marketer in exchange for delayed generic entry, or they might involve deterring Paragraph IV certifications with respect to other products in the portfolio that are likely to face generic entry at a later date.

Table 3-9 presents the estimated effect that introducing an AG has on the brand-name firm's revenues during exclusivity. The regressions control for how the number of manufacturers and their type affect the relative expenditures on both products of the brand-name firm (the brand-name product and the AG). The model specifications are very similar to those in Table 3-8.

Table 3-9 reports how the introduction of an AG affects the revenues of the brand-name firm as a percentage of what it would have earned had the AG not been introduced. For example, the "Effect of Adding an AG to ANDA-Only" figure reported in column (i), 21.0%, implies that introducing an AG to a market with only an ANDA-generic competitor increases the brand-name firm's revenues by 21%, compared to what it would have earned without introducing an AG. All four models in Table 3-9 report that revenues of brand-name firms that introduce AGs are higher on average than revenues of brand-name firms that do not. The estimated AG effects range between slightly less than 6% and 21%. However, despite the large magnitude of some of the estimates, the results are not always statistically significant.[151] Although not all of our specifications allow us to conclude that brand-name firms earn more revenues in markets with an AG than in markets without an AG, none of the estimates provides evidence that brand-name firms lose revenues as a result of introducing an AG. Consequently, based on the quantitative data, brand-name firms may be introducing an AG either as part of a short-run strategy or a long-term strategy. The long-term strategy may include an entry-deterrence element, as well as more benign, revenue-maximizing activities. Chapter 4 explores the brand-name firms' objectives and strategy from additional perspectives.

IV. Conclusion

The analyses presented in this chapter establish several important points. First, firms' decisions to enter, or attempt to enter, markets for specific products can depend on the characteristics of those markets; specifically, Paragraph IV challenges and AG launches are significantly more common with respect to large-market products than small-market products. Second, the introduction of an AG into a market is associated with lower retail and wholesale prices for generic versions of that product. Third, based on estimates of wholesale expenditures first-filer generics make considerably less revenue when an AG enters the market. Finally, while sales of brand-name products are lower when an AG is launched, revenue losses on brand-name products may be offset by revenues from AGs. The data do not suggest that brand-name firms' overall revenues are diminished.

These results paint a very important part of the picture, but leave some portions blank. Empirical analysis in Chapter 6 will demonstrate that the impact of an AG extends beyond the exclusivity period. Those post-exclusivity results play a part in the analysis, and any overall quantitative assessment of the impact of AGs on generic firms' decisions must be deferred until that later discussion.

Table 3-9. Effect of AG Entry on Brand-Name Firm Revenues (Brand-Name Product and AG)

	Unweighted		Sales Weighted	
	(i) No Controls	(ii) Full Controls	(iii) No Controls	(iv) Full Controls
Effect of Adding an AG to ANDA-Only (Standard Error)	21.0%** (10.4%)	5.9% (10.4%)	20.7%* (12.4%)	18.0% (13.6%)
ANDA-Only Mean Relative Expenditures	0.49		0.44	
Sample Size	673	673	673	673

*Statistically different from zero at the 10% level; ** at the 5% level.

4. The Marketing of Authorized Generics: Brand-Name Firms' Objectives and Strategies

Some critics of authorized generic drugs have asserted that brand-name companies market AGs primarily to deter generic firms' challenges to patents. For example, comments submitted by the Generic Pharmaceutical Association (GPhA) in the course of the FTC's study argue:

> There are . . . no legitimate business reasons for authorized generics launched during the generic exclusivity period. Rather, the sole purpose of such products is to undercut and devalue legitimate generic entry. The sale of authorized generics during the generic exclusivity period reduces the value of the 180-day exclusivity and consequently reduces the incentive for generic drug companies to challenge questionable patents.[152]

Similarly, comments filed "on behalf of one of the largest generic pharmaceutical companies in the United States" maintain that "no brand name company launches an authorized generic during the 180-day exclusivity for the comparatively negligible profits associated with such licensing. Brand-name companies release authorized generics to undermine the incentives granted by Congress to generic companies to challenge and invent around patents."[153]

This chapter explores information on brand-name firms' strategies and objectives regarding authorized generic drugs. Specifically, it looks for evidence that brand-name firms view AGs as a way to compete and maintain a revenue stream after generic entry and for evidence that brand-name firms view AGs as a way to undermine generic competitors' incentives to challenge brand-name firms' patents.

For some AGs – those marketed when there is no exclusivity – the AG cannot be a strategic device to limit the incentives to challenge patents. For AGs marketed during exclusivity periods, the evidence suggests a mixture of motivations. Indeed, the same 180-day exclusivity period that may be crucial to generic profitability offers brand-name firms their best opportunity for enhanced revenue, so that entry-deterring and revenue-enhancement objectives cannot be easily distinguished and separated. Thus, brand-name firm documents show an expectation that AGs will increase brand-name firm revenues after generic entry but also recognize that launching an AG during the exclusivity period may undermine generic incentives to challenge questionable patents.

This chapter explores the facts surrounding branded companies' marketing of AGs. It notes the steep decline in brand-name firms' sales that follows the onset of generic competition and explores the role of AGs in maintaining a brand-name firm's revenue stream following generic entry, as described in the brand-name firms' internal documents. It observes that those documents also show clear recognition that AG competition during 180-day exclusivity may diminish incentives for ANDA-generic entry via patent challenges. Finally, the chapter examines brand marketing practices – including AG launch timing and post-exclusivity marketing and AG pricing and profit-splits – that shed additional light on brand-name firm objectives.

I. Authorized Generics and Revenue Enhancement

A. The Use of Authorized Generics to Maintain a Revenue Stream

In recent years, the brand-name industry has been affected by substantial growth in the market share of generic drugs and the speed at which they are adopted. Continuing a trend that began with enactment of the Hatch-Waxman Amendments in 1984,[154] generics' overall share of prescriptions increased from 49 percent in 2000 to 74 percent in 2009.[155] The speed of generic penetration also increased during this period. Until about 2000, studies reported that six months after generic entry, the brand retained 40–70 percent of market share.[156] By contrast, recent observations suggest that for many drugs, brand share at six months is less than 20 percent,[157] and in some cases brand share may fall even more rapidly.[158]

Based on their internal documents, many brand-name firms regard authorized generics as a way to recapture some of the lost revenue. For example, one major brand-name firm used a subsidiary to launch AG products, with the stated goal of maximizing returns after loss of exclusivity ("LOE").[159] The AG subsidiary continues to be the "cornerstone" of the firm's strategy to capture value after its brand-name drugs lose exclusivity.[160] Another large brand-name firm justified decisions to launch AGs based on the "incremental profits" available from "captur[ing] a share of the generic market without cannibalizing the branded business."[161]

The documents suggest that brand-name companies are particularly interested in marketing during 180-day exclusivity for the same reasons that generic companies are – with limited competition and the ability to sell at a relatively high price, the exclusivity period offers the greatest profit opportunity.[162] Thus, while marketing an AG during exclusivity necessarily reduces ANDA-generic returns on patent challenges, it also provides the brand the highest return. For example, one brand-name company explained that when one of its products loses exclusivity, its AG subsidiary blunts the loss because it:

> can also market during the lucrative 180 day period of limited competition. This practice of using an AG to participate in the high margin 180 day exclusivity period has now become standard throughout the industry. . . . Due to the success of this

practice, we anticipate that every product with annual brand sales in excess of $50 million will have an AG launched with a Para IV loss of exclusivity.[163]

Another brand-name firm projected that an AG would add $60–$65 million of incremental business unit contribution in one year "[a]ssuming that the 180-day exclusive period is maintained" but would yield only "marginal" benefit without exclusivity.[164]

The brand-name firms' keen interest in the revenues arising from AGs and their intense concern with any impact of the AG on branded sales are reflected in their extensive forecasting and sales analysis documents. Virtually every brand-name company in the study that had marketed an AG produced multiple forecasts and revenue analyses in response to the FTC Special Orders.[165] The forecasts were incorporated into different phases of company decision-making, including decisions to market an AG, select an external distributor, determine launch timing, and project how much to manufacture.[166] After launch of an AG, companies closely monitored actual revenues, price, and market share to facilitate adjustments based on market conditions.[167]

A key conclusion of the brand-name firms' analyses is that AGs can generate incremental revenue when a branded product loses exclusivity.[168] This is supported by the study's data analysis. Wholesale expenditures during 180-day exclusivity on the brand-name firm's combined products (brand plus any AG) were higher under all models when an AG was present than when only the brand-name product and an ANDA generic competed.[169] This is consistent with a brand-name firm objective of maintaining a revenue stream following generic entry.

B. The Use of Brand-Name Discounting to Maintain a Revenue Stream

In theory, instead of marketing an AG, a brand-name company might try to retain market share after generic entry by cutting the price of its brand-name product to a level directly competitive with generic drugs. Typically, however, brand-name firms have not employed full "price equalization" strategies.[170] This section explores possible reasons why brand-name companies that seek to defend their revenues after generic entry might turn to AGs.

Selling AGs at the ANDA-generic price and brand-name products at a higher price is a form of price discrimination. If customers can be segmented by their willingness to pay a premium for a branded product, such price discrimination affords an opportunity for the brand-name manufacturer to reap greater revenues.[171] Market segmentation indeed appears possible.

The brand will be attractive to purchasers buying under "dispense as written" prescriptions and to consumers who are willing to pay more for brand-name products.[172] The generic is an option for the more price-sensitive customers.

In contrast, reducing price on the brand potentially has some economic and strategic disadvantages. Such discounting entails a loss of residual brand sales at full margin.[173] Moreover, a brand-name firm analysis cautions that a price discount might effectively become permanent, to the brand-name firm's detriment.[174] For example, if the brand cuts price when a generic enters at risk, it may be difficult to restore full price upon a favorable appellate decision.[175] And the same firm's analysis indicates that cutting price on a core branded product could make it more difficult for the brand-name firm to justify the price of any line extensions.[176]

Other considerations sometimes cited in analyzing the choice between offering an AG and reducing brand price across the board upon generic entry include state generic substitution laws and Medicaid mandates for generic substitution.[177] Brand-name firm analyses also note that drug plans encourage generic substitution through their co-payment schedules[178] and that pharmacies typically earn greater profit margins with generic substitution and, along with PBMs, have policies and/or incentives that favor generic substitution.[179]

In sum, the price of brand-name drugs typically remains significantly above generic levels. For the various reasons noted, it appears plausible that reliance on AGs could be the most effective means for brand-name firms to retain revenues following the onset of generic competition.

II. Authorized Generics and Impact on Generic Firms' Incentives

Revenue considerations, however, are not the whole story. Brand-name firm documents produced for this study reveal a clear understanding that the marketing of AGs during 180-day exclusivity periods may have some impact on generic firms' incentives to challenge patents.[180] Of course, the fact that a company recognizes that an authorized generic could deter future generic entry does not necessarily mean that the company employs the strategy to achieve that outcome.

For example, the operating plan for one brand-name firm notes that the ability to launch an AG "during 180 day exclusivity period may make paragraph IV challengers think twice before attacking [brand-name company] brands, due to reduced financial rewards."[181] Another brand-name firm recognizes AGs' potential to "[d]iscourage future paragraph IV litigation by devaluing the 180 days exclusivity period"[182] and to "modestly diminish value of first-to file generics" but adds, "overall financial attractiveness for first to file ANDA is still relatively high."[183] A document from a third brand-name firm emphasizes the disincentive effect over revenue generation with regard to a specific AG: "Financially speaking, [the AG is] not a particularly attractive proposition, but . . . strategically we may want to send a message . . . that [the brand] will launch authorized generics . . . and thereby hopefully reduce future Gx competition for subsequent . . . products coming off patent."[184]

Overall, the document production reflects that brand-name companies see authorized generics as a strategy to maintain revenue but recognize that AGs could deter future patent challenges. It provides no clear basis for deeming one consideration more important than the other and only rarely isolates a single rationale for particular AG marketing decisions. We next examine brand-name firms' practices, finding behavior patterns consistent with maximization of combined brand and AG revenues rather than a sacrifice of revenue to maximize impact on generic competition.

III. Evidence from Brand Marketing Practices

A. Relationship to Exclusivity; Timing of Launch and Withdrawal

Marketing during 180-day exclusivity: Although AGs frequently are marketed during an ANDA-generic's 180-day exclusivity, as would be expected if AGs were launched to deter patent challenges, most AGs are not associated with exclusivity periods. As noted above, about two-thirds of the 119 AGs identified in this study were not marketed during an exclusivity period.[185] Moreover, nearly half of the brand-name drugs for which AGs were launched were subject only to Paragraph I, II, or III certifications and thus were not associated with drugs that had been subject to patent challenges.[186] The fact that brands often introduce AGs in circumstances that are unlikely to have any long-term impact on future patent challenges strongly suggests that AGs have value as a competitive response unrelated to any reduction of incentives to challenge patents.

Launch timing: Brands almost always launch AGs simultaneously with or shortly after ANDA-generic entry. This is consistent both with strategies based on retaining revenues and with strategies premised on deterring patent challenges. As explained below, launching AGs prior to ANDA-generic entry might support claims that aspects of AG marketing serve the sole purpose of devaluing 180-day exclusivity, but this has not been the pattern observed.

Launching an AG before ANDA-generic entry would give the AG a first-mover advantage by which it could gain and keep market share,[187] thereby "[d]ilut[ing] the value of the 180 exclusivity to the ANDA holder."[188] Early launch, however, "cannibalizes" sales of the brand-name product, starting their decline before ANDA-generic entry has occurred.[189] Brand-name firms have chosen to tightly control the timing of AG launch to avoid unnecessary loss of brand sales and other disadvantages.[190] Launch even a short time before confirmation of ANDA-generic entry is disfavored, and AG supply agreements often include strict penalty provisions or financial terms that enforce launch timing.[191] Accordingly, at least apart from settlement contexts, AGs generally are launched immediately upon confirmation of ANDA-generic entry, so as to achieve the highest level of AG sales without unnecessarily eroding brand-name sales.[192] Figure 4-1 illustrates this point; for the 88 drugs/strengths covered by AGs and associated with exclusivity periods during the 2001–2008 period, AG launch occurred within five days of generic entry 76% of the time; AG launch preceded generic entry by more than five days roughly one percent of the time.[193]

This, of course, does not preclude a rationale based on deterring patent challenges; marketing an AG beginning with the 180-day exclusivity period simultaneously raises brand-name firm revenues and decreases revenues of the first-filer. The data do suggest that brand-name firms have not sacrificed combined AG and brand revenues in order to maximize impact on the first-filer. If brand-name firms frequently began AG marketing before generic entry, a long-term strategy, such as deterring Paragraph IV certifications or encouraging settlements that delay generic entry, would have been indicated, but this has not been the case. All in all, the launch timing data are consistent with the presence of both revenue-driven and entry-deterring objectives.

Market withdrawal: Contrary to assertions that AGs are marketed only during exclusivity and are removed from the market almost immediately afterwards,[194] almost all AGs marketed during exclusivity continue to be marketed for an extended period, often for many years.

Indeed, of the 25 oral-solid AGs launched between 2001 and 2006 and associated with a 180-day exclusivity period, 23 continued to be marketed two years after the beginning of exclusivity; by the end of 2009, three to eight years after the start of the exclusivity periods, 16 remained on the market.[195] This is consistent with brand-name firms' statements that they continue to market AGs "after the 180-day period expires, if it is commercially desirable to do so."[196]

In sum, quantitative information shows that brand-name firms market AGs both with and without exclusivity; typically launch AGs on schedules that forgo maximum impact on ANDA-generic rivals while avoiding cannibalization of brand sales; and generally continue marketing AGs after 180-day exclusivity has ended. These facts all point to use of AGs as a revenue-enhancing technique, but the data are also consistent with the use of some AGs as a disincentive to patent challenges by generic firms.

B. Pricing, Market Share, and Profit-Splits

As described above in Chapter 2, AG marketing follows two principal routes; brand-name companies or their subsidiaries distributed 44 percent of the AGs covered by this study; independent licensees distributed the remaining 56 percent. When AG marketing is handled in-house, the brand-name company can exercise direct control. In contrast, pricing decisions by outside licensees typically are independent of the brand.[197] In both cases, however, material produced for this study suggests that brand-name firms shy away from maximizing impact on generic competitors, while enhancing brand-name firm revenues.

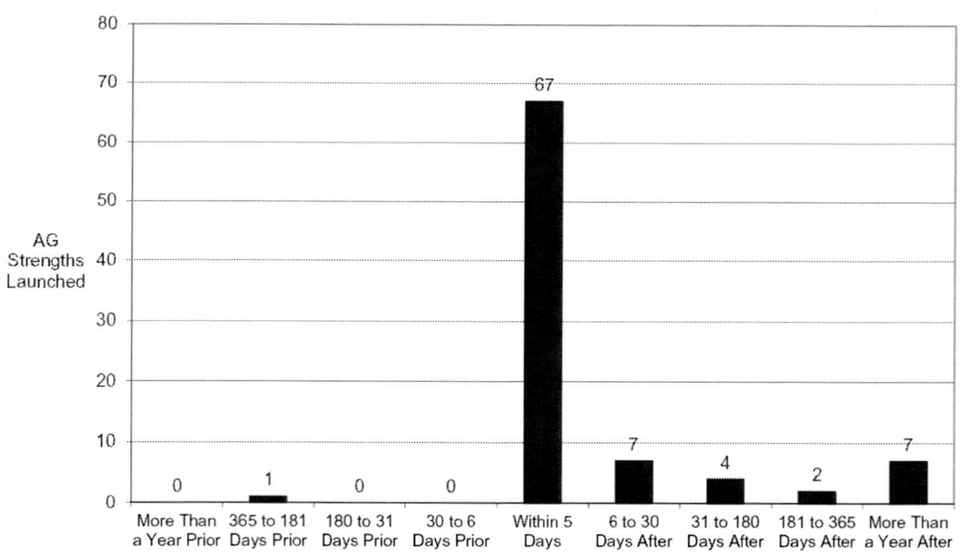

Figure 4-1. Authorized Generic Drug Launch Timing Compared, Strength by Strength, to Entry of Corresponding ANDA-Generics with 180-Day Exclusivity (2001-2008).

Brands that market in-house generally do not appear to aggressively reduce the price of AGs during 180-day exclusivity, even though such discounting might capture a larger share of the market and thereby diminish generic firms' incentives to challenge patents. At least one major brand-name company recognized that lowering AG prices would tend to "[r]educe[] financial incentives to file Para IV ANDAs"[198] but rejected that approach.[199] Indeed, documents explaining the pricing practices of brand subsidiaries often assert that an AG should be a price follower, not a price leader, to avoid driving price down, especially during exclusivity.[200] These documents articulated many drawbacks to aggressive AG pricing during 180-day exclusivity, including loss of the high margin available during that period and possible acceleration of brand erosion.[201] Similarly, brand-name firms' documents suggest that they generally seek to capture a large but measured portion of the market because seeking more would require substantial price cuts.[202] Again, this indicates that brands generally have not attempted to maximize the deterrent value of AGs by acquiring market share at the expense of profitability.

Marketing through independent distributors has followed a similar approach. AGs as a whole were priced similarly to the competing ANDA generics at wholesale, and there was no statistically significant difference between the pricing of AGs marketed by independent licensees and the pricing of AGs marketed by brand-name firm subsidiaries.[203] Describing its criteria for evaluating the effectiveness of competition by a generic marketing partner, one brand-name firm expressly opted for a "[p]rofit maximizing rather than a sales maximizing approach."[204] Indeed, many AG supply agreements specify that the distributor cannot use the AG as a loss leader or price it differently from the way it prices its ANDA-generic products.[205]

Profit-splits, i.e., the percentage of profits that the AG distributor must pay to the brand, are also consistent with the brand's interest in the revenue stream arising from an AG. Apart from contexts where AG marketing rights derive from patent litigation settlements, marketing agreements generally require AG distributors to pay the brand a large percentage of profits on the AG, typically from 50–92 percent.[206] In sum, neither the pricing terms nor the profit splits of arrangements with independent marketers suggest that brand-name firms have maximized AGs' deterrent value without regard to impact on brand-name firm revenues.

IV. Conclusion

Review of documents and data accumulated for this study suggests that brand-name firms understand that authorized generics have two principal effects. Plainly, they are aware that AG marketing during the 180-day exclusivity period could cause potential generic entrants to think twice before adopting strategies based on patent challenges and early, exclusive entry. Claims that this is the sole purpose of AG marketing, however, appear overstated and inconsistent with the marketing strategies that brand-name companies adopt with regard to authorized generics. Marketing an AG is a way for a brand-name firm to preserve a revenue stream after the onset of generic competition. That this marketing frequently occurs during the generic's 180-day exclusivity period is no surprise: that is when maximum profits are available, for the brand-name firm as well as the generic. Moreover, AG marketing typically persists beyond the end of 180-day exclusivity, and most AGs are not marketed during exclusivity periods.

Moreover, while AG marketing substantially impairs generic firms' revenue opportunities, brand-name firms have not sacrificed combined AG and brand revenues in order to maximize impact on the first-filer. Thus, AG marketing typically is timed to begin simultaneously with or follow immediately after generic entry, forgoing a first-mover advantage that would harm generics but also cannibalize brand sales. And AGs usually are price followers, not competitors that undercut generic rivals in ways that would inflict the most harm.

Analysis of brand-name firms' documents and marketing practices consequently provides a mixed picture, one consistent with both revenue-generating and entry-deterring objectives. In subsequent chapters we look to additional sources of evidence in order to examine AGs' likely effects on generics' long-run incentives.

5. The Marketing of Authorized Generics: Generic Firm Perceptions and Decision-making

In Chapter 4 we examined AGs from the perspective of brand-name companies. In this chapter we consider AGs from the perspective of generic pharmaceutical firms, based largely on the documents they submitted in response to the Commission's Generic Company Special Order.[207] In Section I we discuss what the documents reveal about generic company concerns regarding, and reactions to, AGs' effects on their revenues. In Section II we turn to the central issue: the extent to which AGs may create disincentives to patent challenges by generic firms, thereby potentially delaying generic entry and diminishing generic competition.

The generic company documents confirm Chapter 3's empirical finding that the sale of an AG during the exclusivity period substantially reduces the revenue of the ANDA generic, thereby reducing the value of the exclusivity gained through a patent challenge. Yet the documents do not reflect consensus on the longer-term impact of AGs. Although some documents express concern with the potential long-run impact of AGs on generic firm incentives and the financial health of the generic industry, these were largely *advocacy* documents articulating for public presentation the position of the generic firms' trade association[208] and of certain of the generic companies that have been at the forefront of challenging the marketing of AGs during 180-day exclusivity periods. By contrast, there were few *internal company* documents discussing (or even alluding to) the disincentive issue, even from those companies focused on securing exclusivities. Indeed, none of the internal company documents expressly discusses AGs as a factor in deciding whether to file a particular patent challenge. The projected effects of AG competition, however, may have resulted in financial forecasts for Paragraph IV entry by some drugs in small markets showing losses, rather than profits.

At the same time the internal company documents submitted by a number of generic companies raise questions regarding contentions that AGs create significant disincentives to patent challenges and seriously threaten the industry's continued ability to develop generic drugs, as some in the industry have argued. As discussed in Chapter 2, different generic companies have adopted different business strategies in the face of AG competition,[209] and those strategies, not surprisingly, appear to be reflected in how they view AGs and their potential long-term impact.

I. The Impact of AGs on Generic Firm Revenues and Profits: Generic Company Concerns and Responses

A. The Nature of Generic Company Concerns

Generic company concerns about AGs are most clearly set out in advocacy documents submitted by several of the generic companies. These materials focus largely on revenue losses experienced by generic firms due to AG marketing during the 180-day exclusivity period. For example, in one generic firm's 2004 powerpoint presentation to the FTC, entitled "The Anticompetitive Threat of Authorized Generics," the firm referenced the example of another generic company that reportedly lost approximately $400 million of expected revenues due to AG competition during the exclusivity period for one drug, which represented as much as three-times its entire annual R&D budget.[210] In another example, the firm contended that it had lost revenues of over $32 million on one drug during the 180-day exclusivity period alone and that that amounted to over 32% of the firm's entire R&D budget for fiscal year 2004.[211] The presentation estimated that, industry-wide, AGs reduced generic revenues by $700 million to $1.2 billion.[212] Thus, it argued, "[a]uthorized generics harm consumers by impairing the ability of generic companies to continue innovating and developing new generic drugs."[213]

Similar concerns about the impact of AGs on exclusivity, using the same examples of lost revenues, are reflected in other advocacy documents produced by the generic firms, including citizen petitions.[214] Another document, urging that a joint letter be sent to the FDA "requesting that the Agency protect the incentives entitled to generic drug companies for the future development of generic drugs," says that "[t]he consequences of authorized generic deals are tremendous: by losing its 180-day head-start on other generic competitors, a first filing generic company faces strikingly reduced profit opportunities."[215]

Non-advocacy documents confirm that the introduction of an AG during the exclusivity period substantially erodes the expected profitability of the ANDA. Thus, one internal company document observes that authorized generics are "here to stay," and "in general cut in half or more the profitability of the value of the 180-day exclusivity."[216] This estimate is consistent with that in an investment advisory letter, which observed that "[d]ue to market share and pricing erosion at the hands of the authorized player, we estimate that the profits for the 'pure' generic during the exclusivity period could be reduced by approximately 60% in a typical scenario."[217] Another company's sales forecasts assume an AG, and, because of that assumption, the "[f]orecast is reduced from 100% market share during 6 months of exclusivity to 60% market share."[218] In fact, various sales and pre-launch forecasts indicate that generic firms routinely assume the presence of an AG, and weave that consideration, along with assumptions about market size, substitution rates, price erosion,[219] and the likely number of competitors, into their projections of sales and profitability of the ANDA-generic drug during the exclusivity period and beyond.[220] Accordingly, the generic company documents underscore Chapter 3's quantitative findings of revenue impacts and indicate that, especially for those firms whose business models focus on obtaining exclusivities via Paragraph IV filings, the adverse financial consequences of AGs may be significant.

Several other internal company documents allude generally to the effect of AGs on the value of 180-day exclusivity. Thus, a 2005 strategic planning document from one generic firm notes that "price erosion is here to stay," that "[e]xclusivity has become elusive;

[a]uthorized generics erodes market share," and that "authorized generics diminish value of exclusivity."[221] Another document, discussing the competitive profile of a rival generic company, observed as one challenge for that company, "Intense competition/Revenues decline with competition; Authorized generics will impair 180 [day] exclusivity."[222]

A March 2005 business plan of one company likewise refers to the threat posed by AGs to at least some generic companies. After observing that innovators had "become more savvy about protecting their intellectual property" and that patent litigation had grown more difficult and costly for generic challengers, increasing their product development risks and reducing their returns, it continued:

> Of specific concern to [the company], as well as other generic manufacturers is the fact, that quite recently several innovators have been making authorized generics available to the market. Pfizer (the innovator behind a number of products that figure prominently in [the company's] pipeline) has been using Greenstone . . . to launch a steady stream of products whose patents have expired/successfully challenged in court. Greenstone's approach of aggressive product pricing and achieving success in retaining substantive market share is a chilling prospect for any generics company that targets Pfizer products for development and market introduction. GSK and J&J have also introduced generic versions of their leading compounds . . . .[223]

Other internal company documents reflect general concerns about competition from AGs but provide few details. For example, one company, in a 2005 business strategy document, identified AGs as one of two "[p]otential near term pricing pressures," the other being "off shore manufacturers (India/China)."[224] Another firm, in a 2005 competitor assessment, identifies as one of three major focuses for the generic industry "[b]eating back authorized generics from big pharma."[225] Still another identified AGs as one of a large number of factors causing increasing competitive pressures in the generic industry, referencing in particular Indian generics, "Buyer consolidation; Industry-wide capacity increases; Authorized generics; Shared exclusivity; [and] Aggressive innovator responses (e.g., scientific challenges, Citizen's Petitions, follow-on products, own Gx operations)."[226] Likewise, a number of third-party investment reports mention AGs as one of a number of factors responsible for increasing competitive pressures in the industry, again, without any detailed analysis.[227]

In short, the generic company document submissions support the contention that introduction of an AG during the 180-day exclusivity period significantly cuts into the expected revenue and profit of the ANDA-generic, and thereby decreases the value of exclusivity. As discussed below, the generic firms have responded to these pressures in varying ways and consequently view AGs from varying perspectives.

B. Differing Generic Company Responses

Chapter 2 explains that different generic companies have adopted different business strategies in the face of widespread AG marketing.[228] Some have continued to emphasize Paragraph IV certifications and pursuit of 180-day exclusivities. Others instead have sought to partner with brand-name firms in marketing AGs.[229] Still other generic companies pursue a mix of ANDA and AG business. As one document quipped, "If you can't beat em, join em."[230]

Unsurprisingly, with variations in strategic response, firms have developed different attitudes toward AGs,[231] and the companies' document submissions reflect those differences. Thus, for example, one generic firm that has emphasized pursuing exclusivity opportunities submitted advocacy and other third-party documents strongly opposing the introduction of AGs during the exclusivity period.[232] On the other hand, many of the generic company document submissions focused, not on the impact of AGs on 180-day exclusivity, but rather on how best to compete for AG business from the brand-name companies, as the generic firms sought to develop business strategies to take advantage of potential market opportunities provided by AGs.[233] The documents show that some generic firms did in fact embark on marketing efforts aimed at encouraging brand-name companies to use them as distributors,[234] and AG distribution arrangements reportedly became important sources of profits for some generic firms.[235]

At the same time, some documents also suggest that AG distribution opportunities for generic firms even as early as 2004 were becoming more difficult to obtain, thereby prompting some to re-visit their AG strategies.[236] As one generic firm document explains:

> AGx opportunities and expected returns have both been substantially reduced in recent months, due to the decision of various brand companies to market more of their products through their own AGx subsidiaries, and increased competition among generic companies for available AGx deals.. . . .
>
> Revenue and earnings shortfalls by many publicly-traded generic companies due to severe pricing competition has made AGs one of the only ways to maintain growth in the short term; The resulting intense competitive bidding for remaining opportunities has made brand companies realize they are in a position to retain most of the economic value of authorized generic versions of their intellectual property; Historically, generic partners received 20–35% of the economics, but this has now been driven down to 10% or less; The reduced value of AG deals for generic companies will hurt the business models of some companies . . . .[237]

In sum, the documents produced by the generic firms reflect different perspectives on AGs depending in large part on their differing business strategies. With this foundation, the following section examines what the generic company document submissions reveal about the long-term impact of AGs on the incentives of generic firms to challenge patents via Paragraph IV filings.

II. The Long-Term Impact of AGs on Generic Firm Incentives to Bring Generic Products to Market via Patent Challenges

Although a few documents register concern with AGs at a general, strategic level,[238] or suggest an increased need to manage the product selection and litigation processes, none of the generic companies' internal documents states that the presence of AGs caused a firm to decide against pursuing early entry through any specific patent challenge.[239] The internal documents do include financial forecasts that, without providing a narrative or stating any conclusions, could be consistent with assertions that expected AG competition has undermined the profitability of patent challenges for some small-market drugs. Taken together, the documents suggest that, even with AG competition, expected financial returns during the 180-day exclusivity period generally remain sufficiently attractive to incentivize generic firms to pursue early entry through Paragraph IV filings, with the possible exception of certain small-market drugs.

A. Documents Suggesting an Impact on Generic Entry through Patent Challenges

The documents produced by the generic companies suggest that the promise of exclusivity provides an incentive for companies to file Paragraph IV ANDAs and that AG marketing during the 180-day exclusivity period detracts from that incentive. The documents submitted, however, are both fewer and weaker than would be expected if AGs had markedly undermined generic firm business models based on Paragraph IV patent challenges.

On the one hand, the documents speak to the importance generic companies place on exclusivity gained through first-to-file opportunities. A number of the generics' internal strategy documents recommend concentrating on first-to-file opportunities.[240] As one generic company put it, "products with a chance to be FTF need special consideration. . . . The difference between profits on FTF product and not-FTF product are significant."[241] Similarly, third-party investment advisory reports highlight exclusivities as an important component of perceived firm value.[242]

In view of the importance of 180-day exclusivity to many generic companies, AG incursions on exclusivity may also be significant, leading to diminished incentives to file Paragraph IV ANDAs, and, at least in theory, fewer patent challenges. One generic firm produced a strategic planning document that questioned whether "Para IV [is] still a viable strategy," noting that the "Generic Landscape has changed: No More True Exclusivity (Authorized Generics); Probability of Success (POS) of litigation may have changed" and "Market Pricing & Share assumptions have changed."[243] The outcome in that instance, however, was not to cease or shift away from Paragraph IV filings. Rather, the document suggests that the company's mix of Paragraph III and Paragraph IV filings be reviewed and that a more rigorous, systematic selection process be implemented ("[w]e must realign cost/risk against potential upsides in our PIV strategy"), with the goal of placing "Increased Focus on Formulation and Product Selection (pursue higher quality [PIV] cases only)."[244] At the same time, the document reveals that the company planned to approach several large brand-name companies with AG marketing proposals, thereby attempting to diversify its revenue sources.[245]

If generic firms were to become more selective in pursuing first-to-file opportunities because of the reduced value of exclusivity, that could reduce the number of patent challenges overall. Likewise, if the firms decided to significantly cut back on their Paragraph IV filings in favor of pursuing AG marketing opportunities, that too could result in fewer patent challenges. The document submissions provide only scattered support for either of these scenarios, however, and suggest that AGs are but one of a number of factors that shape generic firms' selections of drugs to face patent challenges.

Four other documents offer opinions consistent with AGs having some long-term detrimental impact, but do not delve into the issue.

- One, a third-party report commissioned by one of the generic companies, simply observes that "[t]he authorized generic erodes the market share, profitability and market price of the Paragraph IV generic during the exclusivity period," and states that "[t]he authorized generic strategy has a long term focus by reducing the funding available for generic manufacturers to challenge brand patents to obtain the 180 day exclusivity period."[246]

- An internal company document from the same generic firm reflects much the same opinion.[247]
- Another third-party report, produced by a different generic firm, similarly observes that "authorized generics have eroded a significant financial incentive for the industry" but does not elaborate.[248]
- One other document, reporting a question-and-answer session with one company's executives, addresses both AGs and exclusivity. Thus, in answer to the questions, "What do you think of authorized generics? Are they pro consumer or anti consumer?" the executive replied:

> It depends on whether your focus is short term or long term. I think in the short term they can be viewed as pro consumer because they lower the price immediately.
> For that segment of the population that's private pay, it makes a difference. For that segment that isn't, I don't think it changes their copay much, if at all. The generic copay is the generic copay. So a lot of consumers may see little if any savings.
> Longer term I do think there's some element of the authorized generic approach that's intended to undermine the generic industry. Over time, that could have an impact on the number and types of products brought into the market.[249]

Yet, when asked whether his firm would "still go after the first-to-file opportunities" if 180-day exclusivity were abolished, the same executive appeared somewhat ambivalent about the importance of exclusivity:

> That's what I'm sitting here trying to think through. Would we go after the same number if we didn't see those controls in the market and in the timing of the entrance into the market? That's probably where I've got the most hesitation. I'm not sure we'd go after as many. I would think we'd be more selective.[250]

Finally, some of the financial forecasts produced by generic companies support assertions that the expectation of AG competition has tipped the balance against proceeding with a Paragraph IV challenge for certain small-market drugs. One generic company produced contemporaneous "new product forecasts" for four drugs,[251] and explained these forecasts in a subsequent interpretive analysis submitted to the FTC.[252] Combining the contemporaneous data with some additional assumptions and assertions regarding the firm's assessment methodology, that analysis concludes that the reduced sales and lower prices attributable to AG competition could have led the firm in these cases to decide against (or to defer) pursuing entry via a patent challenge.[253] Indeed, the analyst's calculations appear to suggest that AG competition may have made a difference in two of the cases, one a drug depicted as having annual sales of approximately $40 million (which nonetheless did draw a Paragraph IV challenge from another firm) and the other a drug with annual sales of about $50 million at the time that ANDA-generic development was put on hold.[254] The findings of potential impact on Paragraph IV challenges in small markets are very much in line with the results of this Report's break-even analysis, *infra* in Chapter 6.

B. Documents Suggesting that Impacts of AGs on Generic Entry through Patent Challenges May be Overstated

Several generic companies produced documents that took issue with the contention that AGs would create significant disincentives to future patent challenges. Thus, the general counsel of one generic firm observed:

> Theoretically the possible availability of an "authorized" generic might make a generic company hesitate in filing and then defending a Paragraph IV litigation. However, will that occur in reality. I tend to doubt that the possibility will deter Paragraph IV litigation. Look at the myriad of suits on the blockbusters and then say that if there were an authorized generic all of the claimants would not have filed their Paragraph IV. However is it fair that after spending millions they have an authorized generic to deal with. Yes, at least in my opinion, it is fair!. Look at the price that the holder of an exclusive generic sells the product for, i.e. say 20% less than the brand. A great profit. If there were an "authorized" generic also, perhaps they will have to discount 30–40% – still a great profit. A profit well worth the expense of the Paragraph IV suit![255]

Moreover, the general counsel shared his concerns with GPhA:

> While I do not wish to be seen as a "rabble rouser" or a malcontent, I do have a few concerns and questions regarding the GPHA position on "Authorized Generics" . . . . [W]hile it is obvious to me that the authorized generic would "skim" some of the profits the first to file would get during a period of generic exclusivity, is there proof that the GPHA position, in the real world, is true, i.e., would many, if not most, Paragraph IV filings not be undertaken if the Paragraph IV filer thought that an authorized generic would be marketed before or during a period of generic marketing exclusivity. Actually I do not believe that is true. . . . I believe that there are many members that are "suspicious" of the GPHA position.[256]

Similarly, a 2004 document produced by a generic company that is a subsidiary of a brand-name company questions the seriousness of the AG threat. After setting out the basic arguments for and against AGs,[257] that document catalogues the benefits of AGs to both brand-name companies and generic companies.[258] It notes that "[g]enerics are perceived as pro-consumer and part of the solution to increasing drug costs";[259] questions whether "the generic industry [is] entitled to have the value of 180-day exclusivity frozen in time as a matter of right";[260] and observes that other factors, including "[c]oexclusivity or patent-by-patent exclusivity" and the forfeiture provisions of the MMA, also may reduce the value of exclusivity.[261] While observing that AGs, along with other factors, had diminished the value of exclusivity,[262] it nevertheless concludes that "P-IVs with AG [Are] Still Valuable to Filer."[263] Hence, it concludes that, "[the] Generic Industry will survive and adapt; Pro-consumer approach with lower costs product consistent with generic industry sense of purpose; P-IV value in the future not as assured as before" and goes on to question, "Is this an issue the industry wants to push? . . . Are there higher priorities?"[264]

Some third-party investor reports produced by generic companies likewise express serious doubts about the significance of any disincentive effect of AGs on patent challenges by generic firms. One such report, while indicating that "authorized generics have eroded a significant financial incentive for the industry,"[265] nevertheless projected substantial profits from the exclusivity opportunities studied "even after adjusting for likely competition from authorized generics."[266] Another, after observing that in theory decreased incentives could make generic companies less willing to pursue at-risk launches, stated, "[w]e can't think of a case where the threat of an authorized generic resulted in a generic company deciding not to launch at risk."[267]

III. Conclusion

The generic company documents confirm that competition from an AG substantially reduces the revenue of ANDA-generics during 180-day exclusivity and speak to the importance some generic companies place on first-to-file opportunities. One generic firm produced contemporaneous financial forecasts and a subsequent interpretive analysis that, together, suggest that an expectation of AG competition tipped the balance against that firm's entry via a patent challenge for two drugs in small markets. On the whole, however, the internal company documents lend little support to the contention that AGs have created significant disincentives to generic firms' filing of Paragraph IV ANDAs. None of the internal company documents expressly discusses AGs as a factor in deciding whether to file a particular patent challenge. The document submissions provide scattered indications that some firms have become more selective in pursuing first-to-file opportunities but no evidence that any firm has substantially abandoned its basic Paragraph IV business strategy because of the proliferation of AGs.

While findings based on the limited evidence derived from generic firms' document productions cannot by themselves yield firm conclusions, they provide another piece of evidence for assessing the competitive impact of AGs. In the next chapter we examine the quantitative data for further insights into their long-term competitive effects.

6. Long-Term Effects of Authorized Generics: Price, Revenue, and Break-Even Effects

This chapter extends the analysis of Chapter 3, which considered the impact of authorized generic drugs during the exclusivity period, to time periods in which generic versions of the drug are on the market but no exclusivity applies. The analysis in this chapter is based on two samples of market outcomes: one drawn from drugs for which an exclusivity period was granted but has expired and another based on drugs for which no exclusivity was ever granted. These two scenarios will collectively be referred to as non-exclusivity situations.

The principal difference between the competitive environment outside of exclusivity, as compared to during exclusivity, is the potential for entry by ANDA-generic firms. Firms with tentative FDA approval that are not first-filers are barred from entry during exclusivity. However, firms with approved ANDAs are free to enter at any time outside the exclusivity period. Only one or two generics are typically on the market during exclusivity. In contrast, the number of manufacturers actively selling a generic version of a drug can range from one to more than fifteen outside of exclusivity. Consequently, one may expect an AG to have a greater impact during exclusivity, when it can be one of only a few competitors, rather than one of many.

Chapter 3 showed that introduction of an AG during exclusivity tended to be associated with lower prices, decreased first-filer revenues, and increased brand-name firm revenues. This chapter presents similar analysis using market data from non-exclusivity situations. In general, the results of the analysis of drugs with expired exclusivity periods are remarkably consistent with the exclusivity-period analysis: prices for generic drugs tend to be lower in markets where an AG was launched than in markets without AGs. For markets in which no generic manufacturer was granted an exclusivity period, the estimated effect on generic price of entry by an AG is not consistently different from the effect of entry by an additional ANDA-generic.

In Chapter 3, the analysis of wholesale expenditures demonstrated that introduction of an AG can substantially reduce the revenue of the first-filer generic manufacturer during exclusivity. The new evidence in this chapter suggests that early generic entrants, whether first-filers or AGs, are able to retain a large portion of their market shares even after potentially many other ANDA-generics enter following the 180-day exclusivity period. This first-mover advantage seems to be an important benefit of introducing a product during the exclusivity period. Because the average first-filer who faced an AG during exclusivity begins post-exclusivity competition with a smaller market share, and thus holds on to a portion of this smaller share, the impact of the AG on first-filer revenues persists beyond the 180 days. This result is important because it will be utilized, along with similar estimates from the exclusivity analysis, to calibrate a simple analysis of how the anticipation of facing AG competition may impact the incentives of ANDA-generic manufacturers to pursue Paragraph IV challenges.

This chapter first reviews prior studies that address some of these same issues. It next discusses data sources and analytical methodology, explaining that the data derive from the same sources as in Chapter 3 but that the analysis needs to be tailored to account for differences between exclusivity and non-exclusivity periods. The chapter then presents an econometric analysis of prices and expenditures. It concludes with analysis focused directly on the impact of AGs on the profitability of filing Paragraph IV challenges.

I. Prior Studies

As summarized below, two studies examined the impact of additional generic competitors on price levels after the 180-day exclusivity period. Both show that the marginal impact of an additional generic, whether an ANDA-generic or an AG, is small when more than four or five generics are already on the market. Furthermore, two additional studies considered the impact of AGs on Paragraph IV challenges. Taken together, they suggest that the increased popularity of AG launches has not substantially deterred Paragraph IV challenges and that whatever effects do exist are likely most important with regard to decisions on relatively small-market drugs.

As discussed in Chapter 3, an IMS Study finds that AGs have large price effects during 180-day exclusivity.[268] It extends analysis beyond the exclusivity period by dividing its 18-drug sample into two groups: one comprised of drugs that had 2–5 generics post exclusivity and another for drugs with six or more generic competitors, post exclusivity. The study finds that when 2–5 generics compete, discounts are larger when an AG is also in the market. However, the study finds no long-term price impact from the presence of an AG in markets with six or more competitors.[269]

Using IMS wholesale price data for all drugs that faced new generic competition between January 1999 and December 2003, Berndt et al.[270] plot the relationship between the ratio of contemporaneous generic to brand prices and the number of competitors at 24 months following initial generic entry. Consistent with earlier literature, the authors discover that at 24 months after generic entry ". . . the impact of an additional generic [entrant] is negligible after the fourth or fifth entrant . . . ."[271] While this does not directly address the specific competitive influence of authorized generics, it does suggest that an AG's long-term impact on prices may be small once regulatory restrictions on entry lapse, and conditions are such that many competitors enter.

To the extent that an AG takes sales away from a first-filer generic, expectations about the likelihood of facing AG competition may impact decisions by ANDA-generics about whether to attempt Paragraph IV challenges. One study summarized here finds no support for this hypothesis when analyzing the number of Paragraph IV challenges over time, while AG launches were becoming more prevalent. A second study, using a break-even analysis, finds that the expectation of AG entry may deter Paragraph IV challenges for small-market drugs.

Berndt, et al.[272] analyze whether the upward trend in AG launches over time has had any apparent impact on the number of Paragraph IV certifications. The authors note: "If incentives to file paragraph IV certifications are reduced to the point that no generic manufacturer files a paragraph IV certification against a drug that otherwise would have been successfully challenged, then generic entry could be delayed."[273] However, the authors go on to note that while the "prevalence of authorized generic entry has increased, there has been little overall change in the number of drugs facing paragraph IV certifications, the number of paragraph IV certifications filed per drug, or the timing of paragraph IV certifications relative to NCE [new chemical entity] approval."[274] The authors, therefore, infer that consumers have not borne higher costs as a result of forgone Paragraph IV challenges.

Another analysis conducted by Morgan Stanley[275] attempted to infer how AGs would alter the minimum market size in which it would be profitable to successfully pursue a Paragraph IV challenge. The analysis concludes that the anticipated introduction of an AG would increase the break-even market from one in which the brand had pre-generic-entry sales of \$48 million to one in which pre-entry brand sales were \$110 million.[276] Hence, the study concludes that to the extent that AGs discourage first entry, they would tend to do so in moderately sized markets. This is consistent with another study that addresses this issue and concludes that the introduction of authorized generics is "least problematic . . . in relatively large markets."[277]

II. Data and Methodological Approach

The data analysis presented below has two main goals. First, it seeks to determine the impact of AGs on important market outcomes, such as prices, in situations where market conditions rather than regulatory constraints (apart from FDA ANDA approval) are likely to be the key determinant of the number of competitors in the market. Second, it picks up where

Chapter 3 left off, by determining the impact of AGs on first-filer generics in the months *following* an exclusivity period.

Because markets for drugs that once had an exclusivity period may evolve very differently from markets that never had an exclusivity period, the analysis separately considers the effect of AG entry for drugs that had an exclusivity period at some point and drugs that never had an exclusivity period. In the first instance, the period of study begins immediately following expiration of the exclusivity period (typically six months after initial entry), and includes the same set of products investigated in Chapter 3. In the second instance, analysis begins on the date that any generic competitor entered the market with positive sales, and includes any products that first faced generic competition from 2003 to 2008, and on which no generic manufacturer ever had an FDA-granted exclusivity period. Because of sample attrition over time, only the first 36 months following generic entry are included in the sample used for the analysis in this chapter.

The analysis outside of exclusivity controls for the number of generic manufacturers providing the product. Table 6-1 summarizes some key statistics related to this variable outside of exclusivity. The table reports the number of observations and the percent of observations with an AG for those products that "Had Exclusivity" and products with "No Exclusivity."[278] It reveals that AGs almost always enter some types of markets, while in other markets AGs are rare. For example, markets with a single manufacturer are the most commonly observed competitive arrangement in the data, accounting for approximately 22% of observations. Relatively few of these markets have an AG in either the "Had Exclusivity" or the "No Exclusivity" sample. However, observations of markets with a large number of manufacturers almost always include an AG. For example, the roughly 7% of observations with more than 10 manufacturers include an AG more than 95% of the time. The observation that AGs are normally present when a large number of ANDA-generic manufacturers have decided to enter outside of exclusivity is probably a reflection that these are simply attractive markets in which to participate, rather than an indication of any causal relationship between ANDA-generic entry and AG entry.

Figures 6-1 and 6-2 provide a graphical representation of how the number of manufacturers is related to product prices for products in the "Had Exclusivity" group. Figure 61 plots the number-of-manufacturers series and the relative price series over time for markets in which an AG was present. Figure 6-2 shows the same information for markets in which no AG was present. The measure of price in these figures is the average wholesale generic relative price, derived, as in Chapter 3, by dividing the generic price by the average price of the branded version of the product in the three months preceding generic entry. The average relative price in Figure 6-1 falls from roughly 0.75 in month 0, the first month of exclusivity, fairly steadily to just over 0.30 in month 20, then oscillates around 0.32 through the 36th month after generic entry.

The price decline observed over this period occurs alongside a fairly steady increase in the number of manufacturers over time. The average number of generic manufacturers, including the AG manufacturer (measured on the right vertical axis in Figure 6-1) increases from two in month zero to almost seven in month 28, before it falls to about five by the end of the sample.[279] Note that the number of manufacturers increases slowly in the first several months, indicating that some exclusivity periods did not cover the full 180 days, perhaps because the first-filer faced some difficulty getting the product to market at the start of the exclusivity period. The number of manufacturers increases very substantially after month 5, which would correspond to the end of a typical 180-day exclusivity period.

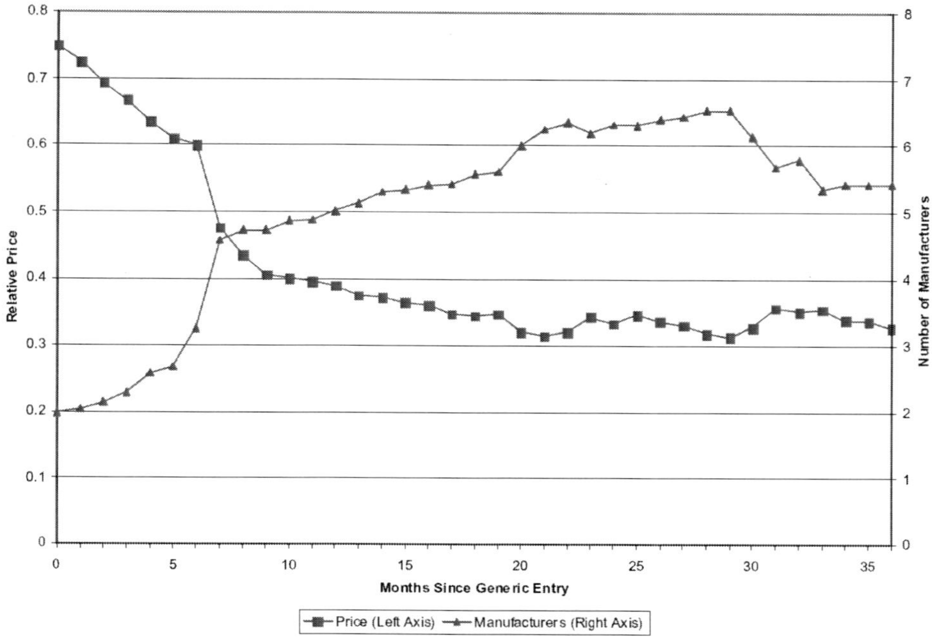

Figure 6-1. Average Generic Wholesale Relative Price and Number of Generic Manufacturers: Products that Had Exclusivity with an AG.

Table 6-1. Summary of Number of Generic Manufacturers and Frequency of AG Launch

Number of Manufacturers	No Exclusivity		Had Exclusivity	
	Number of Observations	Percent with AG	Number of Observations	Percent with AG
1	1,241	5.2%	430	7.9%
2	1,092	30.3%	302	85.1%
3	651	74.3%	336	50.9%
4	566	59.5%	286	84.3%
5	289	58.1%	154	100.0%
6	282	83.0%	136	97.1%
7	400	74.8%	96	87.5%
8	172	52.3%	96	62.5%
9	92	51.1%	160	95.6%
10	210	51.0%	92	94.6%
>10	371	95.4%	124	97.6%
Total	5,366	46.9%	2,212	67.5%

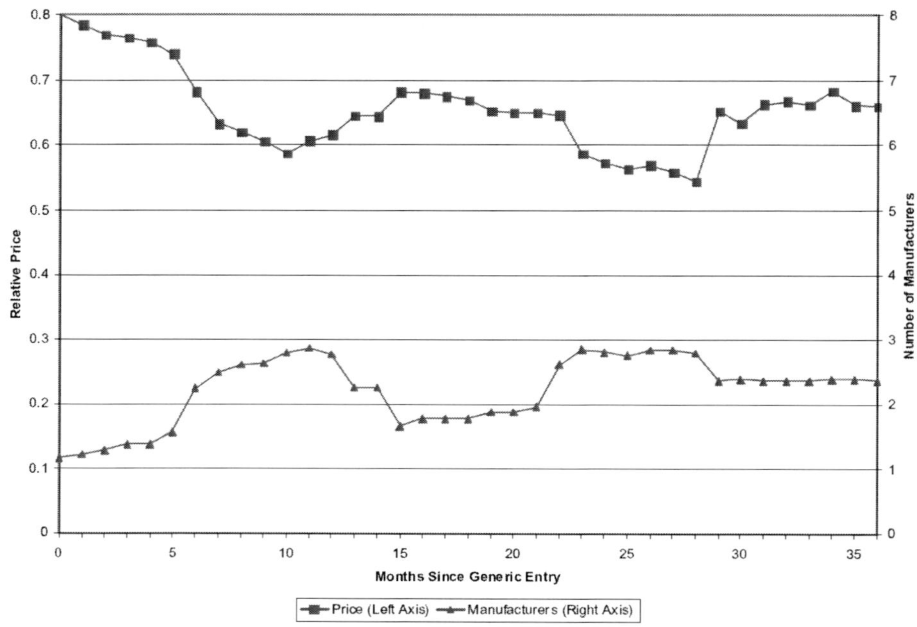

Figure 6-2. Average Generic Wholesale Relative Price and Number of Generic Manufacturers: Products that Had Exclusivity without an AG.

By contrast, the average relative price in Figure 6-2, which depicts markets without an AG, starts just above 0.8 and declines slowly down to about 0.65 by month 36. It would be erroneous to attribute the differences between the price series in these two figures as being caused entirely by the presence or absence of an authorized generic. Notice that the average number of manufacturers in Figure 6-2 starts out just a little above one, climbs almost to three after the exclusivity periods have expired, but never rises above three, whereas the number of manufacturers in Figure 6-1 climbs to almost seven. The econometric analysis presented below attempts to disentangle the effect of an AG from the effect of the level of competition provided by varying numbers of generic competitors.

These graphs also suggest that the question about the impact of an AG needs to be framed somewhat differently in the non-exclusivity analysis. In Figure 6-1, the number of manufacturers in the first several months was a little above two, whereas in Figure 6-2, it was just greater than one. This difference is easily explained by the AG itself accounting for the one additional manufacturer in Figure 6-1. In exclusivity, it was appropriate to think of the AG as an additional competitor. However, outside of exclusivity, ANDA-generic manufacturers can observe the presence or absence of an AG,[280] and can adjust their entry decisions accordingly.[281]

Consequently, instead of considering the AG to be an additional competitor outside of exclusivity, the analysis will essentially assume that the AG displaces an ANDA-generic manufacturer.[282]

The analysis of market outcomes outside of exclusivity reported here rests on one basic model. This model accounts for the direct effect of the number of manufacturers by flexibly allowing prices to vary with the number of competitors, but it assumes that the marginal impact of switching one of those manufacturers from an ANDA-generic competitor to an AG is the same regardless of the number of generic competitors. The results provide an estimate of the average AG effect.[283] The regressions reported in this chapter employ the full set of controls utilized in Chapter 3, namely months since generic entry, dosage form, and therapeutic class.

III. Market Prices of Generic Drugs

The analysis outside of exclusivity begins by considering price effects of AG competition. Using the same IMS data sets discussed in Chapter 3 and described in detail in Appendix I, this section analyzes both wholesale and retail prices under several different methodologies. As in Chapter 3, the price measure is relative price, constructed as the generic price of an extended unit normalized by the average price of the brand-name version of the product during the three months preceding generic entry.

A. Retail Prices

Table 6-2 displays estimates of the effect of an AG on relative generic retail price outside of the exclusivity period. This table reports the percentage change in relative price due to substitution of an AG for an ANDA. The first two columns, labeled (i) and (ii), report estimates based on products that never had an exclusivity period; the last two columns, (iii) and (iv), report estimates based on data for products that previously had an exclusivity period. Two regressions are run on each of these data sets. The Unweighted regression treats each monthly observation of an average generic price equally. The Sales Weighted regression weights each observation proportionate to the sales of the brand-name product prior to generic entry.

The estimated effect is the percentage change in generic relative prices due to substituting an AG for an ANDA-generic competitor. A concern that might arise from the relationship between the brand and the AG is that the AG may be a less fierce competitor than an ANDA-generic firm. In such a case, the price of generic products would be higher in markets where an ANDA-generic is replaced by an AG. The results provide little evidence supporting this concern. The AG effect estimates are negative in three of the four models, implying that prices would be lower in a market with an AG than in a market without an AG, holding the total number of generics on the market fixed. For products that had exclusivity, the estimates are between -10.8% and -10.0%. These estimates are large and statistically different from zero at the 1% level. Only the sales-weighted model for products without an exclusivity period finds that markets with AG competitors have higher prices than markets without AG competitors. Neither estimate for the sample without exclusivity is statistically significant at even the 10% level. This is evidence that consumer benefits from AG introduction during exclusivity periods persist beyond the first 180 days, but that there is no similar benefit when an AG is launched outside of exclusivity.

Table 6-2 also reports estimated mean relative prices for ANDA-Only markets. As in Chapter 3, where similar counterfactual means were calculated, these are estimated by starting with the average relative prices in AG markets, then pulling out the impact of the AG using the regression parameter estimates of AG impact to arrive at the counterfactual No-AG price in these markets. Again, the reason for estimating the counterfactual relative prices is to focus the analysis on markets in which AGs have been introduced, and to estimate the market impact of an AG not being present in those markets. For example, the ANDA-Only mean relative price reported in column (iii) is 0.76. The AG Effect reported in that column is -10.8%, which means that replacing one of the ANDA competitors with an AG would cause the average relative price to fall from 0.76 to 0.68 (=0.76×(1-0.108)).

B. Wholesale Prices

Using the same model and sampling strategy as with the retail data, the competitive effects of AGs on wholesale relative prices are estimated. The goal is to allow a valid comparison of the prices plotted in Figures 6-1 and 6-2 by controlling for the differences between markets that experienced an AG launch and those that did not.

Table 6-3 summarizes the results for wholesale data. The estimates of AG effects on wholesale prices match the direction of the estimates from each corresponding regression in Table 6-2. The AG Effect is statistically significantly different from zero in only the Unweighted regression using data for No Exclusivity drugs, in which case the presence of an AG lowers the average generic price by 19.6%.

Table 6-2. Average Effect of Substituting an AG for an ANDA on Retail Relative Price Outside of Exclusivity

	No Exclusivity		Had Exclusivity	
	(I) Unweighted	(ii) Sales Weighted	(iii) Unweighted	(iv) Sales Weighted
AG Effect (Standard Error)	-2.3% (3.0%)	2.1% (2.3%)	-10.8%*** (3.0%)	-10.0%*** (3.3%)
ANDA-Only Mean Relative Price	0.66	0.59	0.76	0.65
Sample Size	5,337	5,337	2,207	2,207

*** Statistically different from zero at the 1% level

Table 6-3. Average Effect of Substituting an AG for an ANDA on Wholesale Relative Price Outside of Exclusivity

	No Exclusivity		Had Exclusivity	
	(I) Unweighted	(ii) Sales Weighted	(iii) Unweighted	(iv) Sales Weighted
AG Effect (Standard Error)	-19.6%** (8.3%)	3.2% (5.7%)	-13.0% (10.8%)	-6.0% (20.4%)
ANDA-Only Mean Relative Price	0.39	0.25	0.39	0.27
Sample Size	5,366	5,366	2,212	2,212

** Statistically different from zero at the 5% level

IV. Wholesale Expenditures

This section presents an analysis of wholesale expenditures, which, as discussed in Chapter 3, serve as a proxy for firm revenues. This analysis extends Chapter 3's discussion of the impact of AG launches on the revenues of first-filer generic companies and brand-name manufacturers beyond the exclusivity period. It starts by looking at the dynamics of expenditure shares as additional generic competitors enter the market. It then presents econometric analysis of the impact of AG entry on post-exclusivity expenditures on first-filer generics, on the brand-name product, and on the brand-name and AG products combined. Because this section primarily focuses on the long-term impact of decisions to launch an AG during exclusivity, it considers only the set of products that had an exclusivity period.

A. Evolution of Revenue Shares in Markets with and without AGs

Figure 6-1 shows that AG markets experience a great deal of generic entry at the end of the exclusivity period. If the first-filer becomes just one typical generic manufacturer in a market filled with many such competitors, it is possible that the short-term effects of AG entry on first-filer revenues reported in Chapter 3 will dissipate after the exclusivity period, as the markets quickly become much more competitive. Another possibility is that the added competition causes the first-filer to lose some proportion of its current sales, and that having faced competition from an AG during exclusivity, the first-filer is simply competing to hold on to an initially smaller share of the pie.

Initial insights flow from considering the dynamics of expenditure shares in markets with and without AGs. Shares of wholesale expenditures are calculated for up to four types of manufacturers – first-filer generic(s); other ANDA-generic(s); an AG, when appropriate; and the brand -- for each product in each month. Then these shares are averaged across products for each month. Figure 6-3 shows the shares of wholesale expenditures for products with an AG from the first month of generic entry through the third year of generic competition.

The average first-filer quickly takes a share of 40%, but that share falls to just over 30% in the months following the end of the exclusivity period, as the share of other generics increases. As seen in Figure 6-1, the number of generic competitors increases from just over two to almost seven roughly two years after first generic entry. In that light, it is perhaps surprising that the first filer retains as much expenditure share as indicated. Apparently, the first-filer has a first-mover advantage, which may derive from establishing itself as the incumbent supplier to purchasers while facing relatively little competition during the exclusivity period.[284]

The average AG also quickly captures significant expenditure share, and holds onto a significant part of it up through month 36. The brand's share, which was obviously 100% prior to generic entry, drops below 30% during the first several months after generic entry and continues to slowly decline over the following months.[285]

Figure 6-4 shows similar wholesale expenditure shares for products without an AG. The average first-filer obtains a large share during the exclusivity period and tends to retain that share following exclusivity. Figure 6-2 demonstrated that between one and two generics entered these markets following the exclusivity period, on average. Figure 6-4 indicates that these additional entrants typically were able to acquire expenditure shares of only around 10%, in contrast to the first-filer generic, which retained between 60% and 70%. In AG markets subsequent entrants were able to obtain an aggregate expenditure share of approximately 20% following exclusivity, but those markets experienced more generic entry than the non-AG markets of Figure 6-4. With regard to brand expenditures, the pattern of expenditure shares is nearly identical in Figures 6-3 and 6-4. Just as in AG markets, brands in non-AG markets saw their average share of expenditures fall to as little as 30% during exclusivity, though this appears to happen somewhat quicker in AG markets, and then the brand share generally hovers in the 20%-30% range in the months following exclusivity.

Taken together, Figures 6-3 and 6-4 indicate that the expenditure shares obtained by generic manufacturers that enter during the exclusivity period, whether first-filer ANDA generics or AGs, tend not to dissipate quickly when the end of exclusivity allows additional generic entry. Consequently, it is possible that AG effects on first-filer and brand expenditures during exclusivity, as estimated in Chapter 3, may extend beyond the exclusivity period. The remainder of this section presents estimates of those effects.

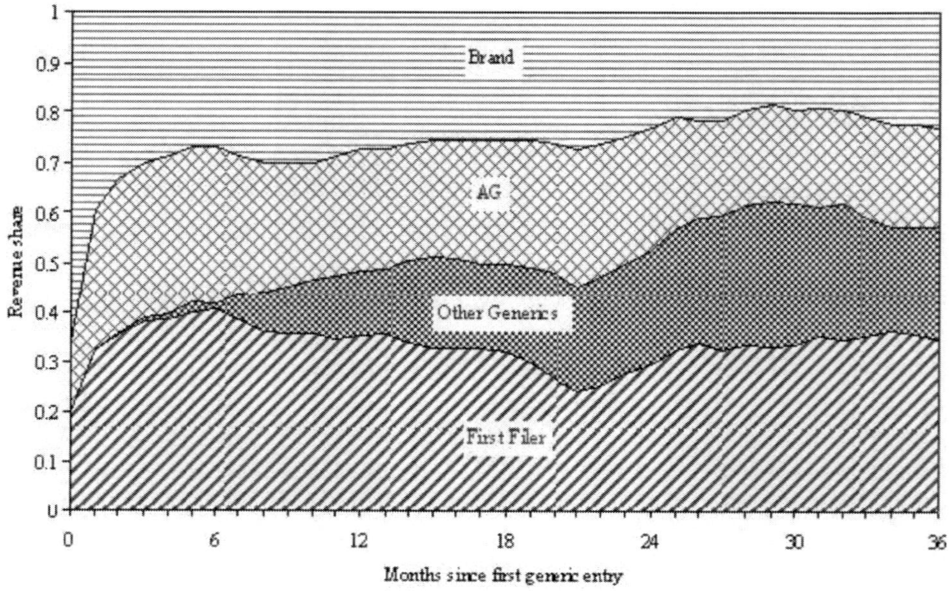

Figure 6-3. Wholesale Expenditure Shares in Markets with an AG.

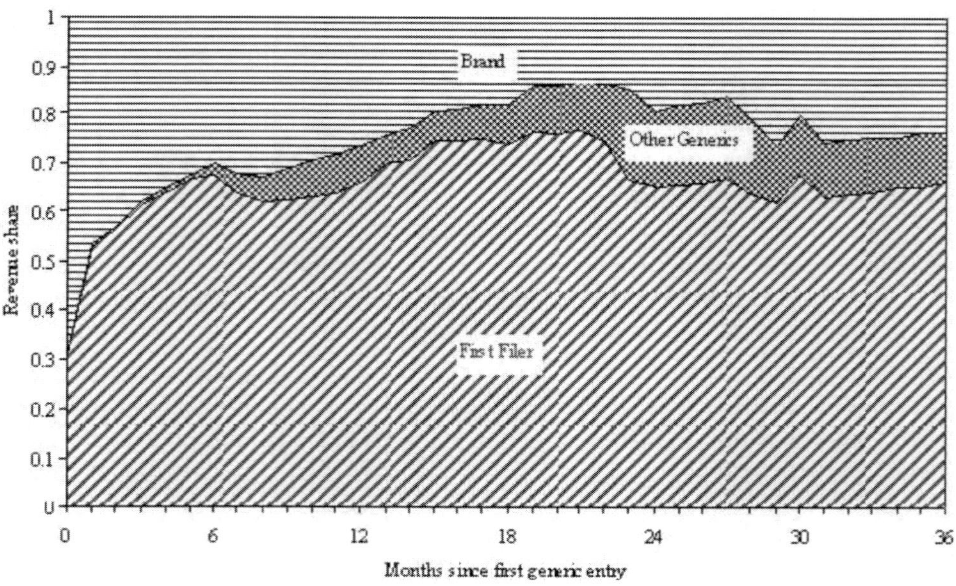

Figure 6-4. Wholesale Expenditure Shares in Markets without an AG.

B. Wholesale Expenditures on the First-Filer's Product

This analysis begins by considering the effect of an AG on first-filer revenues.[286] Although the extra revenue earned during the180-day exclusivity period is likely the primary motivation of a Paragraph IV application, a secondary motivation could be the higher revenues outside of exclusivity that the successful applicant might gain from a first-mover advantage. This advantage may be undercut if an AG is introduced, reducing the incentives of an ANDA-generic firm to bring patent challenges.

The analysis focuses on the relative wholesale expenditure on the products of first-filers, which are calculated as the expenditures on the first-filer product in a given month divided by the average expenditures on the corresponding brand-name product in the three months prior to generic entry. This is the same measure of relative expenditures utilized and described in Chapter 3. The average AG impact on relative expenditures is estimated using the same model employed to analyze prices in Section III.

Table 6-4 shows the estimated average AG effect on first-filer expenditures in the months following the 180-day exclusivity period. The estimate from the Unweighted regression should be interpreted to mean that the presence of an AG, on average, is associated with a 52.5% reduction of wholesale expenditures on the first-filer's product. This estimate is statistically significant at the 5% level. When weighting by pre-entry brand sales, the magnitude of the estimated effect increases, to 62.3%. This table also presents estimates of the counterfactual first-filer relative expenditures by using the regression results to predict what those expenditures would have been in AG markets if an AG had not been introduced. The unweighted average mean relative expenditure is 0.31 and the sales weighted average is 0.24. These may seem low relative to the expenditure shares in Figures 6-3 and 6-4, but those graphs depict the revenue shares of the current market, whereas this table reports relative expenditures. Relative expenditures are measured relative to the pre-entry brand sales, so as the market shifts to the lower priced generics, the total relative expenditures on the brand, AG, and ANDAs will be substantially less than one because the pie is shrinking.

These results imply that the impact of AG entry on first-filer revenues persists beyond the exclusivity period. This is consistent with the story told by Figures 6-3 and 6-4, which show first-filers holding on to market share even when faced with more generic competitors after exclusivity, but starting out with a lower baseline market share when having to compete with an AG during exclusivity.

C. Wholesale Expenditures on the Brand-Name Firm's Products

The analysis now shifts to consideration of the brand-name firm, first estimating the effect of an AG launch on expenditures on the brand-name product itself, then considering the combined impact on the brand and the AG. This enables exploration of whether there is evidence that launching an AG is in the near-term interest of the brand-name company. If combined revenues declined, one explanation might be that the brand-name company is pursuing an unprofitable strategy in order to punish generic companies that pursue Paragraph IV challenges and thereby deter future challenges.

Table 6-5 reports the estimates for brand-name product revenues. The AG Effect estimates are negative, and large in magnitude, but smaller than the estimated impact on first-filer revenues. The estimates range from -21.8% to -15.9%, though the standard errors are quite large, so that one cannot conclude that the real impact is different from zero at any reasonable level of significance. The very large standard errors on the estimated AG Effect imply that brand-name product wholesale relative expenditures vary substantially, and that controlling for the presence of an AG does not consistently account for this variation. Although the estimated impact of negative 21.8% reported in column (I) may appear large, the estimate implies that rather than earning revenues equivalent to 11% of pre-entry brand revenues when no AG was launched, the brand-name product earned revenues equivalent to 8.6% of pre-entry brand revenues when an AG was launched. The main finding here is that brand-name product revenues are much lower than they were prior to generic entry, and the presence of an AG has no statistically significant impact on that result.

Table 6-6 shows the estimates of AG effects on brand-name firm revenues, i.e., the combined revenues from brand-name products and AGs. Average AG effects are large and positive, ranging from 33.3% to 54.1%, though they are not precisely estimated and are not statistically different from zero. The positive results suggest that marketing an AG that substitutes for an ANDA-generic increases the brand-name firm's revenue on average, but the large standard errors suggest that this impact varies substantially across products. This is in line with our prior analysis of brand-name firm wholesale expenditures during exclusivity, which also found positive, but sometimes statistically insignificant, effects of AG introduction.[287]

Table 6-4. Average Effect of Substituting an AG for an ANDA on First-Filer Wholesale Relative Expenditures

	(I) Unweighted	(ii) Sales Weighted
AG Effect (Standard Error)	-52.5%** (22.8%)	-62.3%** (29.5%)
ANDA-Only Mean Relative Expenditure	0.31	0.24
Sample Size	2,070	2,070

** Statistically different from zero at the 5% level

Table 6-5. Average Effect of Substituting an AG for an ANDA on Brand-Name Product Wholesale Relative Expenditures

	(I) Unweighted	(ii) Sales Weighted
AG Effect (Standard Error)	-21.8% (23.9%)	-15.9% (23.0%)
ANDA-Only Mean Relative Expenditure	0.11	0.07
Sample Size	2,077	2,077

This analysis, along with corresponding results from the exclusivity period presented in Chapter 3, allows for a very rough approximation of the magnitude of the impact of AG introduction on brand-name company revenues relative to the revenue stream generated over the life-span of a brand-name drug. Figure K-3 in Appendix K demonstrates that the average number of years between NDA approval and the first generic entry for brand-name drugs that experienced generic entry by 180-day exclusivity from 2001 through 2008 was roughly ten years, during which time the brand-name company would earn relative expenditures of 1.0 per year. When a brand-name drug faces generic competition during a 180-day exclusivity period, it has the option to launch an AG. Table 3-9 reported that the brand-name firm's relative expenditure averages 0.49 when no AG is launched and increases by 5.9% to 0.52 with an AG. Following exclusivity, Table 6-6 reports the brand-name firm's average relative expenditure in ANDA-Only markets is 0.11 and increases by 54.1% to 0.17 with the introduction of an AG. This effect was estimated using only the data up through 36 months following the first generic entry, so the analysis below also stops at that same time. It is possible that the impact of the AG could persist longer than that, so this may understate the impact somewhat. Table 6-7 adds up these relative expenditures over the first thirteen years after introduction of the brand-name product. The difference between the values in the "Total" column indicates that launching an AG gives the brand-name company the equivalent of an additional 0.16 years (or 1.9 months) of pre-entry brand revenues, which is a 1.5% increase over the first thirteen years the brand-name drug is on the market.[288]

Table 6-6. Average Effect of Substituting an AG for an ANDA on Brand-Name Firm (Brand plus AG) Wholesale Relative Expenditures

	(I) Unweighted	(ii) Sales Weighted
AG Effect	54.1%	33.3%
(Standard Error)	(34.4%)	(38.1%)
ANDA-Only Mean Relative Expenditure	0.11	0.07
Sample Size	2,077	2,077

Neither effect is statistically different from zero at the 10% level.

Table 6-7. Impact of AG Introduction on Brand-Name Firm Revenues

Year:	**1**	**2**	**3**	**4**	**5**	**6**	**7**	**8**	**9**	**10**	**11**	**12**	**13**	**Total**
No-AG	1	1	1	1	1	1	1	1	1	1	**0.49/2 + 0.11/2**	**0.11**	**0.11**	10.52
AG	1	1	1	1	1	1	1	1	1	1	**0.52/2 + 0.17/2**	**0.17**	**0.17**	10.68
											Generic Competition			

V. Incentives to File Paragraph IV Challenges

The estimated effects of AG launches on first-filer generic expenditures, presented above and in Chapter 3, suggest that anticipation of AG competition during exclusivity might substantially impact a generic company's calculus about whether to pursue a Paragraph IV challenge. This section uses those estimates in a simple break-even analysis to gauge that potential impact. It first presents a calculation of the expected profits for a first-filer from pursuing a Paragraph IV challenge. This is a model of whether to pursue a Paragraph IV challenge when the only resolution of such a challenge is via litigation; agreements to settle the dispute are not considered. This model is calibrated using the estimates from this chapter and Chapter 3 to investigate the impact of AG entry on the decision to file a Paragraph IV challenge. Such decisions, however, are highly idiosyncratic, and it will never be possible to identify from averages and regression estimates how changed expectations regarding the launch of an AG would have affected decisions regarding any particular drug.

A. The Profit Calculation

The model assumes that the potential Paragraph IV challenger expects that if it spends a certain amount of money to pursue a patent challenge on a particular drug, it will win the challenge with some probability, where a win means that the generic is given approval to immediately market a generic version of the drug during a 180-day exclusivity period. The level of anticipated legal expenses and the probability of winning the challenge could certainly vary across drugs, but this analysis will start by thinking in terms of a given drug for which these numbers could readily be estimated by the generic company. Independent of the legal costs, the company also must pursue research and development in order to be in position to file and win approval of its ANDA. In the event that the Paragraph IV challenge fails, this R&D will still allow the challenger to enter, only not with an exclusivity period, and not until the brand no longer has patent protection.

The expected profit of a Paragraph IV challenger can be written as follows:

Profit of Challenge) = P(win)[(Profit during Exclusivity)+(Profit Post-Exclusivity)]
+ [1-P(win)](Profit of Non-Exclusive Entry)
-(Legal Costs) - (ANDA Costs)

Each of the profit terms on the right side of this equation needs to be estimated. One potential problem with trying to analyze this equation is that it rests on estimates of profits, and as noted in Chapter 3, this Report produces only estimates of revenues through the expenditure analysis. An estimate of operating profits is derived by applying a calibration similar to one used in the Morgan Stanley analysis[289] to estimates of relative prices and expenditures. Legal costs and ANDA costs are estimated based on the generic manufacturers' responses to Special Order specifications that called for data on legal expenditures related to Paragraph IV challenges and on R&D expenditures associated with ANDA filings.[290]

The operating profit of a successful Paragraph IV challenger during the exclusivity period can be calculated using some of the estimates presented in Chapter 3, plus an assumption about profit margins. Assuming constant marginal costs, the operating profits during exclusivity are simply the price of the first-filer generic minus its marginal cost, times the quantity it sells during exclusivity, or $(p_g-c_g)q_g/2$, where quantity is measured in annual sales. An unreported parameter estimate from the wholesale price regressions underlying Table 6-5 is used to estimate the marginal costs of generic manufacturers. The parameter estimates the generic relative price when the number of manufacturers exceeds ten. Assuming that generic prices decline toward marginal costs as the number of competitors grows, the parameter provides a crude estimate of the marginal cost. Depending on model specification, the wholesale relative price with a large number of manufacturers is generally near 0.10, which implies a pre-entry brand profit margin of 90%.[291] The results of this analysis, in any case, are not very sensitive to the assumed marginal cost.

Using this approximation of marginal cost, and some algebraic manipulation, profit can be rewritten as

$$\frac{(\hat{p}_g - 0.1) \times \hat{r}_g \times r_b}{2 \times \hat{p}_g}$$

where the p and r variables are measures of price and revenue, the g and b subscripts indicate whether the generic or pre-entry brand level of the variable is being measured, and anything with a hat on top of it is measured relative to pre-entry brand levels.[292] So the expression for first-filer profits during exclusivity can be re-written as a proportion of pre-entry brand sales, where the proportion is a function of the generic relative price and the generic relative revenue during exclusivity, both of which were estimated in Chapter 3.

Similar algebra yields the following estimate for the first filer's profit during the 2.5 years[293] after the exclusivity period:

$$2.5 \times \frac{(\overline{p}_g - 0.1) \times \overline{r}_g \times r_b}{\overline{p}_g}$$

where variables covered with a bar represent estimated relative statistics from outside of exclusivity, which were estimated previously in this chapter.

Finally, the profitability of entering the market without an exclusivity cannot easily be derived from statistics estimated in this Report. Initially, it is assumed that the patent challenge succeeds with certainty, so this term drops out of the expected profit calculation. However, some of the analysis that follows considers the possibility of unsuccessful challenges. For those situations, a zero-profit entry condition is employed, meaning that outside of exclusivity, generic firms enter until the net present value of the profits from entering equals the costs of obtaining the ANDA, which may include opportunity costs of the manufacturer's time and effort in addition to actual R&D and regulatory filing expenditures. This assumption implies that the expectation of the (Profit of Non-Exclusive Entry) term is equal to the (ANDA Costs) term.

With regard to the cost of Paragraph IV challenges, many respondents to the Special Orders indicated that they did not track these costs on a drug-by-drug basis or could not report the information for similar reasons. For responses that were provided at the drug level, the mean expenditure on a Paragraph IV challenge was approximately $5 million. Expenditures ranged from very low amounts to many multiples of the $5 million mean, and the inter-quartile range was roughly $2 million to $6 million. Similarly, responses to information equests regarding expenditures on R&D and other expenses related to filing an ANDA often were not sufficiently detailed to be useful. However, the responses that did lend themselves to this analysis showed relatively little variation. The inter-quartile range goes from $900,000 to $1.2 million, with a mean of approximately $1 million. Estimates of these costs can vary. An analysis submitted to the FTC by Howrey LLP on behalf of PhRMA utilized an estimate of $5.5 million for litigation costs and $2.5 million in development costs.[294] The robustness of the results to different cost estimates will be explored.

Given estimates of the legal challenge and ANDA costs and the relative prices and relative expenditures estimated previously in this Report, the expected profitability of a Paragraph IV challenge can be expressed entirely in terms of the pre-generic-entry brand sales of the drug and the probability of winning the Paragraph IV challenge. The next section presents break-even analyses focused on these variables.

B. Break-Even Analysis

Suppose a potential Paragraph IV challenger knew with certainty that a challenge would succeed and an exclusivity period would be granted if the company invested \$5 million on the challenge in addition to \$1 million on developing the ANDA. How big would the market for the drug need to be to make such a challenge profitable? How would that market size change depending on whether or not the challenger expected to face AG competition? To start to answer these questions, the profit function developed above is calibrated with estimates based on the expectation of no AG entry.

1. Markets without an AG

The first step is to insert estimates derived from the regression analyses of this chapter and Chapter 3 into the expression representing profit during exclusivity.[295] Table 3-2 reported that the average wholesale generic relative price for a drug in a non-AG market during exclusivity is 0.80; which will serve as the estimate of the relative price of the generic during exclusivity, $\hat{p}_g$. Similarly, Table 3-7 reports that, without an AG, the average wholesale relative expenditure on the first-filer's product during exclusivity is 0.70. Plugging these numbers into the expression for profit during the exclusivity period yields

$$\frac{(0.80 - 0.1) \times 0.70 \times r_b}{2 \times 0.80} = 0.31 \times r_b.$$

As reported in Table 6-3, the average ANDA-Only wholesale relative price post-exclusivity is 0.39, and the average ANDA-Only wholesale relative expenditure post-exclusivity is reported to be 0.31 in Table 6-4. Thus, the profits of the first-filer in the 2.5 years following the exclusivity period are

$$2.5 \times \frac{(0.39 - 0.1) \times 0.31 \times r_b}{0.39} = 0.58 \times r_b.$$

This implies that the first filer revenues in the exclusivity period are a little over half of the sum of their revenues over the 30 months that follow.

The expected profit calculation can now be expressed entirely in terms of the pre-entry brand sales:

(Profit of Challenge) = P(win)[(Profit during Exclusivity)+(Profit Post-Exclusivity)] + [1-P(win)](Profit of Non-Exclusive Entry) -(Legal Costs) - (ANDA Costs)
$=1.0\times(0.31 \times r_b + 0.58 \times r_b) - \$5$ million - \$1 million
$=0.88 \times r_b - \$6$ million.

If the challenger is expected to just break even on the patent challenge, the annual revenues of the brand-name drug would need to be \$6.8 million. If instead of the \$5 million estimate of the cost of pursuing a Paragraph IV challenge a \$10 million estimate was used, expected profits of the first filer would need to total \$11 million instead of \$6 million, and the break-even brand market size would be \$12.5 million.

2. Markets with an AG

Alternatively, a Paragraph IV challenger might expect to face AG competition, both during the exclusivity period and in the years that follow. Table 3-2 reports that the addition of an AG causes average generic wholesale relative prices to fall by 12.8%, so the average relative price during the exclusivity period would be the 0.80 used above times (1 - 0.128), or 0.70. Table 3-7 estimates that average relative expenditures fall by 52.0% when an AG is launched, so the average relative expenditure during exclusivity would be the 0.70 used above times (1 0.52), or 0.34.

Similarly, the presence of an AG causes the post-exclusivity relative price to fall by 13.0%, according to Table 6-3, so the mean relative price falls to 0.34. Table 6-4 indicates that the post-exclusivity relative expenditures on the first-filer's drug fall by 52.5% when an AG is present, so relative expenditures fall to 0.15. Plugging these estimates into the expected profit formulas yields:

$$\text{(Profit of Challenge)} = 1.0 \times (0.14 \times r_b + 0.26 \times r_b) - \$5 \text{ million} - \$1 \text{ million}$$
$$= 0.40 \times r_b - \$6 \text{ million}.$$

The pre-entry brand revenues would need to be \$14.9 million in order for the challenger to have expected profit of exactly zero. Using the \$10 million estimate of challenge expenses, break-even market size increases to \$27.3 million.

Two observations warrant emphasis. First, the estimated break-even market is more than twice as large when the first filer must compete with an AG. This is not surprising: the AG takes share from the first filer during the exclusivity period, that effect persists after exclusivity, and prices are lower in the presence of an AG. Second, break-even levels are satisfied by very low-sales drugs. The break-even market sizes reported here are much smaller than the break-even market sizes estimated by Morgan Stanley. The main reason for this difference is that the Morgan Stanley analysis only accounted for the benefits of a successful Paragraph IV challenge that accrue during the exclusivity period. The analysis of this chapter suggests that the benefits from being a first-filer persist well after the end of the exclusivity period, thus making challenges in smaller markets more attractive.[296]

Comparing these market sizes to the market sizes of the drugs[297] included in the empirical analysis of this chapter puts this result into perspective. Suppose that all drugs first experiencing generic entry in 2003 through 2008 are ranked from the drug with the smallest annual brand sales, or market size, prior to generic entry to the drug with the largest. Then for each drug, add up the total market size attributable to that drug and all smaller drugs, and divide by the sum of market sizes for all drugs, which is \$68 billion. This produces what is referred to in Figure 6-5, on the vertical axis, as the cumulative density of market size, measured as annualized wholesale expenditures on the brand-name product prior to generic entry. The horizontal axis, for instance, indicates that 10% of the drugs have sales of \$5.4 million or less. The graph shows that these 10% of drugs account for a negligible portion of the total market share; less than 0.01%. The median drug has annual pre-entry brand sales of approximately \$129 million, which is indicated in the exact center of the horizontal axis. Since this is the median, 50% of the products in the sample have pre-entry annual brand sales below $129 million, and these account for only 3.3% of the cumulative market size in the sample, as indicated by the curve. Continuing along the curve to the right, the smallest 70% of drugs (with sales of up to $454 million) account for only about 12% of the dollars. Even the smallest 90% of the drugs (with sales of up to $1.8 billion) account for less than half (49%) of the dollars.

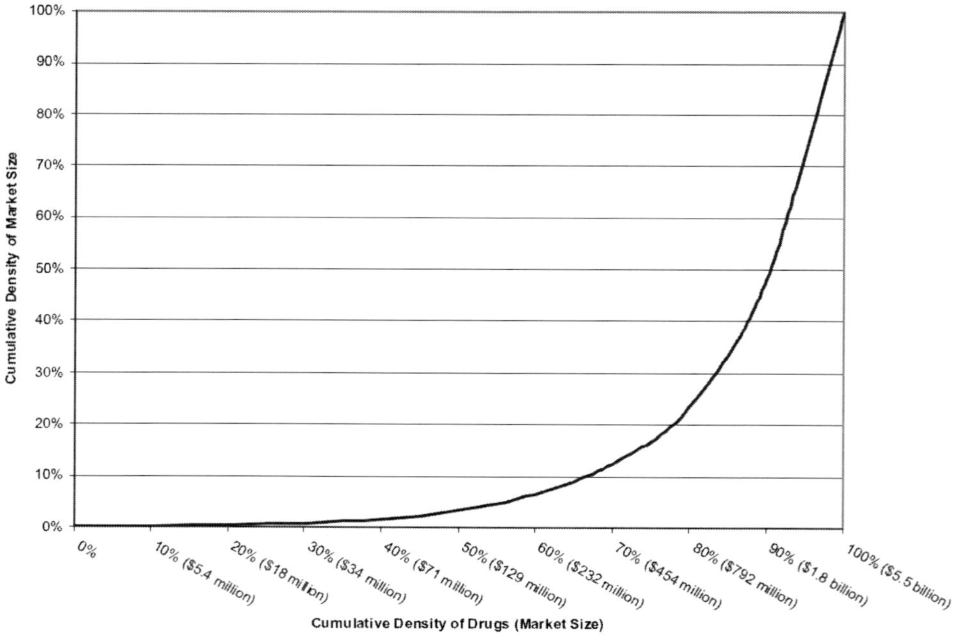

Figure 6-5. Cumulative Share of Pre-Entry Wholesale Sales For Drugs Experiencing First Generic Entry from 2003 through 2008.

Using the higher cost estimates, the break-even analysis above identifies drugs with sales below $27.3 million as those for which an expectation of an AG would deter a Paragraph IV challenge. Figure 6-5 indicates that drugs of this magnitude constitute between 20% and 30% of the drugs in the sample, but account for less than 1% of the total sales. Using the lower cost estimates, expected AG entry would deter Paragraph IV challenges affecting drugs with sales below roughly $15 million, representing a little under 20% of the drugs in the sample but less than 1% of total sales.[298] However, this analysis was based on the presumption that the Paragraph IV challenge will succeed with certainty. Challengers, of course, almost never are 100% certain to succeed. The analysis below further explores the relationship between market size and probability of winning the Paragraph IV challenge.

3. Effect on Threshold Probability of a Successful Challenge

Another way to think about the effect of AG competition on the decision to bring a Paragraph IV challenge is to fix the drug's market size and to consider how the probability of winning the challenge necessary to justify pursuing it changes when an AG is launched. As noted above, this analysis must account for the impact on profits when the challenge is unsuccessful and the generic enters only in a non-exclusivity situation. Given that any generic firm can pursue the R&D to enter in a non-exclusivity market, we impose a zero profit entry condition implying that the operating profit from entering a non-exclusivity market must equal the cost of obtaining the ANDA. Plugging the estimated relative prices and revenues from the markets without AGs into the expression for expected profit from a Paragraph IV challenge yields:

(Profit of Challenge) = P(win)[(Profit during Exclusivity)+(Profit Post-Exclusivity)] + [1-P(win)](Profit of Non-Exclusive Entry) -(Legal Costs) - (ANDA Costs)
= P(win)×(0.31 × r_b + 0.58 × r_b) + [1-P(win)]($1 million) - $5 million - $1 million
= P(win)× (0.88 ×r_b - $1 million)- $5 million.

Setting this expected profit to zero implies a relationship between the probability of winning the challenge and the pre-entry brand sales of the drug. Figure 6-6 plots this relationship, along with the corresponding relationship calibrated with price and revenue information from AG markets. This graph again assumes a $5 million cost for the patent challenge and $1 million for obtaining the ANDA.

To understand this graph, start by considering a challenge that has 100% chance of success. The "No AG" curve crosses 100% at a market size of $6.8 million – exactly the break-even market size calculated above for markets without an AG under the assumption that the challenge would be successful. Similarly, the "AG" curve crosses 100% at a market size of $14.9 million, which is the break-even AG market calculated above.

The new question this graph answers is how much the presence of an AG would change the calculus surrounding a Paragraph IV challenge that may or may not succeed. For example, consider a drug with pre-generic-entry brand sales of $130 million, which is about the median market size for drugs that faced first generic entry from 2003 through 2008, as depicted in Figure 6-5.[299] The "No AG" curve on the graph shows that at $130 million, the challenger would have to believe it has at least a 4% chance of winning in order to expect the challenge to be profitable even if an AG will not enter. If the challenger thinks it has less than a 4% chance of being successful, this model suggests the challenge would not be profitable regardless of whether an AG enters. The AG curve in this graph shows that for a $130 million drug, that chance of winning has to increase to approximately 10% in order for the challenge to be profitable, in expectation, when it is anticipated that an AG will enter. If the challenger believes it has better than a 10% chance of winning, this model suggests the challenge is expected to be profitable regardless of whether an AG enters. If the challenger thought it had between a 4% and a 10% chance of winning a Paragraph IV challenge on a $130 million drug, the expected profitability of the challenge would depend on the likelihood of AG entry. More generally, the area between these two curves depicts the situations where the perceived likelihood of AG entry can impact whether or not a Paragraph IV challenge can be expected to be profitable.

Without data on how generic companies perceive their probabilities of success for Paragraph IV challenges, it is not possible to determine how many additional challenges would be pursued if expectations shifted from expecting an AG to not expecting one, though consideration of a few examples can be instructive. For the median drug, it was shown above that the range of probabilities over which an AG could impact whether a challenge is expected to be profitable or not is narrow. However, for some drugs just below the median, the range can be quite substantial. For instance, the 30th percentile drug shown in Figure 6-5 has $34 million in annual sales. For a drug of that size, Figure 6-6 shows that expectation of an AG launch can be pivotal for success probabilities from 17% to 39%. Although a substantial number of drugs of this approximate size are on the market, Figure 6-5 indicates that these drugs account for less than 1% of the dollars. On the other hand, drugs the size of the 70th percentile drug or larger, with annual sales in excess of $454 million, account for 87% of the expenditures. For this 70th percentile drug, the AG is pivotal only for success probabilities between 1.3% and 2.7%, and that range shrinks for even larger drugs. For these bigger drugs, the 180-day exclusivity period is so profitable, even if shared with the AG, that the probability of success need not be very high for a challenge to be profitable in expectation.

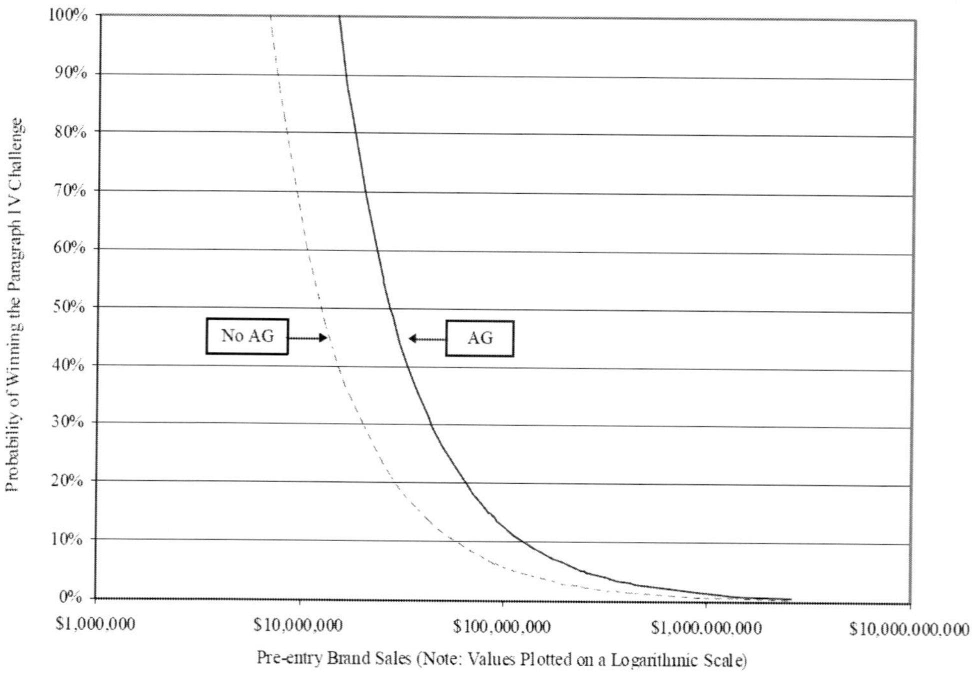

Figure 6-6. Break-Even Market Sizes for Varying Probabilities of Successful Paragraph IV Challenge.

At stake, however, is not the number of generic challenges but an authorized generic's potential to reduce or delay actual competition. Although many factors affect a decision to file a Paragraph IV ANDA, Figure 6-6 provides a rough sense of when the expectation of an authorized generic could deter actual generic competition. For example, on the median-sized drug, with annual sales of about $130 million, the expectation of AG competition would deter a generic challenger with a four to ten percent chance of winning the patent litigation.[300] The only challenges that would be deterred by expectation of an AG *and* have a reasonably large probability of being successful are on the relatively small drugs.[301] If a challenger anticipates a 50 percent chance of success, an expectation of AG competition could tilt the balance against bringing a patent challenge in markets with brand sales between $12 million and $27 million, a range that accounts for 13 percent of drugs, but, given their low sales, approximately one percent of total prescription drug expenditures.

VI. Conclusion

This chapter reports analysis of the impact of authorized generics outside of 180-day exclusivity periods. The results are generally consistent with those obtained in Chapter 3 for the exclusivity periods. To the extent that AG presence in a market had an impact on prices, it tended to be associated with lower prices in markets where an exclusivity period had expired. No consistent price effect of replacing an ANDA-generic with an AG was found when no generic had entered the market with an exclusivity period. Across both types of markets, none of the estimated effects provided statistically significant evidence of AG entry causing higher prices. Furthermore, there was strong evidence that first-filer generics continued to earn less revenue in markets where an AG had been launched. Brand-name companies tended to make greater revenues when they launched an AG, though this result was not statistically significant.

Given that an AG launch has a large and lasting impact on the revenues of first-filers, it is perhaps not surprising that analysis of incentives to file Paragraph IV challenges finds that the expectation of AG competition could potentially influence some marginal challenge decisions.

These effects appear unlikely to impact decisions on high-sales drugs, but could potentially play a role in decisions to challenge small and medium market drugs. The only challenges that would be deterred by expectation of an AG *and* have a reasonably large probability of being successful are on the relatively small drugs.

7. Assessing the Impact of AG Competition from Patent Challenge Data

The financial analyses of Chapters 3 and 6 show that AG marketing during exclusivity has a large and lasting effect on the revenues of first-filers that could influence some marginal decisions as to whether to challenge a patent. This chapter examines whether there have been fewer patent challenges since 2003, as AGs have become more common.

In particular, this chapter examines (1) the relationship between patent challenges and the sales levels of brand-name drugs;[302] (2) trends in the prevalence of such challenges, as manifested by ANDA filings and by drugs for which patent challenges were or were not made; and (3) generics' willingness to bring patent challenges under circumstances when they are likely to share exclusivity with ANDA generic competitors (i.e., situations analogous to sharing exclusivity with an AG).

Some caveats are important. To begin with, the chapter identifies relationships between various factors and the levels of patent challenges, but does not demonstrate cause and effect. Indeed, many factors may influence a generic company's decision to file an ANDA or to challenge a patent, and the measures of the prevalence of patent challenges in this chapter reflect their aggregate force. For example, it is possible that disincentives to patent challenges arising from the marketing of AGs during exclusivity might be masked by other factors that encouraged such challenges. Moreover, the data cannot directly answer whether there would have been more challenges in the absence of authorized generics. Finally, although this chapter quantifies challenges in various ways, it does not purport to address the appropriate level of incentives or to determine whether the number of challenges is normatively sufficient or appropriately matched to the set of drugs available for such challenges.

With these caveats, the chapter presents analyses that consistently find that despite AGs and other trends that could reduce a generic's revenues from 180-day exclusivity, patent challenges have increased in recent years for both large- and small-revenue drugs. This evidence is inconsistent with the concern that AG competition has deterred Paragraph IV challenges.

I. Patent Challenges by Sales Level

Concern regarding the possible impact of AGs on patent challenges has focused most intensely on smaller drugs. Generic companies might have sufficient incentive to challenge patents on high-sales drugs regardless of whether an AG might be marketed, because the returns from 180-day exclusivity could still be substantial. However, the profits from marketing a generic version of a small-market drug could be insufficient to cover the costs of filing an ANDA and litigating an infringement suit, especially if an AG reduces the generic's profits.[303] Thus, in theory, if AGs have a deterrent effect on patent challenges, it likely would be greatest for drugs with low sales.[304]

Table 7-1. Number of Drugs Subject to First Patent Challenges, by Sales Level

Year	<$50M	$50-100M	$100-500M	>$500M
2003	2	1	7	10
2004	2	3	10	8
2005	6	3	11	7
2006	6	7	9	6
2007	8	5	19	9
2008	6	11	15	7
SUM	30	30	71	47

The table shows, by sales level, the number of drugs for which the first Paragraph IV certification was made from 2003–2008. Limited to tablet and capsule dosage forms.

A. Challenges to Patents on Low-Sales Drugs

Analysis shows that generic companies challenged patents covering drugs with both large and small markets, including drugs with sales below $50 million. Tables 7-1 and 7-2 present data on sales levels for the year that the first Paragraph IV certification was made for a particular drug (i.e., the year that the drug was "subject to a first patent challenge").[305] Table 7-1 shows the number of brand-name drugs subject to a first patent challenge from 2003 through 2008, by the level of the brand's retail sales at the time of the challenge.[306] Twenty-six percent of such drugs had sales above $500 million, while 17% had sales below $50 million.

Indeed, as shown in Table 7-2, for each year from 2003 through 2008, the low end of sales of drugs subject to first patent challenges was less than $25 million.

The finding that patent challenges for brand-name drugs with sales below $50 million were relatively common was not anticipated in view of prior break-even studies suggesting that the minimum market size necessary to profitably pursue a successful patent challenge is approximately $50 million, and even more when an AG is present.[307] It appears more consistent with the finding in Chapter 6 that break-even levels for entry via a patent challenge that the generic believes it has a 50% probability of winning may be satisfied in markets with annual sales of $27.3 million when an AG is anticipated, and $12.4 million without an AG.[308] AGs have been very uncommon for drugs with sales of less than $50 million[309] and consequently may have played a reduced role in decisions regarding patent challenges for such drugs.

The sales-level data thus suggest that many low-sales drugs receive patent challenges, notwithstanding potential AG competition. This is not to say that patent-challenge incentives are adequate for all small-market drugs. Nor does it suggest that patent challenges are as *likely* for small-revenue drugs as for large-revenue drugs.[310] Indeed, as a general matter, the reverse is true.[311] The challenges to some small-revenue drugs could be explained by factors that made the drug more valuable to the company than the brand's sales level would suggest. For example, challenges may have occurred in settings where the generic company anticipated a future increase in the drug's sales[312] or had a special interest in a particular drug because of its therapeutic class, or where the generic company was already challenging the same patent with respect to another drug or perceived infringement litigation (or successful infringement litigation) to be unlikely.

Table 7-2. Sales Level of Drugs Subject to a First Patent Challenge

Year	Mean	Median	High	Low
2003	$843,642,560	$552,932,201	$2,744,362,983	$14,233,749
2004	$516,485,864	$263,147,176	$2,660,862,609	$19,038,498
2005	$638,065,023	$140,743,745	$4,586,054,348	$6,062,011
2006	$470,661,254	$139,450,992	$4,104,412,829	$898,843
2007	$393,678,636	$176,808,691	$2,865,218,782	$3,796,938
2008	$358,240,772	$130,728,844	$2,769,467,688	$22,304,549

Mean, median, high, and low sales of drugs for which the first Paragraph IV certification was made from 2003–2008. Limited to tablet and capsule dosage forms.

To explore this issue, we examined the circumstances for challenges regarding the twelve drugs during the 2003–2008 time frame for which sales were under $20 million. For eight of the twelve low-sales drugs, the first ANDA with a Paragraph IV certification was filed within three years of NDA approval, and anticipated growth in sales might have been a factor.[313] For three drugs, the therapeutic class of the low-sales drugs may have contributed to the companies' interest in pursuing a challenge.[314] In several instances economy of litigation appears to have been a factor: the generic company challenged the same patents with regard to a related drug with a larger market, thus reflecting an overall financial incentive greater than that of the smaller drug.[315] In other instances, the generic company might have believed that it was unlikely to be sued. Thus, for one low-sales drug, the generic company might have thought that litigation was unlikely because the brand-name company had not filed an infringement suit when another generic firm challenged the same patent with regard to a different product.

Together, these facts suggest that generic companies may be more selective with regard to low-sales drugs, bringing challenges under conditions that they consider favorable. The combination of factors in such cases supports patent challenges even in small markets. But that may not always be the case, and it is possible that a perception that AG competition is likely could tilt the balance against a patent challenge in some instances.

B. Trends in Sales Levels of Drugs Subject to Challenge

The trends in 2003–2008 sales levels of brand-name drugs for which patent challenges were made provide no suggestion that AG marketing has inhibited challenges with regard to low-sales drugs. Table 7-2 shows the mean, median, and range of the sales of brand-name drugs subject to a first patent challenge from 2003 through 2008. While there is some year-to-year variation, during this period the mean and median sales level of drugs subject to a first challenge clearly show no increase. Rather, in 2003, the mean sales level of drugs subject to a first patent challenge was $844 million; in 2008, the mean was $358 million. The median sales level declined 76 percent between 2003 and 2008, from $553 million to $131 million.[316]

If challenges below a certain sales level were unprofitable, one would anticipate that a generic company would not undertake such challenges, and that AGs would elevate the breakeven point. All else being equal, if AGs inhibited patent challenges on small-market drugs, one would also expect an *increase* in the mean and median sales levels of drugs subject to a first patent challenge during the period under study. The declining sales levels from 2003 through 2008 thus provide no suggestion that patent challenges have diminished in smaller markets with the presence of AG competition.

II. The Prevalence of Patent Challenges and Drugs Subject to Patent Challenges

Increases in both the number of ANDAs with Paragraph IV certifications and the number of drugs for which an ANDA includes such certifications also suggest that, in aggregate, patent challenges did not decrease after AGs became common.

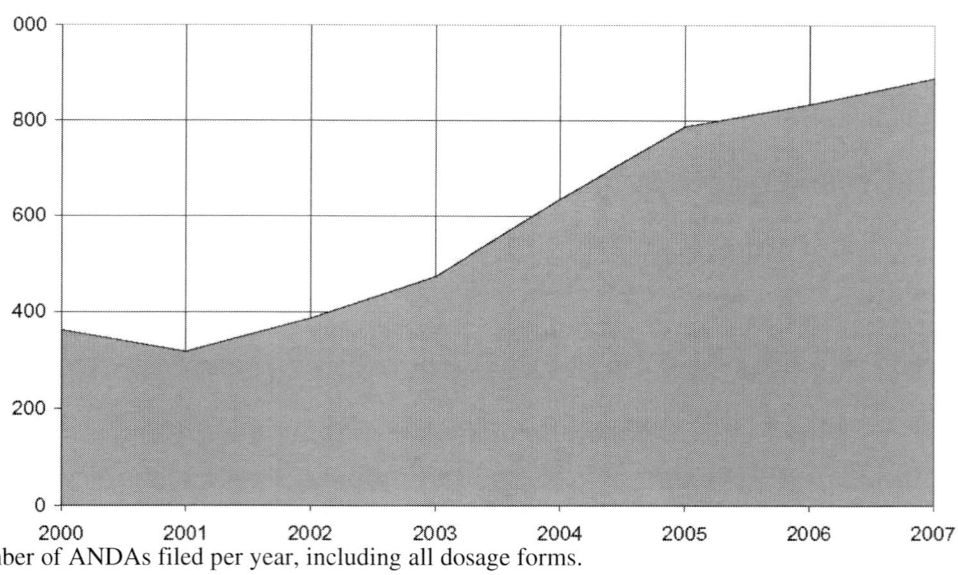

Number of ANDAs filed per year, including all dosage forms.

Figure 7-1. Number of ANDAs Filed per Year, 2000-2007.

A. ANDA Filings and Paragraph IV Certifications

Figures 7-1 and 7-2 show trends in ANDA filings and patent certifications from 2000 through 2007.[317] Figure 7-1 shows that the total number of ANDAs filed per year increased steadily from 362 in 2000 to 887 in 2007. The increase in ANDA filings likely reflects both greater utilization of prescription drugs[318] and growth in the market share of generic drugs, which rose from 47% in 2000 to 67% in 2007.[319]

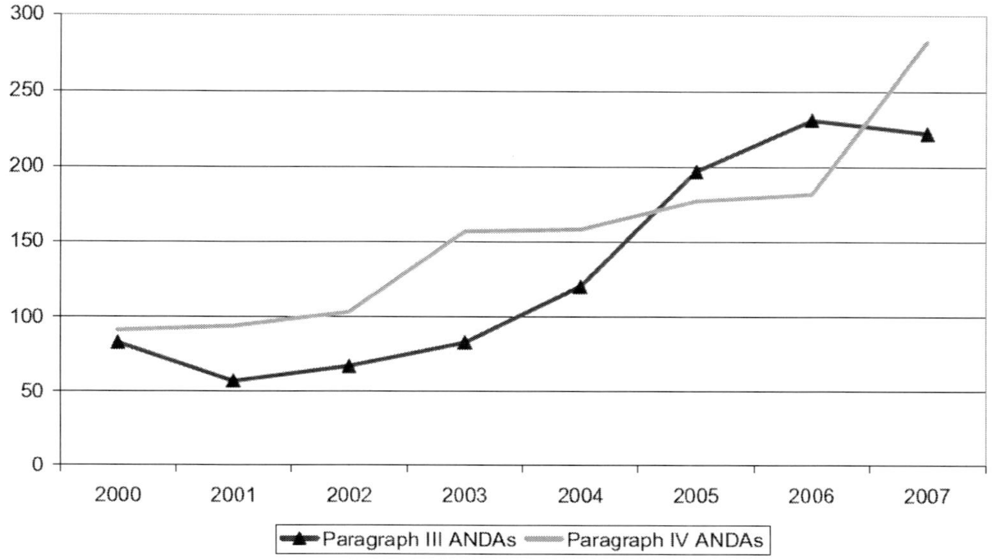

Numbers of ANDAs filed per year for which the highest patent certification was Paragraph III or Paragraph IV. Includes all dosage forms.

Figure 7-2. Paragraph III and Paragraph IV ANDAs Filed per Year, 2000-2007.

The trends in ANDAs filed with respect to patent-protected drugs are similar to the overall increase in ANDAs. As explained above, a company that files an ANDA for a drug for which patents are listed in the Orange Book must certify whether it intends to wait until patent expiration to market its generic product (a "Paragraph III" or "PIII" certification) or whether it seeks entry before patent expiration by challenging the patent on the basis of invalidity or non-infringement (a "Paragraph IV" or "PIV" certification).[320] As shown in Figure 7-2, Paragraph III and IV ANDAs increased roughly in parallel from 2000–2007, although the total increase in PIV certifications was somewhat greater than that of PIIIs. The substantial increase in PIVs after 2004, when AGs had become common, is another piece of evidence consistent with the conclusion that authorized generics have not noticeably deterred Paragraph IV challenges.

B. Drugs Subject to ANDAs with First PIV and PIII Certifications

We next examined both the number of drugs for which a first ANDA with a PIV certification was filed and the number for which companies chose to make a PIII certification and wait until patent expiration before entering.[321] This analysis suggests that despite the likelihood that an AG will be marketed during 180-day exclusivity, companies have not opted to enter after patent expiration rather than to pursue a patent challenge.[322]

Indeed, as illustrated in Figure 7-3, the number of drugs subject to a first patent challenge approximately doubled between 2003 and 2008. This increase appears as steady growth between 2003 and 2006 and a large increase in 2007.[323]

The increase could be attributed to any number of factors, and analysis of causation lies beyond the scope of this study. For present purposes, we merely recognize that during the period in which AGs became common and disincentive effects might have been observed, the number of drugs for which companies challenged patents increased.

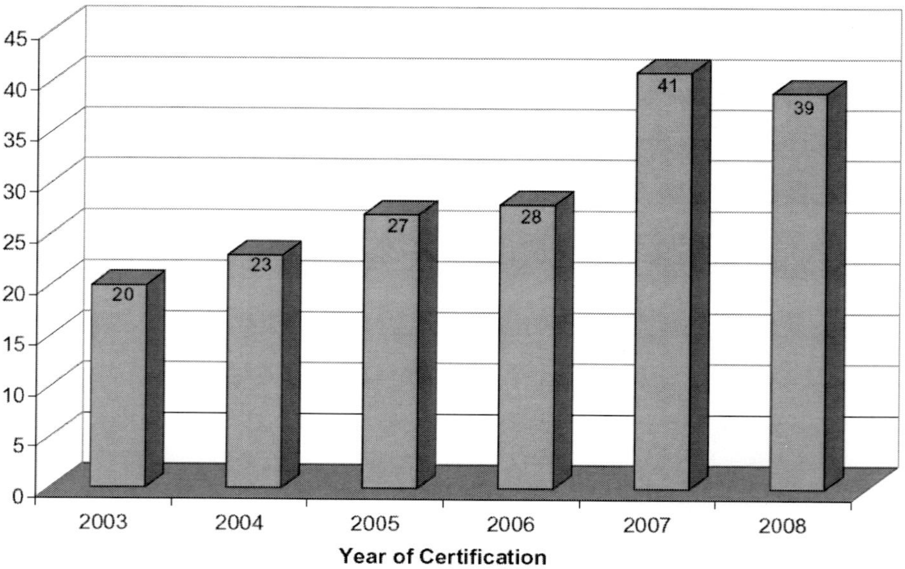

Number of drugs per year for which an ANDA included a first Paragraph IV certification. Limited to tablet and capsule dosage forms.

Figure 7-3. Number of Drugs Receiving A First Paragraph IV Certification.

Table 7-3. Number of Drugs with First Paragraph III and IV Certifications, by Year

Year	Number of 1st-PIIIs	Number of 1st-PIVs
2003	1	20
2004	5	23
2005	8	27
2006	2	28
2007	2	41

Number of drugs per year for which an ANDA included a first Paragraph III certification, and no ANDAs with Paragraph IV certifications were filed; and number of drugs per year for which an ANDA included a first Paragraph IV certification. Limited to tablet and capsule dosage forms.

While Paragraph IV certifications increased overall after AGs became common, it does not eliminate the possibility that for some drugs, AG competition might have led generic companies to defer entry until patent expiration rather than to challenge a questionable patent. To obtain additional insight into generic companies' decision-making, we examined the relative numbers of drugs subject to patent challenges and drugs subject only to ANDAs with PIII certifications. Specifically, for the period from 2003 through 2007, we identified drugs for which a first ANDA with a PIII certification was filed, and no ANDA made a PIV certification (a "PIII drug"), and drugs for which a first ANDA with a PIV certification was filed ("PIV drugs").[324]

Table 7-3 shows that PIII drugs were very uncommon, both in absolute and relative (percentage) terms.

From 2003 through 2005, there were fourteen PIII drugs, compared to 70 PIV drugs. From 2006 through 2007, the most recent period analyzed, there were only four PIII drugs, in contrast to 69 PIV drugs.[325] Thus, during 2006–07, only five percent of the 73 patent-protected drugs for which a first ANDA was filed were PIII drugs.[326] Accordingly, for most patent-protected drugs for which generic companies filed ANDAs from 2003 through 2007, at least one company chose to make a PIV certification, despite the possibility of competition from an AG.[327]

The few drugs for which companies filed only ANDAs with PIII certifications could not be fully explained on the basis of inadequate financial incentives. On the one hand, Table 7- 4 shows that both average and median sales of PIII drugs were substantially less than those of PIV drugs.[328]

Yet a significant fraction of both PIII and PIV drugs had relatively small markets. As shown in Figure 7-4, both PIII and PIV drugs appear with some frequency in the categories involving sales of less that \$50 million, \$50–100 million, and \$100–500 million.[329]

Thirty-one percent of PIV drugs had sales under \$100 million, compared to 50% of PIII drugs. Moreover, for all low sales levels, the number of PIV drugs greatly exceeded the number of PIII drugs. Thus, factors other than low revenues – i.e., factors that would not have been affected by AGs, such as patent strength – may have contributed to companies' decisions to forgo a patent challenge on the PIII drugs.

In sum, these data suggest that under recent market conditions, and in spite of the possibility that an AG might substantially reduce a generic's revenues during 180-day exclusivity, most patent-protected drugs for which an ANDA was filed were subject to at least one ANDA with a PIV certification. This is consistent with the finding of PIV certifications for drugs with low sales levels reported in Table 7-1, and with the apparent decrease in recent years of the mean and median sales levels of drugs subject to a first patent challenge (Table 7-2). While the results cannot pin down why patent challenges increased after the marketing of AGs became common, they indicate that in the aggregate, patent challenges did not decline after AGs became common. Seemingly, if a drug warrants developing an ANDA and there is a credible basis for a patent challenge, the drug likely warrants making a PIV certification rather than a PIII, despite the burden of litigation that a patent challenge might entail.

III. Patent Challenges Leading to Shared Exclusivity: New Chemical Entities

To better understand how the possible entry of an AG during 180-day exclusivity affects generic companies' willingness to challenge patents, this section considers patent challenges under circumstances in which multiple first-filers of ANDAs are likely to compete during 180-day exclusivity. The possibility of such "shared exclusivity" is analogous to the possibility of AG entry during exclusivity; in both instances the ANDA-generic must consider whether to proceed with a patent challenge despite the prospect of enhanced price competition, reduced market share, and diminished revenue.[330] Shared exclusivity, however, is more amenable to study because of the ability to identify a set of drugs likely to exhibit shared exclusivity and to predict when the relevant patent challenges might occur.

Shared exclusivity occurs most frequently for challenges to patents on drugs that have New Chemical Entity (NCE) exclusivity, a five-year marketing exclusivity granted by the FDA with regard to approximately 25% of all brand-name drugs.[331] The purpose of NCE exclusivity is to encourage development of innovative drug products based on new active ingredients.[332] Unlike other marketing exclusivities, NCE exclusivity bars not only the approval of an ANDA, but also the *filing* of an ANDA during the first five years after NDA approval. There is an exception for ANDAs with a PIV certification, however – ANDAs with PIV certifications may be filed after four years.[333] Thus, a generic company that seeks 180-day exclusivity has a strong incentive to file an ANDA with a PIV certification after four years have elapsed, on the first day such a filing is allowed.[334]

Since 2003, the FDA has required the sharing of 180-day exclusivity among all filers that make a PIV certification on the first day.[335] This sharing of exclusivity should reduce a generic firm's return on a patent challenge, similar to the sharing of exclusivity with an AG. Accordingly, we have analyzed first-day Paragraph IV certifications for drugs with NCE exclusivity as a model of generic company decision-making under circumstances when shared exclusivity with a competitor is likely.[336]

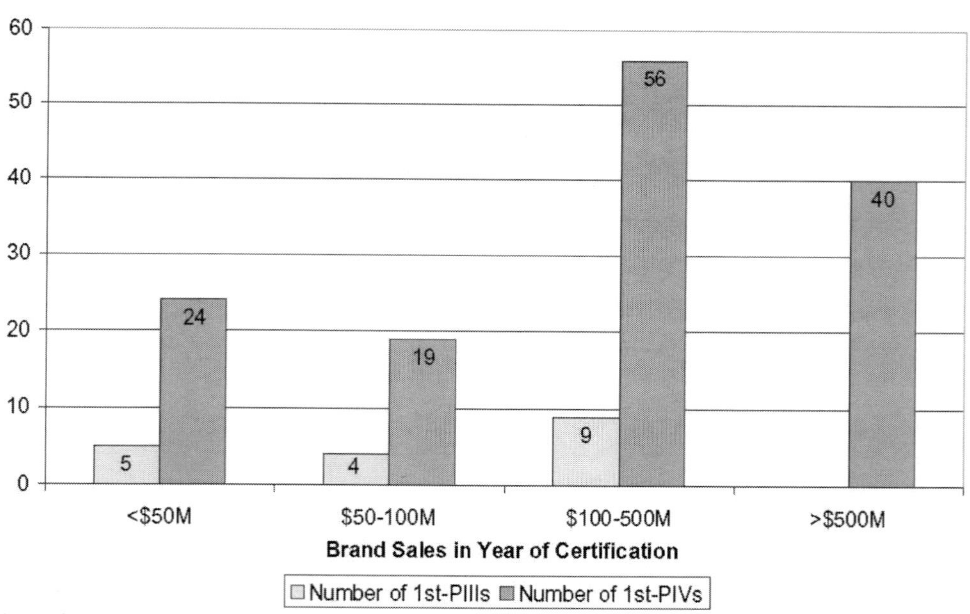

Number of PIII and PIV drugs by sales level of the brand-name drug in the year of the first such certification (2003–2007). Limited to tablet and capsule dosage forms.

Figure 7-4. Number of Drugs with First Paragraph III and Paragraph IV Certifications from 2003-2007, by Brand Sales.

Although shared exclusivity among first-day ANDA filers could substantially reduce the revenues available to any given filer, first-day PIVs have become common. Generic companies' willingness to make PIV certifications under circumstances in which they likely will share exclusivity with other ANDA filers provides further evidence that they may be willing to challenge patents notwithstanding potential AG competition.

Table 7-4. Sales Levels of Drugs with First Paragraph III and IV Certifications

	Sales of 1st-PIIIs	Sales of 1st-PIVs
Mean	$136,245,673	$541,720,294
Median	$96,476,032	$196,760,152
High	$475,445,072	$4,586,054,348
Low	$1,735,383	$898,843

Mean, median, high, and low sales of PIII and PIV drugs for the year of the first such certification (2003-2007). Limited to tablet and capsule dosage forms.

Figure 7-5 presents data on the extent to which ANDAs with PIV certifications were filed on the first possible day for NCE drugs between 2002 and 2008, a period that includes about a year and a half before the implementation of shared exclusivity in 2003. The number of NCE drugs eligible for challenge, those for which four years had elapsed since NDA approval, varied. The number of eligible NCEs was highest in 2002-2003, when there were 17-19 such drugs per year. From 2004 through 2008 the number was lower, ranging from nine to twelve per year. Because of this variation, Figure 7-5 presents the data in both numerical and percentage form.

First-day patent challenges were relatively uncommon at the beginning of the period under study, and became more frequent at the end. Although many NCEs covered by patents were available for challenge in 2002–2003, most did not draw Paragraph IV certifications on the first day. Only one out of 17 faced a first-day challenge in 2002, and seven out of 19 in 2003. From 2004 through 2007, the number of NCE drugs subject to a first-day challenge ranged from three to five per year, and eight such challenges occurred in 2008. While 12–16 NCEs per year were *not* subject to a first-day patent challenge in 2002 and 2003, only three did not experience such a challenge in 2008.

Accordingly, the percentage of NCEs subject to an ANDA with a first-day PIV certification rose from a low of 6% in 2002 to 27–45% in 2003–2007, and reached a high of 73% in 2008.[337] While the yearly sample size is small, the data suggest that the possibility of sharing exclusivity has not deterred generic companies from making patent challenges.

Furthermore, as shown in Table 7-5, the average number of first-day patent challenges for a given NCE was particularly high in most years beginning in 2005.[338] That year recorded an average of eleven ANDAs with first-day PIV certifications per NCE, and the numbers were also relatively high in 2007 and 2008; some NCEs have been subject to as many as sixteen first-day ANDAs with PIV certifications.

The data in Table 7-5 and Figure 7-5 indicate that companies have been willing to undertake patent challenges despite the known likelihood of sharing 180-day exclusivity with other ANDA filers.[339] By analogy, the data provide some indication that companies may be willing to undertake patent challenges despite the prospect of sharing exclusivity with an AG.

IV. Conclusion

Analysis of a number of measures of the frequency and scope of challenges to pharmaceutical patents suggests that patent challenges continue to be induced for most drugs, even though AGs substantially diminish generic revenues during 180-day exclusivity. Despite concerns that challenges to patents on small-market drugs might be inhibited, such challenges do occur, and the surge in AG marketing has not been accompanied by any observed increase in the sales level of drugs for which patents are challenged.

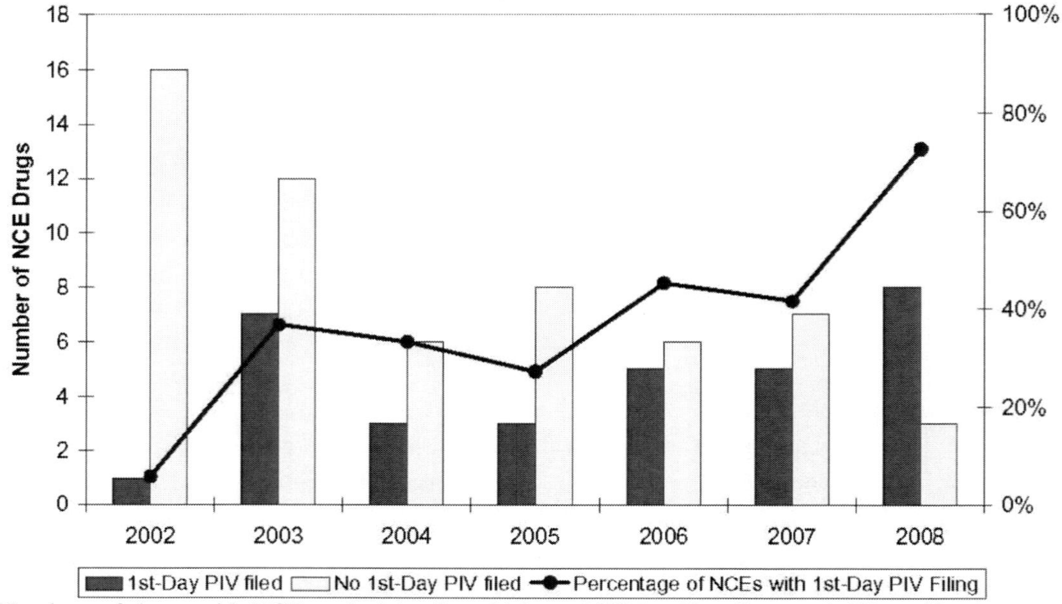

Numbers of drugs with NCE exclusivity for which an ANDA with a Paragraph IV certification was filed on the first day such a filing is allowed (after four years of NCE exclusivity have elapsed). The figure also shows the percentage of NCE drugs for which an ANDA with a Paragraph IV certification was filed on the first possible day. The figure includes all patent-protected drugs for which four years of NCE exclusivity elapsed between Jan. 1, 2002 and Dec. 31, 2008.

Figure 7-5. NCE Drugs with a Paragraph IV Certification Filed on the First Possible Day.

Table 7-5. Mean Number of ANDAs with PIVs Filed on the First Possible Day, Per NCE

Year	Mean Number of First-Day PIV ANDAs Per NCE
2002	4.0
2003	3.0
2004	3.3
2005	11.0
2006	4.0
2007	8.8
2008	5.8

For patent-protected drugs for which four years of NCE exclusivity elapsed between Jan. 1, 2002 and Dec. 31, 2008, the table reports the mean number of ANDAs with Paragraph IV certifications filed on the first day such filing was allowed. The table does not include NCEs for which no ANDA was filed on the first day.

In addition, the number of ANDAs with Paragraph IV certifications rose dramatically in recent years, and the number of drugs with such certifications also increased. By contrast, generic companies rarely have chosen to wait until patent expiration to enter the market; drugs for which only ANDAs with Paragraph III certifications are filed have been very uncommon in recent years. And even at the lowest sales levels, the number of Paragraph IV drugs greatly exceeds the number of Paragraph III drugs. Moreover, examination of the analogous situation posed by first-day Paragraph IV certifications for new chemical entities, for which the generic company is likely to share exclusivity with other ANDA applicants, suggests that generic companies are nonetheless willing to undertake patent challenges. Thus, a variety of findings point to the conclusion that generic firms continue to bring patent challenges for most drugs, even though AGs are now common.

8. The Use of Authorized Generics in Patent Litigation Settlement Agreements

As reported in Chapter 3, AG competition typically reduces an ANDA-generic's revenues during the 180 days of marketing exclusivity by approximately 50 percent. To prevent this loss of revenue, the ANDA-generic may be willing to delay its entry in return for a brand's agreement *not* to launch an authorized generic during the generic's 180 days of marketing exclusivity.

Such agreements can harm consumers in two ways:

- First, generic entry, and the accompanying discounts, would not be available to consumers as soon as otherwise would be the case. Because generic drugs often are priced substantially below the price of brand-name drugs,[340] overall prescription drug costs could be significantly higher with just a few additional months without generic competition in a large market.
- Second, consumers would lose the benefit of additional price discounting resulting from AG competition during the 180-day marketing exclusivity, as discussed in Chapter 3, Section III.A. This consumer harm arises because the brand has agreed not to compete against the ANDA-generic during the exclusivity period, i.e., from the *absence* of competition between the AG and the ANDA-generic.[341]

Analysis shows:

- About one-quarter (75 out of 333) of the final patent settlements filed with the FTC under the Medicare Prescription Drug, Improvement, and Modernization Act of 2003 ("MMA") between FY 2004 and 2010 contained provisions that involved AGs in ways that raised potential competitive concerns.
- Of the 333 final patent settlements filed during this period, 157 were with first-filer generics.[342] About one-quarter (39 out of 157) of those involved (1) an explicit agreement by the brand not to launch an AG to compete against the first-filer, combined with (2) an agreement by the first-filer generic to defer its entry. On

average, the entry date specified in the agreement was 37.9 months after the settlement date.

- Annual brand sales of the affected products ranged from $7.1 million to $5.3 billion, with an average market size of $616 million and a median market size of $245 million. Seven settlements covered products with annual brand sales between $1 billion and $5.3 billion.
- Over the seven years studied, settlements that combined deferred entry with "No AG" promises governed the sales of drugs with a total market exceeding $23 billion.

This chapter describes and analyzes the various types of agreements that involved AGs in ways that raised potential competitive concerns.

I. The Problem of Anticompetitive Brand-Generic Patent Settlement Agreements

Under Hatch-Waxman, patent litigation between a brand and a generic typically occurs when a generic seeks entry *prior to* expiration of the patents on a corresponding brand-name drug by alleging that such patents are invalid or not infringed by the generic's drug product. The parties often settle rather than litigate the case to its conclusion. Such settlements do not necessarily raise concerns under the antitrust law. For example, if the brand and generic settle the litigation simply by agreeing on a time for generic entry that is prior to patent expiration but later than immediate entry without any compensation, such a settlement most likely reflects the parties' views on the likelihood of success of their respective patent challenges and patent defenses, as well as their respective tolerances for risk. These types of simple settlements, with no other provisions, generally do not raise competition concerns.

Settlements in this context can raise serious competition concerns, however, when they involve compensation from the brand to the generic to delay generic entry beyond the time of a simple compromise date along the lines described above (hereinafter, the "simple compromise date"). The FTC has challenged a number of these settlements as anticompetitive. Such settlements, known as "exclusion payment" or "pay-for-delay" settlements,[343] thwart the goal of the Hatch-Waxman Amendments to encourage generic companies to challenge questionable patents and promptly "make available more low cost generic drugs," while simultaneously protecting legitimate patent claims covering innovator drugs.[344] Settlements potentially raising "exclusion payment" issues are now common.[345] Congress is now considering a variety of legislative proposals regarding "pay-for-delay" settlements, and the Commission supports restricting such settlements.

In recent years, a number of brand-generic patent settlement agreements filed under the MMA appear to use provisions relating to authorized generics – instead of direct monetary payments – to compensate a generic in return for a generic's agreement to delay its entry beyond the simple compromise date. Moreover, material produced in connection with the FTC's study of authorized generics confirms that a brand-name company may agree to refrain from offering a competing AG to maximize the net present value of both the brand-name and generic products. Documents from a brand-name firm show how an agreement not to compete with an AG increases the revenues of both the brand-name and generic companies. The brand-name company's revenues increase because generic entry and the accompanying drop in brand revenues occur later than they would without the brand's promise not to market an AG; the generic's revenues increase because its ANDA-generic product does not face competition from an AG.[346] Indeed, the brand-name company's documents show that if it launched an AG to compete with the first-filer generic during its 180 days of marketing exclusivity, the net present value of the generic's product would decline by nearly a third. If, however, the brand agreed not to offer an AG, and the generic agreed to further delay its entry in exchange for that agreement, the combined net present value of both companies' products would be maximized.[347] Thus, the company's documents confirm that a "No AG" provision can serve to compensate a generic for delaying entry. Indeed, "No AG" agreements may be simply another form of pay-for-delay in which the compensated-for deferral of generic competition benefits the settling companies at the expense of consumers.

The combination of documents such as this, along with the proliferation of MMA filings containing provisions relating to AGs, prompted staff to examine the role of AGs in Hatch-Waxman settlements.[348]

II. The Possible Use of AGs to Compensate Generics for Deferring Generic Entry

A. Agreements Involving AGs

To examine the role of AGs in Hatch-Waxman settlements, staff categorized the final patent settlement agreements that the FTC has received under the MMA for fiscal years 2004 through 2010, along with one additional agreement received outside the MMA framework.[349] Seventy-five final patent settlement agreements from FY 2004 through FY 2010 contained provisions that involved AGs in ways that raised potential competitive concerns.[350] These agreements fall into four basic categories:

(1) For the product whose patents are being litigated by the brand and the generic, the brand expressly agrees not to use an AG to compete against the first-filer generic for a period of time, and the generic agrees to defer entry (39 agreements);
(2) For the litigated product, either (a) there is no explicit promise not to compete, but the agreement creates incentives discouraging the brand from launching an AG that would compete against the first-filer (11 agreements), or (b) the brand explicitly agrees not to engage in AG competition, but the generic is not eligible for the 180-day exclusivity period (5 agreements);
(3) For the litigated product, the brand appoints a subsequent-filer generic as an AG marketer in competition with the first-filer (8 agreements); or
(4) For a *different* product – one that was not the subject of the underlying patent litigation – the brand appoints the generic as the AG marketer (12 agreements).

Figure 8-1 breaks down these agreements by type of AG provision.

B. Type (1) Agreements: Explicit Commitments Not to Compete with an AG

Thirty-nine settlement agreements with a first-filer during the period between FY 2004 and FY 2010 involved an explicit commitment by the brand not to use an AG to compete with the first-filer for all or some portion of the first-filer's 180 days of marketing exclusivity, combined with a restriction on the generic's ability to market its product.[351] Agreements with first-filers are particularly attractive to the brand because the actions of the first-filer may substantially affect the timing of generic competition.[352] As noted above, Type (1) agreements may be based on a promise by the generic to delay entry, which increases the period of time that consumers are deprived of the benefits of brand-generic competition. In addition, such agreements also deprive consumers of AG-ANDA competition whenever generic competition does begin for the litigated product.

These thirty-nine settlements involving explicit brand promises to refrain from marketing a competing AG for at least some period during the exclusivity were not evenly distributed over the seven-year period. Like other settlements potentially involving pay-for-delay, "No AG" agreements have become commonplace. Of the 39 agreements from FY 2004 to FY 2010, 24 were made between FY 2004 and FY 2009 (an average of four per year), while 15 were in FY 2010. The 15 agreements in FY 2010 in which brand-name firms agreed not to introduce an AG were nearly 60% of the 26 agreements that year containing payments to a first-filer and a restriction on that firm's ability to market its product. "No AG" agreements thus have become a recognized mode of compensation to generics for restrictions on entry. Figure 8-2 presents the data for each fiscal year.

The detailed terms of settlements involving a restriction on the first-filer's ability to market its product and an explicit promise by the brand not to launch or sponsor an authorized generic varied.

- Slightly more than two-thirds – 27 out of 39 – allowed the generic to offer its own product without facing competition from the brand's AG for some period of time. In the other twelve cases, either the brand agreed exclusively to supply the generic with the AG, or the generic could choose whether to market its own product or the AG. In either case, the result would be no competition between an AG and the first-filer's generic product for a certain period of time.
- The length of time during which the brand agreed not to launch or sponsor an AG ranged from 10 days to 45.5 months. The average length of the restriction on the brand's ability to offer a competing AG was 9.6 months, and the median was six months. Indeed, for about half of the agreements (20 out of 39), the restriction was six months, i.e., the length of the 180-day exclusivity period.[353]
- Brand-name sales of the affected products ranged from $7.1 million to $5.3 billion, with average market sales of $616 million and median market sales of $245 million.[354] Seven settlements between FY 2004 and FY 2010 covered products with annual sales between $1 billion and $5.3 billion. Over the seven years studied, settlements that combined deferred entry with "No AG" promises governed the sales of drugs with a total market exceeding $23 billion. In 2010 alone, such settlements involved drugs with a total market size of $4.6 billion.
- Many agreements not to offer a competing AG governed products with relatively low sales; a few of these precluded a competing AG for two years or more. In larger markets, the restriction on AG competition rarely lasted more than six months.[355] Figure 8-3 plots the duration of agreements not to offer competing AGs against sales levels.

- The length of time between the settlement and the date when generic entry was allowed to commence ranged from 0.75 months to 101.75 months. For 12 products, the time from settlement to allowable entry was more than four years.[356] Under the terms of 17 agreements, generic entry was prohibited for at least three years. The average interval from settlement to allowable generic entry was 37.9 months, and the median was 31.3 months.

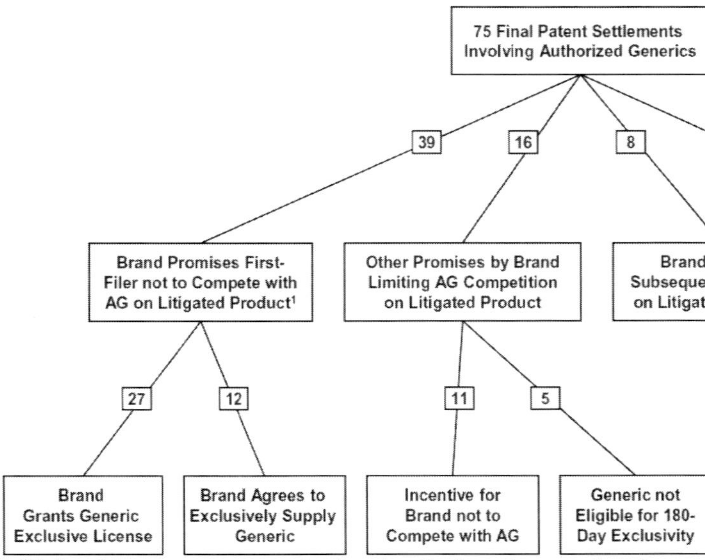

1. Eight of these agreements also involve the brand appointing the generic as an AG on another product, and are not counted in the 12 agreements in that category.
2. One of these agreements also involves the brand appointing the generic as an AG on another product, and is not counted in the 12 agreements in that category.
3. Only agreements providing for the marketing or possible marketing of an AG by a subsequent filer during a first-filer's 180-day exclusivity are included. Nine other agreements with subsequent filers provided for the marketing of an AG, but only after the expiration of 180-day exclusivity.

Figure 8-1. Overall Breakdown of Final Patent Settlement Agreements Involving Provisions on Authorized Generics: Fiscal Years 2004-2010.

Eight of the Type (1) agreements filed under the MMA also included an additional AG provision, providing for AG competition on a *different* product (that is, not the product at issue in the underlying patent litigation). In these agreements, the brand agreed not to compete with an AG against the first-filer's generic product, and in addition the brand contracted with that generic firm to market an AG version of a different product. Such agreements typically offer the generic a certain percentage of the revenues from sales of the AG for the other product.

These revenues can provide additional value to persuade a generic to delay its entry on the litigated product. For example, in one situation a brand allowed the generic to launch the AG for the product strength for which the generic was not the first-filer, in addition to agreeing that the brand would not market a competing AG for the strengths for which the generic was the first-filer. This agreement ensured that the generic would have sole 180-day exclusivity on the two strengths for which it was the first-filer and that it could compete with the company that was the first-filer on the third strength during that first-filer's 180-day exclusivity. Thus, the settling generic would be able to enter at the time of generic entry for each of the three strengths, giving it a competitive advantage relative to the first-filer on the third strength, which was required to wait until 181 days after generic entry to launch the two strengths for which it was not the first-filer.

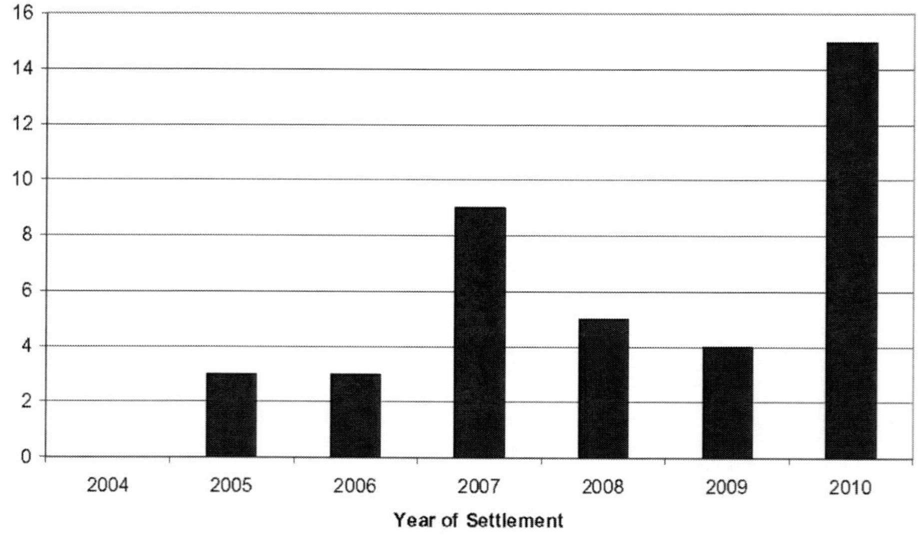

Figure 8-2. No Authorized Generic Promises in Brand/First-Filer Patent Settlement Agreements.

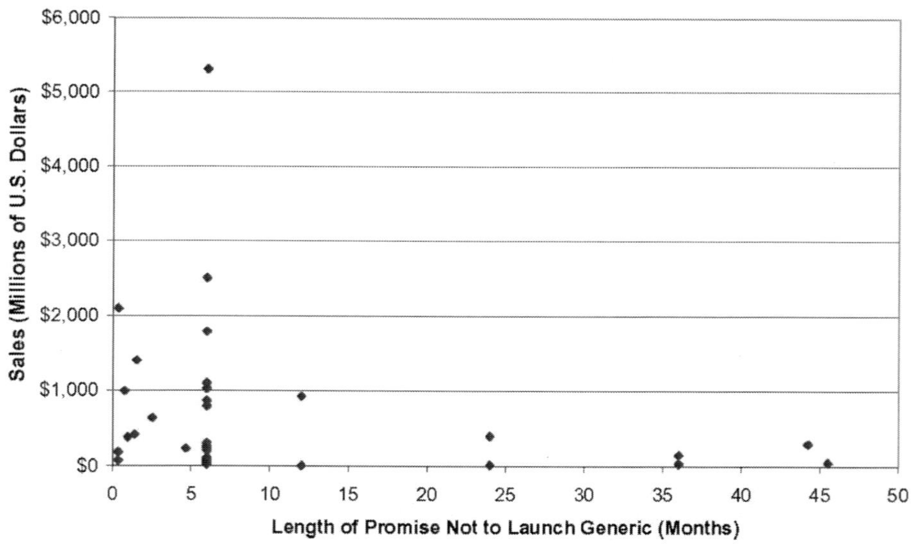

Figure 8-3. Final Patent Settlement Agreements with First-Filers.

Another arrangement found in several Type (1) agreements involves drugs with two dosage forms; the generic is allowed to enter shortly after settlement with an AG or ANDA-generic version of one product, but entry is deferred on the other. The second product usually has much higher sales.[357] Such a package of commitments could induce the generic to defer entry on the higher-sales product by promptly providing it with revenues on the lower-sales product and shielding it from a competing AG with respect to one or both of the products.

C. Type (2) Agreements: Other Promises by Brands Limiting AG Competition on the Litigated Product

Type (2) agreements encompass two categories of AG provisions that in some cases may operate in a manner similar to Type (1) "No AG" arrangements. The effect of these agreements, however, is more difficult to determine from the face of the agreement alone. First, in eleven agreements there was no explicit brand promise to a first-filer to refrain from marketing a competing AG, but there were provisions that could create an incentive for the brand not to market a competing AG. These provisions either provided that royalties due to the brand would drop significantly if the generic faced competition on the drug at issue within a specified period of time or appeared otherwise to discourage the brand from offering a competing AG.[358] These agreements effectively could operate as promises by the brand not to launch or sponsor an AG for a period of time.

The second category of Type (2) agreements consists of five agreements that contain an explicit promise by the brand not to compete with an AG, but (unlike the Type (1) agreements) at the time of settlement the generic did not have the right to 180-day exclusivity. In some instances, the generic was pursuing approval under a regulatory framework that does not provide a 180-day exclusivity period.[359] In others, the generic had forfeited its exclusivity, selectively waived its exclusivity in favor of a business partner, or settled after having triggered its exclusivity by an at-risk launch. The impact of the "No AG" provisions in these situations is less predictable than in Type (1) settings. But in some cases an inquiry into the surrounding facts might reveal an effect similar to the Type (1) scenario because no other generic rivals were in a position to compete. For example, in one instance the first-filer no longer had the right to exclusivity because it had waived its rights to another generic with which it had a contractual relationship. The settlement agreement indicated that the parties expected that the latter firm would be the only competitor during the 180day period.

D. Type (3) Agreements: Brand Appoints a Subsequent Filer as an AG for the Litigated Product

From FY 2004 through FY 2010, there were eight Type (3) settlement agreements providing for the marketing or possible marketing of an AG version of the litigated product by a subsequent filer during the first-filer's 180-day exclusivity.[360] If the brand-name company would have marketed the authorized generic (by itself or with another distributor), the settlement does not alter the competitive dynamic. These agreements raise complex issues. If no AG otherwise would have been marketed, such agreements have the potential to reduce prices to consumers through AG competition during the 180-day exclusivity period. At the same time, they might prolong the period without generic competition by affecting the timing of generic entry by the first-filer.

One way that an agreement with a subsequent filer could affect the timing of generic entry is by eliminating a patent challenge that could have precipitated generic competition. By continuing to litigate, a subsequent filer might obtain a court decision of patent invalidity that would allow the first-filer to market its product,[361] or a court decision of invalidity or non-infringement that would trigger the first-filer's exclusivity period or its forfeiture.[362] The Federal Circuit has recognized that brand-name companies may seek to settle with subsequent filers because brand-name firms "have a strong incentive to avoid litigation that would trigger the first Paragraph IV ANDA filer's exclusivity period and allow the FDA to approve subsequent . . . ANDAs 181 days" thereafter.[363]

Agreements with subsequent filers also might affect the timing of generic entry through provisions that make the subsequent filer's right to market an AG during the first-filer's 180-day exclusivity contingent on whether the first-filer launches at risk or has not settled its litigation with the brand. Such agreements allow the subsequent filer to market an AG for the litigated product during the first-filer's exclusivity, but *only if* the first-filer launched at risk or had not settled its litigation. Otherwise, the subsequent filer can market the AG 181 days after the first-filer's launch. By ensuring that the relevant terms, though normally kept confidential, become known by the first-filer, the brand-name firm may induce the first-filer to delay entry, in order to avoid triggering the subsequent filer's right to enter as an AG during the first-filer's 180 days of marketing exclusivity.[364] The first-filer could settle the lawsuit, accepting delayed entry to avoid AG competition, or it could refrain from launching at risk.

Four of the eight Type (3) agreements with subsequent filers were of this type. For example, one agreement provided that if the first-filer launched its ANDA-generic product without settling with the brand, the subsequent filer would be allowed to market the AG during the first-filer's 180-day exclusivity.[365] However, if the first-filer settled with the brand and launched its ANDA-generic pursuant to a license under the brand's patents, the subsequent filer could not market the AG until 181 days after the first-filer's launch. The brand and the first-filer subsequently entered a settlement that deferred ANDA-generic entry for about three years and confirmed that the first-filer would not face a competing AG during its 180-day exclusivity.[366]

Firms can make the terms of agreements with subsequent filers known to the first-filer through a variety of means – by publicly announcing the relevant terms of the agreement; by using the agreement as a tool in settlement negotiations with the first-filer; or even by making the agreement available in a public forum. Indeed, a similar agreement was made publicly available in the brand-name firm's 8-K filing with the Securities and Exchange Commission.[367]

E. Type (4) Agreements: Brand Appoints Generic as AG on Another Product

In twelve agreements, the brand appointed the generic as the AG marketer for another product.[368] If the brand-name company would have marketed an AG on the other product regardless of the settlement, the settlement would not affect the competitive dynamics. Type (4) agreements, however, can provide AG competition, and lower prices, when there is a 180-day marketing exclusivity period for another product – not the product whose patents are being litigated by the brand and generic – and the brand would not otherwise have marketed an AG. At the same time, if the generic is a first-filer on the litigated product, the agreement may serve to compensate the generic for delaying its entry on that product. Thus, Type (4) agreements can act as "side-deals" to compensate a generic for deferring entry on the litigated product. Also, a Type (4) agreement might affect the timing of generic entry for the other product in a manner similar to a Type (3) agreement by making the settling generic's right to market an AG of the other product during the exclusivity period of the first-filer for that product contingent on whether the first-filer launches at risk or has not settled with the brand.[369]

III. Conclusion

A review of recent brand-generic settlements reveals that agreements not to compete with ANDA-generics through an AG have become a recognized mode for a brand to provide compensation to generics and, therefore, can be used as exclusion payments in patent settlement agreements. The empirical analyses in Chapters 3 and 6 suggest that the probable presence of AGs is likely to reduce the compensation a first-filer can command because it will anticipate considerably lower revenues when facing AG competition; such revenue impacts are well known to both brand-name firms and their generic rivals. A promise not to launch an AG could be an attractive and convenient way to transfer the value of this revenue impact from the brand to the first-filer; negotiations over terms may be particularly easy because the cost to the brand and the benefit to the generic are proportional to the size of the market and estimable by both. However, numerous alternative forms of compensation exist, so it is likely that alternative settlement terms could be reached in many circumstances, even if the parties could not have used a "No AG" clause as a form of compensation. Any restrictions on pay-for-delay agreements should account for all viable forms of brand-generic payments to delay entry, including an agreement not to compete with an AG.

Appendix A. Letter from Senators Leahy, Grassley, and Rockefeller

May 9, 2005

Chairman Deborah Platt Majoras
Federal Trade Commission
600 Pennsylvania Avenue, NW
Washington, DC 20580
Dear Chairman Majoras and Commissioners:

It has come to our attention that the practice of "authorized" generic drugs may produce anti-competitive results and, thus, present an issue worthy of study by the Federal Trade Commission.

The amendments to the Hatch-Waxman Act of 1984, enacted as part of the Medicare Modernization Act (Title XI, PL 108-173), provide that, in general, a generic company that successfully challenges the patent of a name brand pharmaceutical company earns 180 days of marketing exclusivity on that generic drug. The legislation was designed to strengthen incentives for generic manufacturers to bring generic drugs quickly to market, and thus promote competition and lower prices for consumers.

We have heard concerns that the practice of "authorized" generics could have a negative impact on competition for both blockbuster and smaller drugs, because the generic industry would be less inclined to invest in their production. Consequently, if the generic industry were to be less incentivized to produce such generic drugs to compete with name brand drugs, it is possible that fewer generic drugs would come to market and the prices for certain drugs would remain high for consumers.

We are interested in determining the short term and long term effects on competition of the practice of "authorized" generics. Consequently, we request, pursuant to § 6(b) of the Federal Trade Commission Act, that the Commission conduct a study on this issue. We ask that this study look into the short term competitive benefits of introduction of "authorized" generics during the 180 day market exclusivity period. We also ask that the study look into the long term impact of the practice of "authorized" generics on competition in the drug market and on the price of drugs, as well as on the viability of the generic drug industry.

If such a study were to prove unfeasible, we hope the FTC will be able to conduct a workshop on this issue in the near future. If you have any questions about this request, please feel free to contact Susan Davies of Senator Leahy's office, Rita Lari Jochum of Senator Grassley's office, or Jocelyn Moore of Senator Rockefeller's office. They can be reached at (202) 224-7703 (Sen. Leahy), (202) 224-5564 (Sen. Grassley), or (202) 224-6472 (Sen. Rockefeller), respectively.

Sincerely,

Patrick Leahy
United States Senator

Chuck Grassley
United States Senator

John Rockefeller
United States Senator

cc: Commissioner Pamela Jones Harbour
Commissioner Thomas Leary
Commissioner Jon Leibowitz
Commissioner Orson Swindle

APPENDIX B. LETTER FROM REPRESENTATIVE WAXMAN

September 13, 2005

Deborah Majoras
Chairman
Federal Trade Commission
600 Pennsylvania Avenue, NW
Washington, DC 20580-0002

Dear Chairman Majoras:

I am writing to request that the Federal Trade Commission conduct a study pursuant to section 6(b) of the Federal Trade Commission Act on the impact of so-called "authorized generics" on competition in the prescription drug marketplace. I recognize that the Commission may also be considering a workshop on this subject, but rise of authorized generics raises serious competitive issues and requires a full study.

As you know, authorized generics are generic drugs that enter the market under aegis of the brand name drug manufacturer. There is evidence that brand name drug companies are increasingly using authorized generics to undermine one of the incentives to increase competition created by The Drug Price Competition and Patent Term Restoration Act of 1984 (Hatch-Waxman Amendments).

The Hatch-Waxman Amendments provide a special incentive to generic companies that challenge patents on the brand name drug – in exchange for undertaking the costs and risks of patent litigation, the successful challenger is given 6 months of marketing without any other generic competition. The purpose of this incentive is to encourage challenges to patents that otherwise would inappropriately block competition. Brand name companies, however, are now increasingly arranging for authorized generics to enter the market during the 6-month period of generic exclusivity, substantially reducing the value of that exclusivity to the generic drug manufacturer who challenged the patent.

As the Commission has documented, there have been a large number of successful patent challenges since enactment of the Hatch-Waxman Amendments, bringing generic drugs to market much earlier than would otherwise have occurred.[370] If the rise in authorized generics causes generic drug manufacturers to stop challenging patents for certain products, generic competition will be significantly delayed, and consumers, businesses, and governments will unnecessarily pay monopoly drug prices for much longer periods.

In 2002, the Commission issued a landmark report detailing tactics then being used by the pharmaceutical industry to delay generic competition months and even years past the time intended by Congress at a cost of billions of dollars.[371] Congress responded to that study by enacting legislation in 2003, closing loopholes in the Hatch-Waxman Amendments. I do not believe it is a coincidence that brand name companies began to exploit the practice of authorizing generics after the closing of those loopholes.

To follow up on the Commission's 2002 report, a study on the impact of authorized generics on competition is urgently needed. Such a study should examine (1) whether the 6-month exclusivity period provided by the Hatch-Waxman Amendments to the first generic drug manufacturer to challenge a patent is a significant incentive for patent challenges; (2) whether the increasing use of authorized generics has reduced, or is likely to reduce, the number of patent challenges or to otherwise delay or decrease generic competition, e.g., by reducing the number of generic drugs brought to market; and (3) whether prescription drug consumers benefit more from the short-term competition offered by authorized generics or by the earlier marketing of generic drugs that are the subjects of successful patent challenges, to the extent that the 6-month exclusivity is responsible for such challenges.

If you have any questions about this request, please contact Ann Witt of my staff at (202) 225-3976.

With kind regards, I am

Sincerely,

HENRY A. WAXMAN
Member of Congress

Appendix C. List of Companies Covered by the Study

Brand Companies

3M Company
Abbott Laboratories
Aqua Pharmaceuticals, LLC
Astellas Pharma US, Inc.
AstraZeneca Pharmaceuticals LP
Bayer HealthCare Pharmaceuticals
Biovail Pharmaceuticals Inc.
Blansett Pharmacal Co., Inc.
Boehringer Ingelheim Corp
Bradley Pharmaceuticals
Bristol-Myers Squibb Company
Celgene Corporation
Cephalon, Inc.
Duramed Pharmaceuticals, Inc. (Barr)
Eisai Corporation of North America
Elan Corporation
Eli Lilly and Company
Forest Laboratories, Inc.
Gate Pharmaceuticals (Teva)
GlaxoSmithKline
Hi-Tech Pharmacal Co., Inc.
Hoffmann-La Roche Inc.
Jerome Stevens Pharmaceuticals
Johnson & Johnson
King Pharmaceuticals, Inc.
K-V Pharmaceutical Co.*
Lannett Company, Inc.
Merck & Co. Inc.
MGI Pharma Inc.
Mission Pharmacal Company, Inc.
Novartis Corporation
Novo Nordisk, Inc.
Organon Inc.
Otsuka America, Inc.
PDL BioPharma, Inc.*
Pfizer Inc.
Procter & Gamble Company, The
Purdue Pharma L.P.
Reliant Pharmaceuticals, Inc.
Salix Pharmaceuticals, Inc.*
Sankyo Pharma Inc. [Daiichi Sankyo, Inc.]
Sanofi-Aventis US LLC
Savient Pharmaceuticals, Inc.
Schering-Plough Corporation
Schwarz Pharma Inc. (UCB)
Sciele Pharma, Inc.
Shire PLC
Sigma-Tau Pharmaceuticals, Inc.*
Solvay America, Inc.
Somerset Pharmaceuticals, Inc.
Stat-Trade, Inc.
Takeda America Holdings, Inc.
Tyco Healthcare Group LP [Covidien]
UCB Pharma Inc.
Valeant Pharmaceuticals International
Warner Chilcott Holdings Company III, Limited
Watson Pharmaceuticals, Inc.
Wyeth
X-Gen Pharmaceuticals, Inc.

Generic Companies

Actavis U.S.
Akyma Pharmaceuticals LLC
Anchen Pharmaceuticals, Inc.
Andrx Corporation (Watson)
Apotex, Inc.
Aurobindo Pharma USA, Inc.
Barr Pharmaceuticals, Inc.
Biovail Pharmaceuticals, Inc.
Blu Pharmaceuticals, LLC
Boca Pharmacal, Inc.
Breckenridge Pharmaceutical, Inc.
Lannett Company, Inc.
Lupin Pharmaceuticals, Inc.
Major Pharmaceuticals, Inc.
Mallinckrodt Pharmaceuticals (Covidien)
Martec Pharmaceutical, Inc.
Mylan Inc.
Paddock Laboratories, Inc.
Par Pharmaceutical Companies, Inc.
Perrigo Company
Prometheus Laboratories, Inc.
Qualitest Pharmaceutical, Inc. & Vintage

Caraco Pharmaceutical Laboratories
Carlsbad Technology, Inc.
Cobalt Laboratories, Inc.
CorePharma LLC
DAVA Pharmaceuticals, Inc.
Deca Pharmaceuticals, LLC
Dr. Reddy's Laboratories, Inc.
Endo Pharmaceuticals
Eurand N.V.
Gedeon Richter USA, Inc
Glades Pharma (Stiefel Labs)*
Glenmark Pharmaceuticals, Inc.

Golden State Medical Supply, Inc.
Hikma Pharmaceuticals Ltd.
Hi-Tech Pharmacal Co., Inc.*
Impax Laboratories, Inc.
Interpharm Holdings, Inc.
Invagen Pharmaceuticals, Inc.
Ivax Pharmaceuticals, Inc. (Teva)
K-V Pharmaceutical Co.
Pharmaceutical, Inc.
Ranbaxy Pharmaceuticals, Inc.
Rising Pharmaceuticals
Roxane Laboratories, Inc. (Boehringer)
Sandoz, Inc. (Novartis)
Spectrum Pharmaceuticals Inc.
Sun Pharmaceutical Industries Inc.
Taro Pharmaceuticals U.S.A. Inc.
Teva Pharmaceuticals USA, Inc.
Three Rivers Pharmaceuticals, LLC
Trigen Laboratories Inc.
UCB, Inc.
United Research Laboratories, Inc. & Mutual Pharmaceutical Co., Inc.
Upsher-Smith Laboratories, Inc.
Versapharm Inc.
Watson Pharmaceuticals, Inc.
Wockhardt USA Inc.
Zydus Pharmaceuticals (USA) Inc.

Authorized Generic Companies

Heritage Pharmaceuticals, Inc.
Prasco Laboratories
*did not receive a Special Order

APPENDIX D. BRAND-NAME DRUG COMPANY SPECIAL ORDER

OMB Control No. 3084-0140
Expires 8/31/2010[372]

United States of America before Federal Trade Commission

Commissioners: Deborah Platt Majoras, Chairman
Pamela Jones Harbour
Jon Leibowitz
William E. Kovacic
J. Thomas Rosch

FTC Matter No. P062105

Order to File Special Report

Pursuant to a resolution of the Federal Trade Commission dated March 28, 2006, entitled "Resolution Directing The Use Of Compulsory Process," a copy of which is enclosed, Company A, hereinafter referred to as the "Company," is ordered to file a Special Report with the Commission containing the information specified herein. The enclosed Authorized Generic Drug Study Federal Register Notice describes the purpose and scope of the information collection.

Please supply the following information, data, and documents, consistent with the Definitions and Instructions contained in Appendix A:

Part I

1. State the full name of the Company and its official address, and its state of incorporation.
2. State whether the Company is a subsidiary company; whether the Company has subsidiary companies; and report the same information specified in Item 1 regarding each parent or subsidiary engaged in research and development, planning and design, production and manufacturing, distribution, or sales and marketing of any drug product.
3. Submit one copy of each organization chart and personnel directory in effect on January 1 of each year since January 1, 2001, (a) for the Company as a whole and, (b) for each of the Company's subsidiaries or divisions involved in the AG drug business, if any.
4. For each drug on "List A" provided by the FTC, state whether any orally administered capsule or tablet form of the drug, at any strength, has been marketed in the United States as an AG drug product (either currently or previously), with a launch date after Jan. 1, 2001, under an NDA for which the Company holds rights or held rights at the time of launch or any time thereafter.
5. For each drug on "List B" provided by the FTC, state whether the specified dosage form and strength of the drug has been marketed in the United States as an AG drug product (either currently or previously), with a launch date after Jan. 1, 2001, under an NDA for which the Company holds rights or held rights at the time of launch or any time thereafter.
6. Submit a list of all of the Company's orally administered prescription AG drug products of any capsule or tablet form launched in the United States after Jan. 1, 2001 (either currently or previously marketed under a NDA for which the Company holds or held the rights), including but not limited to the drugs on the lists provided by the FTC, and provide the following information regarding marketing in the United States: (a) proprietary/trade name of the AG, if any; (b) proprietary/trade name of the brand-name drug for which the NDA authorizes the marketing of the AG; (c) active ingredient; (d) dosage form; (e) NDA number of the brand-name drug that authorizes the marketing of the AG (5 digits, no letter); (f) dosage strength; (g) date of approval of the NDA for each strength; (h) the AG's 9-digit National Drug Code (NDC) number for each strength (labeler and product code separated by a hyphen); (i) the date of launch for each NDC number; (j) the date of discontinuance for each NDC

number, if any; (k) the name of the firm/business entity associated with each NDC labeler code; (l) the relationship (or former relationship) of each labeler code firm/entity to the Company, e.g., current or former division, subsidiary, affiliate, licensee, contractor; (m) the address and phone number of the firm/business entity associated with each NDC labeler code.

7. For each AG on the list provided by the Company in response to Item 6, state whether the marketing entity is part of the Company, so that the Company will coordinate with the marketing entity in providing complete answers to the requests in Part III, Items 10, 15, 18, 21, 24, 27, 28, and 30 below or whether the marketing entity is not part of the Company, so that the FTC will need to contact the AG marketing entity identified in Item 6(k).

Part II

8. Submit to the FTC by Jan. 31, 2008 a list of any additional AGs launched in the United States by Dec. 31, 2007 and the information requested in Item 6.
9. For changes in the information provided to the FTC in response to Item 6 that occur by Dec. 31, 2007, submit updated information to the FTC by Jan. 31, 2008.

Part III

10. For each AG drug on the list the Company provided to the FTC in response to Item 6, state the date of the first public announcement of the marketing or intended marketing of the AG in the United States.
11. For each AG drug on the list the Company provided to the FTC in response to Item 6, state whether marketing of the AG occurred pursuant to a litigation settlement agreement between the Company and an ANDA-generic company, or whether at any time the Company entered into a litigation settlement agreement not to market the AG or to market it after a specified date more than 30 days after execution of the agreement. If so, state the names of the parties, court, case number, date that the litigation was filed, and the date of the settlement agreement.
12. For each brand-name drug on the list the Company provided to the FTC in response to Item 6(b) (brand-name versions of AGs), provide the following information in regard to marketing in the United States: (a) proprietary/trade name of the brand-name drug; (b) active ingredient; (c) dosage form; (d) NDA number (5 digits, no letter); (e) dosage strength; (f) date of approval of the NDA for each strength; (g) the 9-digit National Drug Code (NDC) number for each strength (labeler and product code separated by a hyphen); (h) the name of the firm/business entity associated with each NDC labeler code; (i) the relationship (or former relationship) of each labeler code firm/entity to the Company, e.g., Company, predecessor company, current or former division, subsidiary, affiliate, licensee, contractor; (j) therapeutic category; (k) pharmacological class; (l) 14-digit GPI (Medi-Span's Generic Product Identifier); (m) date of entry by the first competing ANDA-generic drug; (n) whether the first ANDA-generic entry occurred pursuant to a 180-day exclusivity period, and if so, provide (o) the names of all ANDA-generic companies that entered during such exclusivity.

13. For all strengths of brand-name drugs on "List B" that were not covered in the response to Item 12 (i.e., brand-name drugs for which no AG was marketed), provide the information requested in Item 12.
14. For all strengths of brand-name drugs on "List B" listed in the response to Item 13 (i.e., brand-name drugs for which no AG was marketed), state whether a litigation settlement agreement between the Company and an ANDA-generic company provided that an AG would not be marketed. If so, state the names of the parties, court, case number, date that the litigation was filed, and the date of the settlement agreement.
15. *Sales of AG drugs, by NDC.* For each AG drug in the list the Company provided to the FTC in response to Item 6, for sales in the United States from Jan. 1, 2001-March 31, 2007, state the (a) applicable month and year; (b) the drug identifying information described in the second paragraph of Instruction (D); (c) the AG=s 11-digit NDC number (including labeler, product, and package size codes separated by hyphens); (d) package size; (e) package type; total monthly sales to all customers, net of discounts, rebates, promotions, returns and chargebacks, in (f) units (as represented by the NDC=s package size code), and in (g) dollars.
16. *Sales of brand-name drugs (AG version marketed), by NDC.* For each brand-name drug on the list the Company provided to the FTC in response to Item 12 (brand-name versions of AGs), for sales in the United States from Jan. 1, 2001-March 31, 2007, state the (a) applicable month and year; (b) the drug identifying information described in the second paragraph of Instruction (D); (c) 11-digit NDC number (including labeler, product, and package size codes separated by hyphens); (d) package size; (e) package type; total monthly sales to all customers, net of discounts, rebates, promotions, returns and chargebacks, in (f) units (as represented by the NDC's package size code), and in (g) dollars.
17. *Sales of brand-name drugs (no AG version marketed), by NDC.* For all brand-name drugs on "List B" that were not covered in the response to Item 16 (i.e., brand-name drugs listed in response to Item 13, for which no AG was marketed), provide the information requested in Item 16.
18. *Total sales/revenues from AG drugs.* For each AG drug in the list the Company provided to the FTC in response to Item 6, for sales in the United States from Jan. 1, 2001-March 31, 2007, state the (a) applicable month and year; (b) the drug identifying information described in the second paragraph of Instruction (D); (c) the Company's total monthly sales/revenues attributable to all strengths and package sizes of the dosage form under consideration, net of discounts, rebates, promotions, returns and chargebacks, in dollars; and (e) the total monthly sales in prescriptions.
19. *Total sales: brand-name drugs (AG version marketed).* For each brand-name drug on the list the Company provided to the FTC in response to Item 12 (brand-name versions of AGs), for sales in the United States from Jan. 1, 2001-March 31, 2007, state the (a) applicable month and year; (b) the drug identifying information described in the second paragraph of Instruction (D); (c) the Company's total monthly sales attributable to all strengths and package sizes of the dosage form of the brand-name drug under consideration, net of discounts, rebates, promotions, returns and chargebacks, in dollars; and (d) the total monthly sales in prescriptions.

20. *Total sales: brand-name drugs (no AG marketed).* For all brand-name drugs on "List B" that were not covered in the response to Item 19 (i.e., brand-name drugs listed in response to Item 13, for which no AG was marketed), provide the information requested in Item 19.
21. *Prices of AG drugs: WAC and AWP.* For each AG drug in the list the Company provided to the FTC in response to Item 6, for sales in the United States from Jan. 1, 2001-March 31, 2007, state the (a) applicable month and year; (b) the drug identifying information described in the second paragraph of Instruction (D); (c) the AG's 11-digit NDC number (including labeler, product, and package size codes separated by hyphens); (d) package size; (e) package type; (f) wholesale acquisition cost ("WAC," see 42 U.S.C. § 1395w-3a(b)(6)(B)); and (g) the average wholesale price ("AWP").
22. *Prices of brand-name drugs (AG version marketed): WAC and AWP.* For each brand-name drug on the list the Company provided to the FTC in response to Item 12 (brand-name versions of AGs), for sales in the United States from Jan. 1, 2001-March 31, 2007, state the (a) applicable month and year; (b) the drug identifying information described in the second paragraph of Instruction (D); (c) 11-digit NDC number (including labeler, product, and package size codes separated by hyphens); (d) package size; (e) package type; (f) WAC; and (g) the AWP.
23. *Prices of brand-name drugs (no AG marketed): WAC and AWP.* For all brand-name drugs listed in the response to Item 13 that have been subject to ANDA-generic competition (i.e., brand-name drugs for which a date of ANDA-generic entry was entered in Item 13(m)), provide the information requested in Item 22 (for the period from Jan. 1, 2001-March 31, 2007).
24. *Prices of AG drugs: AMP.* For each AG drug in the list the Company provided to the FTC in response to Item 6, for sales in the United States from Jan. 1, 2001-March 31, 2007, state the (a) applicable quarter and year; (b) the drug identifying information described in the second paragraph of Instruction (D); (c) the AG=s 9-digit NDC number (including labeler and product codes separated by a hyphen); and (d) the average manufacturer price ("AMP") as defined by, and reported to, the Centers for Medicare and Medicaid Services (CMS).
25. *Price of brand-name drugs (AG version marketed): AMP.* For each brand-name drug on the list the Company provided to the FTC in response to Item 12 (brand-name versions of AGs), for sales in the United States from Jan. 1, 2001-March 31, 2007, state the (a) applicable quarter and year; (b) the drug identifying information described in the second paragraph of Instruction (D); (c) 9-digit NDC number (including labeler and product codes separated by a hyphen); and (d) the AMP as defined by, and reported to, the CMS.
26. *Prices of brand-name drugs (no AG marketed): AMP.* For all brand-name drugs listed in the response to Item 13 that have been subject to ANDA-generic competition (i.e., brand-name drugs for which a date of ANDA-generic entry was entered in Item 13(m)), provide the information requested in Item 25 (for the period from Jan. 1, 2001-March 31, 2007).
27. Submit all documents that were prepared by or for any officer(s) or director(s) of the Company and/or, if applicable, the marketing entity, or that are in the files of any current or prior Company (and/or marketing entity) senior vice president (or

equivalent position) with product line responsibility (during all or part of the period from January 1, 2003-April 3, 2006) for an AG and/or a brand-name drug in the list the Company provided to the FTC in response to Item 6 (or, in the case of unincorporated entities, individuals exercising similar functions), as follows. (a) For each AG/brand-name pair identified in the list the Company provided to the FTC in response to Item 6, submit planning, decisional, or strategy documents prepared from Jan. 1, 2002 to April 3, 2006, including studies, surveys, analyses, and reports (both internal and external), that evaluated, considered, or analyzed (but did not merely refer to) the marketing or possible marketing of an AG or AGs (as a response to current or future generic competition or for other reasons), including but not limited to whether or not to license or otherwise market a brand-name drug product as an AG drug product; reasons for marketing an AG and/or refraining from marketing an AG; the timing of AG launch relative to a 180-day exclusivity period; the marketing of an AG during 180-day exclusivity; the marketing of an AG in the context of paragraph IV
certifications and settlements of litigation; the marketing of AGs upon expiration of patents or marketing exclusivities claiming a brand-name drug product or its use; and the profitability or other benefits of marketing an AG drug. (b) With respect to AGs in general, submit documents as described in (a) of this Item.

28. For each AG drug identified in the list the Company provided to the FTC in response to Item 6, submit copies of any public announcements, e.g., press release(s) of the planned marketing or launch of the AG in the United States.
29. If the Company licensed or otherwise authorized the marketing by another entity of an AG drug product in the list the Company provided to the FTC in response to Item 6, submit the agreement that authorized marketing (including agreements between the Company and any business entity acquired after the agreement was executed).
30. Submit planning, decisional, or strategy documents dated Jan. 1, 2006-April 29, 2007 that discuss the effect(s) or possible effect(s) of the enactment of Section 6003 of the Deficit Reduction Act of 2005, P.L. 109-171,[373] on the marketing of AGs after Jan. 1, 2007.

By direction of the Commission.

Deborah Platt Majoras
Chairman

SEAL

Date of Order: September 26, 2007

Appendix A. General Instructions

A. Organization of Resp[onses and Due Dates of Parts

The Special Report consists of three parts, a Preliminary Report as specified in Part I, which must be filed by November 5, 2007, or within 30 days of receipt of this Special Order, whichever is later; an Updated Preliminary Report as set forth in Part II, which must be filed by Jan. 31, 2008; and a Detailed Report as set forth in Part III, which must be filed by January 4, 2008.

B. Responses to Questions

The Special Report should be entered into the Excel spreadsheets provided with this Order whenever possible. The FTC has entered the question numbers and the information that must be provided in the header row of each column. To efficiently enter the requested information, companies may wish to electronically "copy and paste" drug identifying or other information that must be entered on more than one row or worksheet. When it is not possible to enter the required answer or information into the applicable worksheet, or no worksheet has been provided, restate the Item and provide the required answer or information. If any question cannot be answered fully, give the information that is available and explain in detail in what respects and why the answer is incomplete.

All responses to Items 1-2 and 4-13 should be submitted to the FTC in both paper and in electronic form (as Excel, Word, or WordPerfect documents) on machine-readable CDs or DVDs.

C. Definitions

The following definitions apply to all Items:

(1) "Active ingredient" means a drug's nonproprietary established name, including the established names for all active ingredients, as defined at 21 C.F.R. § 299.4 and used in the Orange Book.[374]

(2) "ANDA" means Abbreviated New Drug Application, as set forth in 21 U.S.C. § 355(j).

(3) "ANDA-generic drug" means a drug marketed or sought to be marketed pursuant an approved ANDA and usually sold under the established name of the active ingredient(s).

(4) "Authorized generic ("AG") drug" means any drug sold, licensed or marketed under an NDA approved by the FDA under 21 U.S.C. § 355(c); and marketed, sold or distributed (directly or indirectly) without using the listed drug=s brand-name and with a different NDC product number or labeler number (or both).[375]

(5) "Brand-name" drug means an innovator drug product marketed pursuant to an approved NDA under a proprietary, trademark-protected name.

(6) "Capsule" means all dosage forms of capsules as set forth in Appendix C of the Orange Book, including capsule; capsule, delayed release (DR); capsule, delayed release pellets (DRP); and capsule, extended release (XR).

(7) "Company" means 3M Company, its domestic and foreign parents, predecessors, divisions, subsidiaries, affiliates, partnerships and joint ventures, and all directors, officers, employees, agents and representatives of the foregoing. The terms "subsidiary," "affiliate," and "joint venture" refer to any person in which there is partial (50 percent or more) or total ownership or control between the company and any other person. As used in this definition, the term "person" includes the company and means any natural person, corporate entity, partnership, association, joint venture, government entity, or trust.

(8) "Documents" means all computer files and written, recorded, and graphic materials of every kind in the possession, custody or control of the Company.

(9) "NDA" means a New Drug Application, as set forth in 21 U.S.C. § 355(b) and approved under 21 U.S.C. § 355(c).

(10) "Tablet" means all dosage forms of tablets as set forth in Appendix C of the Orange Book, including tablet; tablet, chewable (C); tablet, coated particles (CP); tablet, delayed release (DR); tablet, delayed release, orally disintegrating (DR OD); tablet, extended release (XR); tablet, orally disintegrating (OD).

D. Data Submissions

Unless modified by agreement in writing with the staff of the Federal Trade Commission, all numerical data submitted in response to Items 15-26 must be submitted in a spreadsheet format both on paper and on machine-readable CDs or DVDs. The Commission will accept database and spreadsheet data in the following formats: MS Excel, MS Access, tab-delimited or fixed width text files. All financial information required to be submitted by this Order should be in whole dollar amounts. For Items 15-26, the applicable month (quarter) and year requested refers to each month and year for which the Company provides the information called for by the given Item. If the information is not kept in the form requested, the Company is encouraged to contact the Commission representative to discuss alternative formats in which the information may be provided.

To identify the drug for which data is being provided, for those Items requesting data on AGs (Items 15, 18, 21, and 24) state on the applicable row or page the (b)(1) proprietary/trade name of the AG, if any; (b)(2) proprietary/trade name of the brand-name drug; (b)(3) active ingredient; (b)(4) dosage form; (b)(5) NDA number (5 digits, no letter); and the (b)(6) dosage strength (except for Item 18). For Items requesting data on brand-name drugs (Items 16-17, 19-20, 22-23, and 25-26), state the previously listed identifying information (b)(1)-(6), omitting (6) for Items 19 and 20.

E. Document Submissions

This Special Order covers documents in the Company's possession, custody or control, wherever the documents are located. However, unless or until the Commission notifies Company otherwise in writing, the Commission will not seek to enforce the Special Order to compel the production of documents that were located outside the United States at the time Company received the Special Order. In order to expedite the receipt of documents reflecting the views of all recipients of Special Orders, the Commission requests your cooperation in producing any such documents on a voluntary basis by the date specified in this Special Order.

Provide two paper copies of each document. All documentary responses should be Bates-stamped.

F. Responsibilities of Company and AG-Marketing Entity Officials

1. Companies that market AGs via entities that are part of the Company as defined in definition (7) are required to coordinate with those marketing entities in the submission of certain information on AGs in Part III, as described in the instructions to individual Items. If the marketing entity identified in Item 6(k) is not part of the

Company, the FTC will also contact the marketing entity, and require it to submit certain information on the AGs it markets. The Company's response to Item 7 merely notifies the FTC, on a drug-by-drug, entity-by-entity basis, whether the Company will contact the marketing entity and coordinate with it, because it is part of the Company or whether the FTC will contact the marketing entity, because the marketing entity is not part of the Company. For most Items, however, the Company and any independent marketing entity (which the FTC will contact separately) will be required to respond. The Company's response to Item 7 does NOT eliminate the Company's requirement to respond to each Item, unless expressly stated in the instructions for an Item.

2. The Special Report is required to be subscribed and sworn to by an official of the Company who has prepared or supervised the preparation of the Special Report from books, records, documents, correspondence, and other data and material in the Company's possession. In addition, if the Company indicates in response to Item 7 that it will coordinate with its AG marketing entity, then Items 10, 15, 18, 21, 24, 27-28, and 30 must be subscribed and sworn to by an official of the subsidiary, or other entity of the Company that markets AGs. Each subscriber to the Special Report is to give his or her full name, title, and contact information in a notarized certification at the end of the Special Report, as set forth in Appendix B.

G. Questions

Any questions you have relating to the scope or meaning of this Order, or suggestions for possible modifications thereto, should be directed to Karen A. Goldman, Federal Trade Commission, Office of General Counsel, 600 Pennsylvania Ave., N.W., Washington, DC 20580, (202) 326-2574, kgoldman@ftc.gov.

H. Submission of Report

The Special Report must be Bates-stamped.

You are advised that penalties may be imposed under applicable provisions of federal law for failure to file Special Reports or for filing false reports.

Two copies of the Special Report shall be filed with the Secretary, Federal Trade Commission, Room H-159, 600 Pennsylvania Ave., NW, Washington, DC 20580 by 5:00 PM on the dates specified herein.

Instructions for Specific Items

Part I

1-3. Self-explanatory.

4. To facilitate the Company's response, the FTC has provided two lists of drugs marketed by the Company in the United States during the relevant time frame. "List A" is a list of drugs for which the available information indicates that an AG was launched by the Company, or with its authorization, after Jan. 1, 2001 (a blank list will be provided if the FTC is not aware of any AGs). Using the Excel spreadsheet containing List A, confirm that at least one orally administered capsule or tablet form

of each drug has been marketed as an AG by entering "yes" in the applicable column. If the Company believes that no orally administered capsule or tablet form of the drug has been marketed as an AG, enter "no."

5. "List B" is a list of the Company's orally administered capsule and tablet dosage forms of drugs for which at least one ANDA with a paragraph IV certification was filed and generic competition began after Jan. 1, 2001, or for which generic competition has not yet begun and at least one ANDA with a paragraph IV certification was filed after Jan. 1, 2001. The list contains only those strengths for which a paragraph IV certification has been made. Some of the drugs on List B may also appear on List A. Using the Excel spreadsheet containing List B, enter "yes" if a particular strength of a drug has been marketed as an AG in the United States, or "no" if it has not.
6. The Company's response to this Item must include all orally administered AGs of any capsule or tablet dosage form launched in the United States after Jan. 1, 2001, for which the Company holds rights to the NDA under which the AG is marketed, or held rights to the NDA when the AG was launched or any time thereafter, regardless of whether the AG is currently marketed by the Company. The response must address, but is not limited to, the drugs on the lists provided by the FTC. Thus, the Company's response must include all orally administered capsule or tablet dosage forms of its AGs, regardless of whether the drug was on either List A or List B, or whether the corresponding brand-name drug was subject only to paragraph I, II, or III certifications. Enter the list of the Company's AG drugs and the required information for each on the spreadsheet provided by the FTC. Enter the specific dosage form, e.g., capsule DR, capsule XR, tablet DR, or tablet XR. Enter each strength for each dosage form on a different row. If more than one entity marketed a particular drug, use different rows to enter the information for each entity.

   Item 6(h), (k), (m). The response to Item 6(h) should include all 9-digit NDC numbers used in the direct or indirect marketing, sale, or distribution of the AG in the United States, whether by the Company or by other entities, e.g., licensees under the Company's NDA. Thus, Item 6(k) should provide a complete list of entities that market the AG, whether the marketing entity is part of the Company or independent of it. Do not, however, include NDC numbers that cover repackaged or relabeled drug products (such as those for use in institutions) that were previously sold under one of the aforementioned NDCs. If the NDCs associated with the AG have changed, e.g., due to marketing by different business entities, provide all NDC numbers that have been used. If there are multiple NDC numbers for a given strength, each should be entered on a different row.

   The address and phone number of the firm/business entity that markets the AG (requested in Item 6(m)) need only be entered the first time that the name of the entity is provided in response to Item 6(k).
7. If an AG is marketed via an entity that is part of the Company as defined in definition (7), the Company must enter "yes" on the applicable spreadsheet column, and it is required to coordinate with the marketing entity in the submission of information on that AG. If an AG is marketed by an entity that is not a part of the Company, such as a contractor or licensee, the Company must enter "no," and the marketing entity will be contacted by the FTC and asked to provide certain

information. A Company's response of "no" to Item 7 does NOT eliminate the Company's requirement to respond to each Item below, unless expressly stated in the instructions for an Item.

Because some manufacturers of brand-name pharmaceuticals also manufacture ANDA-generic drugs, the FTC reserves the right to request additional information from the Company, and directly from marketing entities that are part of the Company, even if the Company has responded to this request or provided a coordinated response to an Item.

Part II

8. This Item requests the basic information in Item 6 on any AGs launched in the United States by Dec. 31, 2007 pursuant to a NDA for which the Company holds rights that were not included in the Company's initial response to that Item. For the purposes of this study, the FTC will not require any information beyond that requested in Item 6 for these AGs.
9. This Item requests updated information on AGs identified by the Company in its initial response to Item 6, including but not limited to, whether the marketing of the AG has been discontinued or otherwise changed (e.g., dosage form or strength, marketing entity).

Part III

10. On the applicable spreadsheet and column, enter the date of the first public announcement by any entity, including but not limited to announcements made by the Company, of the intended marketing of each AG. Documentation of the first announcement is requested in Item 28.
11. On the applicable spreadsheet and column, enter "yes" if the marketing of the AG occurred pursuant to a settlement agreement, or if the Company entered into a settlement agreement not to market the AG or to market it after a specified date more than 30 days after execution of the agreement; enter "no" if there were no such agreements. If "yes," restate Item 11 on a separate document, identify the AG, and provide the required information about the litigation.
12. For identification and informational purposes, Item 12(a)-(f) repeats information provided in Item 6(b)-(g). Each strength should be listed in a separate row, followed by the rest of the requested information. If there are multiple NDC numbers for a given strength, each should be entered in a different row.

    Item 12(j), (k). State the therapeutic category and pharmacological class as set forth in the U.S. Pharmacopeial Convention, Inc., U.S.P. Medicare Model Guidelines, Version 2, Feb. 6, 2006.[376]

    Item 12(l). When entering the 14-digit GPI, separate the two-digit fields with dashes.

    Items 12(m), (n), (o). If the brand-name drug has not been subject to ANDA-generic competition, enter "none" in response to Item 12(m), and do not respond to Items 12(n) and (o).
13. Enter the required information for each brand-name drug on "List B" that was not covered in the response to Item 12 on the spreadsheet provided by the FTC. Enter the

specific dosage form, e.g., capsule DR, capsule XR, tablet DR, or tablet XR. Enter each strength, and each 9-digit NDC number related to a particular strength, in a different row. If the NDCs associated with the drug have changed, provide all NDC numbers that have been used. With respect to therapeutic category and pharmacological class, follow the instructions in Item 12. If the brand-name drug has not been subject to ANDA-generic competition, enter "none" in response to Item 13(m), and do not respond to Items 13(n) and (o).

14. On the applicable spreadsheet and column, enter "yes" if a litigation settlement agreement between the Company and an ANDA-generic company provided that an AG would not be marketed, and if not, enter "no." If "yes," restate Item 14 on a separate document, identify the drug, and provide the required information about the litigation.
15. Item 15 requests monthly net sales data for AGs for all 11-digit NDCs arising from the 9-digit NDCs provided in response to Item 6(h), i.e., including all package size codes for those NDCs. If the Company answered "yes" to Item 7 with respect to a particular drug, the Company must coordinate with its marketing entity in providing the information requested in Item 15. If the Company is not coordinating with its marketing entity with respect to a particular drug, i.e., it answered "no" in response to Item 7 for that drug, the Company should only submit data for Items 15(a)-(f). In such cases, the FTC will ask the marketing entity to provide the information requested in Items 15(g).
16. Include sales for each strength provided in response to Item 12(e). Thus, the response to Item 16 should include sales for all 11-digit NDC codes arising from the 9-digit codes provided in response to Item 12(g).
17. Include sales for all 11-digit NDC codes arising from the 9-digit codes provided in response to Item 13.
18. Responses to this Item represent the Company's combined sales or revenues from all strengths and NDC numbers.
19. If the Company answered "yes" to Item 7 with respect to a particular drug, the Company must coordinate with its marketing entity and provide the net sales for the Company (including the marketing entity) with respect to that drug. However, the Company must respond to Item 18 even if the Company answered "no" to Item 7 and is not coordinating with the marketing entity. In such cases, the Company should provide its revenues (including royalties, license fees, and transfer payments) arising from sales in the United States, not the sales of the independent marketing entity. In calculating its net revenues, the Company should include its own discounts, rebates, promotions, returns and chargebacks (if any), not those of the independent marketing entity.
20. Responses to these Items represent the Company's combined sales from all strengths and NDC numbers.
21. The referenced 11-digit NDCs should have been listed in response to Item 15(c).
22. The referenced 11-digit NDCs should have been listed in response to Item 16(c).
23. The 11-digit NDCs should be a subset of those listed in response to Item 17. Provide data for the entire requested period, regardless of whether the drug was subject to ANDA-generic competition for the entire time.

24. Item 24 requests the quarterly Average Manufacturer Price ("AMP," *see* 42 U.S.C. § 1396r-8(k)(1)), for each AG listed by the Company in response to Item 6, for all 9-digit NDCs provided in response to Item 6(h).

    If the Company answered "yes" to Item 7 with respect to a particular drug, the Company must coordinate with its marketing entity in providing the information requested in Item 24. If the Company is not coordinating with its marketing entity with respect to a particular drug, i.e., it answered "no" in response to Item 7 for that drug, the Company should not respond to this Item. In such cases, the FTC will ask the independent marketing entity to provide the AMP.
25. The Company must provide the information requested in Item 25, regardless of its response to Item 7 and whether it is coordinating with the marketing entity.
26. The 11-digit NDCs should be those listed in response to Item 23. Provide data for the entire requested period, regardless of whether the drug was subject to ANDA-generic competition for the entire time.
27. When responding to Item 27(b), do not duplicate documents provided in response to Item 27(a).

    If the Company answered "yes" to Item 7 with respect to a particular drug, the Company must coordinate with its marketing entity in responding to Item 27(a) with respect to that drug. In responding to Item 27(b) in regard to documents generally about AG drugs, the Company must coordinate with its marketing entity if it answered "yes" to Item 7 with respect to any drug. However, the Company must respond to Items 27(a) and 27(b) even if it answered "no" in response to Item 7 and is not coordinating with the marketing entity. In such cases, the marketing entity will be asked to respond to Items 27(a) and 27(b), in addition to the Company.

    Group the documents by drug product, and if applicable, segregate the documents obtained from the Company from the documents obtained from the marketing entity. For each document, indicate the name of the person from whose files the document came and whether the document was generated within the Company or externally; if generated externally, provide the name of the source of the document.
28. If the Company answered "yes" to Item 7 with respect to a particular drug, the Company must coordinate with its marketing entity in responding to this Item with respect to that drug. Group the documents by drug product.
29. The Company must respond to Item 29 with respect to all AGs for which the Company answered "no" in response to Item 7, and is not coordinating with the marketing entity. Group the documents by drug product, and indicate the name of the person from whose files the document came.

    If an agreement authorizing the marketing of an AG was previously submitted to the FTC pursuant to the Medicare Prescription Drug, Improvement, and Modernization Act of 2003,[377] do not provide another copy of the agreement. Provide the names of the parties, the date of the agreement, and the date that the agreement was submitted to the FTC.
30. The Company must respond to this Item, and if the Company answered "yes" to Item 7 with respect to any drug, the Company must coordinate with its marketing entity in responding to this Item. For each document, indicate the name of the person from whose files the document came.

Appendix B. Certification

This Special Report, together with any and all appendices and attachments thereto, was prepared and assembled under my supervision in accordance with instructions issued by the Federal Trade Commission in its Special Orders for the Authorized Generic Drug Study. Subject to the recognition that, where so indicated, reasonable estimates have been made because books and records do not provide the required information, the information is, to the best of my knowledge, true, correct, and complete. Where copies rather than original documents have been submitted, the copies are true, correct, and complete.

____

Type or Print Name and Title

____

Type or Print Company Name and Address

____

Type or Print Phone Number and E-Mail Address

____

(Signature)

Subscribed and sworn to before me at the City of ______________________________, *State of* ________________________, *this*_________ *day of*__________, *20*____.

____

(Notary Public)

My Commission Expires: ________________

APPENDIX E. GENERIC DRUG COMPANY SPECIAL ORDER

OMB Control No. 3084-0140
Expires 8/31/2010[378]

United States of America before Federal Trade Commission

Commissioners: Deborah Platt Majoras, Chairman
Pamela Jones Harbour
Jon Leibowitz
William E. Kovacic
J. Thomas Rosch

FTC Matter No. P062105

Order to File Special Report

Pursuant to a resolution of the Federal Trade Commission dated March 28, 2006, entitled "Resolution Directing The Use Of Compulsory Process," a copy of which is enclosed, Company A, hereinafter referred to as the "Company," is ordered to file a Special Report with the Commission containing the information specified herein. The enclosed Authorized Generic Drug Study Federal Register Notice describes the purpose and scope of the information collection.

Please supply the following information, data, and documents, consistent with the Definitions and Instructions contained in Appendix A:

1. State the full name of the Company and its official address, and its state of incorporation.
2. State whether the Company is a subsidiary company; whether the Company has subsidiary companies; and report the same information specified in Item 1 regarding each parent or subsidiary engaged in research and development, planning and design, production and manufacturing, distribution, or sales and marketing of any drug product.
3. Submit one copy of each organization chart and personnel directory in effect on January 1 of each year since January 1, 2001, (a) for the Company as a whole and, (b) for each of the Company's subsidiaries or divisions involved in the AG drug business, if any.
4. For each AG drug on the list of AG drugs provided by the FTC, state the (a) proprietary/trade name of the AG, if any; (b) proprietary/trade name of the brand-name drug for which the NDA authorizes the marketing of the AG; (c) active ingredient; (d) dosage form; (e) NDA number of the brand-name drug that authorizes the marketing of the AG (5 digits, no letter); (f) dosage strength; (g) 14-digit GPI (Medi-Span's Generic Product Identifier); (h) the AG's 9-digit National Drug Code (NDC) number for each strength (labeler and product code separated by a hyphen); (i) name of the firm/business entity associated with each NDC labeler code; (j) date of launch for each NDC number; (k) date of discontinuance for each NDC number, if any; (l) date of the first public announcement of the marketing or intended marketing of the AG; and (m) whether at any time the Company marketed the drug as an ANDA-generic drug.
5. Submit a list of the Company's orally administered prescription AG drug products of any capsule or tablet form that were launched after Jan. 1, 2001, but are not on the FTC's list of AG drugs (if any), and provide the information requested in Item 4.
6. For each AG drug addressed in Items 4 and 5, state whether marketing of the AG occurred pursuant to a litigation settlement agreement between the Company and a brand-name company. If so, state the names of the parties, court, case number, date that the litigation was filed, and the date of the settlement agreement.
7. For each drug on the list of ANDA-generic drugs provided by the FTC and any ANDA-generic drugs identified in response to Item 4(m), state the (a) brand-name of the reference listed drug (RLD); (b) NDA number of the RLD; (c) active ingredient; (d) dosage form; (e) ANDA number (5 digits, no letter); (f) dosage strength; (g) the ANDA-generic's 9-digit National Drug Code (NDC) number for each strength

(labeler and product code separated by a hyphen); (h) name of the firm/business entity associated with each NDC labeler code; (i) date of launch for each NDC number; (j) date of discontinuance for each NDC number, if any; (k) whether entry of the Company's ANDA-generic drug product occurred pursuant to a 180-day exclusivity period; and if entry occurred pursuant to 180-day exclusivity, the (l) date the exclusivity period began, the (m) date of expiration of the exclusivity period, and the (n) names of any other ANDA-generic companies that entered during the exclusivity period.

8. For each ANDA-generic drug addressed in Item 7, state the (a) active ingredient; (b) dosage form; (c) ANDA number (5 digits, no letter); (d) dosage strength; (e) date of ANDA filing; (f) date of ANDA approval for each dosage strength; (g) 14-digit GPI (Medi-Span's Generic Product Identifier); (h) patent numbers of patents for which the Company made a patent certification under 21 U.S.C. § 355(j)(2)(A)(vii); (i) paragraph number of the certification for each patent number; (j) date of each patent certification; (k) paragraph number of any amended patent certifications; and the (l) date of amendment of the patent certification.
9. *Sales of AG drugs, by NDC.* For each AG drug addressed in Items 4 and 5, for sales in the United States from Jan. 1, 2001-March 31, 2007, state the (a) applicable month and year; (b) the drug identifying information described in the second paragraph of Instruction (D); (c) the 11-digit NDC number (including labeler, product, and package size codes separated by hyphens); (d) package size; (e) package type; total sales to all customers, net of discounts, rebates, promotions, returns and chargebacks, in (f) units (as represented by the NDC's package size code), and in (g) dollars.
10. *Sales and costs of ANDA-generic drugs, by NDC.* For each ANDA-generic drug addressed in Item 7, for sales in the United States from Jan. 1, 2001-March 31, 2007, provide the information requested in Item 9, and (h) the cost to manufacture, including all direct and indirect labor, material, and overhead expenses. If the Company does not manufacture a drug, provide the cost of purchasing it in response to (h), and indicate that the stated amount is the cost of purchase.
11. *Total sales of AG drugs.* For each AG drug addressed in Items 4 and 5, for sales in the United States for the period from Jan. 1, 2001-March 31, 2007, state the (a) applicable month and year; (b) the drug identifying information described in the second paragraph of Instruction (D); (c) the Company's total sales attributable to all strengths and package sizes of the dosage form under consideration, net of discounts, rebates, promotions, returns and chargebacks, in dollars; and (d) the total sales in prescriptions.
12. *Total sales of ANDA-generic drugs.* For each ANDA-generic drug addressed in Item 7, for sales in the United States from Jan. 1, 2001-March 31, 2007, provide the information requested in Item 11.
13. *Prices of AG drugs: WAC and AWP.* For each AG drug addressed in Items 4 and 5, for sales in the United States from Jan. 1, 2001-March 31, 2007, state the (a) applicable month and year; (b) the drug identifying information described in the second paragraph of Instruction (D); (c) the 11-digit NDC number (including labeler, product, and package size codes separated by hyphens); (d) package size; (e) package type; (f) wholesale acquisition cost (AWAC," *see* 42 U.S.C. § 1395w-3a(b)(6)(B)); and (g) the average wholesale price ("AWP").

14. *Prices of ANDA-generic drugs: WAC and AWP.* For each drug on the list of ANDA-generic drugs addressed in Item 7, for sales in the United States from Jan. 1, 2001-March 31, 2007, provide the information requested in Item 13.
15. *Prices of AG drugs: AMP.* For each AG drug addressed in Items 4 and 5, for the period from Jan. 1, 2001-March 31, 2007, state the (a) applicable quarter and year; (b) the drug identifying information described in the second paragraph of Instruction (D); (c) the 9-digit NDC number (including labeler and product codes separated by a hyphen); and (d) the average manufacturer price ("AMP") as defined by, and reported to, the Centers for Medicare and Medicaid Services (CMS).
16. *Prices of ANDA-generic drugs: AMP.* For each ANDA-generic drug addressed in Item 7, for the period from Jan. 1, 2001-March 31, 2007, provide the information requested in Item 15.
17. *Cost data and documents.* For each ANDA-generic drug addressed in Item 7, state the (a) active ingredient; (b) dosage form; (c) ANDA number (5 digits, no letter); (d) research and development costs; (e) the costs of filing the ANDA; (f) the costs for patent-related litigation (if any). Also, submit (g) any documents sufficient to show the identified product's research and development costs, costs to file the ANDA, patent-related litigation costs (if any), and any other sunk costs allocated to the drug. In those cases in which the Company is not the sole defendant, describe how litigation expenses have been distributed among the defendants.
18. Submit documents that were prepared from Jan. 1, 2003 to April 3, 2006, by or for any officer(s) or director(s) of the Company, or that are in the files of any current or prior Company (or marketing entity) senior vice president (or equivalent position) with product line responsibility (during all or part of the period from January 1, 2003-April 3, 2006) for any specific ANDA-generic drug (or, in the case of unincorporated entities, individuals exercising similar functions) (a) that considered, evaluated, analyzed, or discussed AGs or the possibility of AGs with regard to whether to file an ANDA and/or make a paragraph III or IV certification with respect to any specific drug (regardless of whether the Company filed such ANDA); (b) that considered, evaluated, analyzed or discussed the impact that entry by an AG drug had or would have on the profitability (during 180-day exclusivity or otherwise) of any specific ANDA-generic drug product marketed by the Company, or for which submission of an ANDA was under consideration; or (c) that comprise planning, decisional, or strategy documents that discuss AGs but not in regard to a particular drug, including documents that discuss AGs in regard to filing ANDAs, making paragraph III or IV certifications, and/or the possible impact of AGs on the profitability of ANDA-generic drugs during 180-day exclusivity or otherwise.
19. For the AG drugs addressed in Items 4 and 5: Submit planning, decisional, or strategy documents, including studies, surveys, analyses, and reports (both internal and external), that were prepared from Jan. 1, 2003 to April 3, 2006, by or for any officer(s) or director(s) of the Company, or that are in the files of any current or prior Company (or marketing entity) senior vice president (or equivalent position) with product line responsibility (during all or part of the period from January 1, 2003-April 3, 2006) for the specified AG drug (or, in the case of unincorporated entities, individuals exercising similar functions), that evaluated, considered, or analyzed the marketing or possible marketing of the AG; the timing of AG launch relative to any

anticipated 180-day exclusivity period; the effect or potential effect of the AG on ANDA-generic competition; the marketing of the AG in the context of settlements of patent-related litigation; the profitability or other benefits of marketing the AG; and/or whether to market an ANDA-generic drug or an AG.

20. For the AG drugs addressed in Items 4 and 5: (a) If the Company and the brand-name company entered into an agreement that licensed or otherwise authorized the marketing of the identified drug product as an AG, submit the agreement. (b) Submit copies of any public announcements, e.g., press release(s), of the planned marketing or launch of each AG.

By direction of the Commission.

Deborah Platt Majoras
Chairman
SEAL
Date of Order: December 10, 2007

Appendix A. General Instructions

A. Organization of Responses and Due Dates of Parts

The Company's Special Report must be filed by March 19, 2008.

B. Responses to Questions

The Special Report should be entered into the Excel spreadsheets provided with this Order whenever possible. The FTC has entered the question numbers and the information that must be provided in the header row of each column. To efficiently enter the requested information, companies may wish to electronically "copy and paste" drug identifying or other information that must be entered on more than one row or worksheet. When it is not possible to enter the required answer or information into the applicable worksheet, or no worksheet has been provided, restate the Item and provide the required answer or information. If any question cannot be answered fully, give the information that is available and explain in detail in what respects and why the answer is incomplete.

All responses to Items 1-2 and 4-8 should be submitted to the FTC in both paper and electronic form (as Excel, Word, or WordPerfect documents) on machine-readable CDs or DVDs.

C. Definitions

The following definitions apply to all Items:

(1) "Active ingredient" means a drug's nonproprietary established name, including the established names for all active ingredients, as defined at 21 C.F.R. § 299.4 and used in the Orange Book.[379]

(2) "ANDA" means Abbreviated New Drug Application, as set forth in 21 U.S.C. § 355(j).

(3) "ANDA-generic drug" means a drug marketed or sought to be marketed pursuant to an approved ANDA and usually sold under the established name of the active ingredient(s).
(4) "Authorized generic ("AG") drug" means any drug sold, licensed or marketed under an NDA approved by the FDA under 21 U.S.C. § 355(c); and marketed, sold or distributed (directly or indirectly) without using the listed drug's brand-name and with a different NDC product number or labeler number (or both).[380]
(5) "Brand-name" drug means an innovator drug product marketed pursuant to an approved NDA under a proprietary, trademark-protected name.
(6) "Capsule" means all dosage forms of capsules as set forth in Appendix C of the Orange Book, including capsule; capsule, delayed release (DR); capsule, delayed release pellets (DRP); and capsule, extended release (XR).
(7) "Company" means Company A, its domestic and foreign parents, predecessors, divisions, subsidiaries, affiliates, partnerships and joint ventures, and all directors, officers, employees, agents and representatives of the foregoing. The terms "subsidiary", "affiliate" and "joint venture" refer to any person in which there is partial (50 percent or more) or total ownership or control between the company and any other person. As used in this definition, the term "person" includes the company and means any natural person, corporate entity, partnership, association, joint venture, government entity, or trust.
(8) "Documents" means all computer files and written, recorded, and graphic materials of every kind in the possession, custody or control of the Company.
(9) "ANDA" means a New Drug Application, as set forth in 21 U.S.C. § 355(b) and approved under 21 U.S.C. § 355(c).
(10)"Tablet" means all dosage forms of tablets as set forth in Appendix C of the Orange Book, including tablet; tablet, chewable (C); tablet, coated particles (CP); tablet, delayed release (DR); tablet, delayed release, orally disintegrating (DR OD); tablet, extended release (XR); tablet, orally disintegrating (OD).

D. Data Submissions

Unless modified by agreement in writing with the staff of the Federal Trade Commission, all numerical data submitted in response to Items 9-17 must be submitted in a spreadsheet format both on paper and on machine-readable CDs. The Commission will accept database and spreadsheet data in the following formats: MS Excel, MS Access, tab-delimited or fixed width text files. All financial information required to be submitted by this Order should be in whole dollar amounts. For Items 9-16, the applicable month (quarter) and year requested refers to each month and year for which the Company provides the information called for by the given Item. If the information is not kept in the form requested, the Company is encouraged to contact the Commission representative to discuss alternative formats in which the information may be provided.

To identify the drug for which data is being provided, for those Items requesting data on AGs (Items 9, 11, 13, and 15) state on the applicable row or page the (b)(1) proprietary/trade name of the AG, if any; (b)(2) proprietary/trade name of the brand-name drug for which the NDA authorizes the marketing of the AG; (b)(3) active ingredient; (b)(4) dosage form; (b)(5) NDA number (5 digits, no letter) of the brand-name drug that authorizes the marketing of the AG; and the (b)(6) dosage strength (except for Item 11). For Items requesting data on ANDA-generic drugs (Items 10, 12, 14, and 16) state on the applicable row or page the (b)(1) active ingredient; (b)(2) dosage form; (b)(3) ANDA number (5 digits, no letter); and the (b)(4) dosage strength (except for Item 12).

E. Document Submissions

This Special Order covers documents in the Company's possession, custody or control, wherever the documents are located. However, unless or until the Commission notifies Company otherwise in writing, the Commission will not seek to enforce the Special Order to compel the production of documents that were located outside the United States at the time Company received the Special Order. In order to expedite the receipt of documents reflecting the views of all recipients of Special Orders, the Commission requests your cooperation in producing any such documents on a voluntary basis by the date specified in this Special Order.

Provide two paper copies of each document. Group the documents by drug product. For each document, indicate the name of the person from whose files the document came and whether the document was generated within the Company or externally; if generated externally, provide the name of the source of the document. All documentary responses should be Bates-stamped.

F. Responsibilities of Company

The Special Report is required to be subscribed and sworn to by an official of the Company who has prepared or supervised the preparation of the Special Report from books, records, documents, correspondence, and other data and material in the Company's possession.

Each subscriber to the Special Report is to give his or her full name, title, and contact information in a notarized certification at the end of the Special Report, as set forth in Appendix B.

G. Questions

Any questions you have relating to the scope or meaning of this Order, or suggestions for possible modifications thereto, should be directed to Karen A. Goldman, Federal Trade Commission, Office of General Counsel, 600 Pennsylvania Ave., N.W., Washington, DC 20580, (202) 326-2574, kgoldman@ftc.gov.

H. Submission of Report

The Special Report must be Bates-stamped.

You are advised that penalties may be imposed under applicable provisions of federal law for failure to file Special Reports or for filing false reports.

Two copies of the Special Report required by this Order should be submitted to the attention of Karen A. Goldman, Federal Trade Commission, Room H-503, 600 Pennsylvania Ave., NW, Washington, DC 20580 by 5:00 PM on the dates specified herein.

Instructions for Specific Items

1-3. Self-explanatory.

4. The FTC has provided two lists of drugs marketed by the Company during the relevant time frame that must be addressed in the Company's Special Report. The first is a list of AG drugs that were first launched in the United States after Jan. 1, 2001 (a blank list will be provided if the FTC is not aware of any AGs). Using the Excel spreadsheet containing this list, enter the information requested in Item 4 with regard to marketing in the United States. Enter the specific dosage form, e.g., capsule DR, capsule XR, tablet DR, or tablet XR. Enter each strength for each dosage form on a different row. When entering the 14-digit GPI, separate the two-digit fields with dashes.

   The response to Item 4(h) should include all of the Company's 9-digit NDC numbers used in the marketing, sale, or distribution of the AG in the United States. Do not include NDC numbers that cover repackaged or relabeled drug products (such as those for use in institutions) that were previously sold under one of the aforementioned NDCs. If the NDCs associated with the AG have changed, provide all NDC numbers that have been used. If there are multiple NDC numbers for a given strength, each should be entered on a different row.

5. Add to the Excel spreadsheet containing the FTC's list of AGs any other AGs that fit the specified criteria but were not on FTC's list. Follow the instructions for Item 4 for entering the requested information on these AGs.

6. On the applicable spreadsheet and column, enter "yes" if the marketing of the AG occurred pursuant to a settlement agreement, "no" if it did not. If "yes," restate Item 6 in a separate document, identify the AG, and provide the required information about the litigation.

7. The second list provided by the FTC is a list of ANDA-generic drugs marketed by the Company (i) for which at least one ANDA with a paragraph IV certification was filed by any company and the first ANDA-generic launch in the United States by any company was after Jan. 1, 2001; and (ii) for which an AG version of the applicable brand-name drug was first launched in the United States by another company after Jan. 1, 2001. Using the Excel spreadsheet containing this list, enter the information requested in Item 7 with regard to in the United States. Add any ANDA-generic drugs identified in response to Item 4(m) to the FTC's list (if they are not already on the list), and enter the information requested in Item 7. Enter the specific dosage form, e.g., capsule DR, capsule XR, tablet DR, or tablet XR. Enter each strength for each dosage form on a different row; enter all strengths marketed by the Company, even if the Company is aware that no AG was marketed for a particular strength.

   The response to Item 7(g) should include all of the Company's 9-digit NDC numbers used in the marketing, sale, or distribution of the ANDA-generic drug in the United States. Do not include NDC numbers that cover repackaged or relabeled drug products (such as those for use in institutions) that were previously sold under one of the aforementioned NDCs. If the NDCs associated with the ANDA-generic drug have changed, provide all NDC numbers that have been used. If there are multiple NDC numbers for a given strength, each should be entered on a different row.

8. Enter each patent number in a separate column, followed by columns with the information requested with respect to each patent. When entering the 14-digit GPI, separate the two-digit fields with dashes.
9. Item 9 requests monthly net sales data for AGs for all 11-digit NDCs arising from the 9-digit NDCs provided in response to Item 4(h) and Item 5, i.e., including all package size codes for those NDCs.
10. Item 10 requests monthly net sales and cost data for all 11-digit NDCs arising from the 9-digit NDCs provided in response to Item 7(g).

11, 12. Responses to Items 11 and 12 represent combined sales from all strengths and NDC numbers.

13, 14. Items 13 and 14 request monthly WAC and AWP for all 11-digit NDCs arising from the 9-digit NDCs provided in response to Items 4(h), 5, and Item 7(g), respectively.

15, 16. Items 15 and 16 request the quarterly AMP (*see* 42 U.S.C. § 1396r-8(k)(1)), for all 9-digit NDCs provided in response to Items 4(h), 5, and Item 7(g), respectively.

17. Self-explanatory.
18. The documents requested by this Item are not limited to those that consider drugs marketed or previously marketed by the Company, nor are they limited to those that discuss drugs identified in the lists provided by the FTC. For example, responsive documents might consider drugs for which the Company filed an ANDA that has not yet been approved; drugs for which the Company considered making a paragraph IV certification, but the ANDA that was filed did not contain a paragraph IV certification; or drugs for which the Company considered filing an ANDA, but ultimately did not.

    Do not duplicate documents when responding to Items 18(a), (b), and (c).
19. Do not duplicate documents submitted in response to Item 18.
20. For press releases, the source of the document need not be provided.

    If an agreement authorizing the marketing of an AG was previously submitted to the FTC pursuant to the Medicare Prescription Drug, Improvement, and Modernization Act of 2003,[381] do not provide another copy of the agreement. Provide the names of the parties, the date of the agreement, and the date that the agreement was submitted to the FTC.

Appendix B. Certification

This Special Report, together with any and all appendices and attachments thereto, was prepared and assembled under my supervision in accordance with instructions issued by the Federal Trade Commission in its Special Orders for the Authorized Generic Drug Study. Subject to the recognition that, where so indicated, reasonable estimates have been made because books and records do not provide the required information, the information is, to the best of my knowledge, true, correct, and complete. Where copies rather than original documents have been submitted, the copies are true, correct, and complete.

____

Type or Print Name and Title

____

Type or Print Company Name and Address

____

Type or Print Phone Number and E-Mail Address

____

(Signature)

Subscribed and sworn to before me at the City of ____________________ , State of____________________________, this _____________ day of_____________, 20 .

____

(Notary Public)

My Commission Expires: ____________________

APPENDIX F. AUTHORIZED GENERIC DRUG COMPANY SPECIAL ORDER

OMB Control No. 3084-0140
Expires 8/31/2010[382]

United States of America before Federal Trade Commission

COMMISSIONERS: Deborah Platt Majoras, Chairman
Pamela Jones Harbour
Jon Leibowitz
William E. Kovacic
J. Thomas Rosch

FTC Matter No. P062105

Order to File Special Report

Pursuant to a resolution of the Federal Trade Commission dated March 28, 2006, entitled "Resolution Directing The Use Of Compulsory Process," a copy of which is enclosed, Company A, hereinafter referred to as the "Company," is ordered to file a Special Report with the Commission containing the information specified herein. The enclosed Authorized Generic Drug Study Federal Register Notice describes the purpose and scope of the information collection.

Please supply the following information, data, and documents, consistent with the Definitions and Instructions contained in Appendix A:

1. State the full name of the Company and its official address, and its state of incorporation.
2. State whether the Company is a subsidiary company; whether the Company has subsidiary companies; and report the same information specified in Item 1 regarding each parent or subsidiary engaged in research and development, planning and design, production and manufacturing, distribution, or sales and marketing of any drug product.
3. Submit one copy of each organization chart and personnel directory in effect on January 1 of each year since January 1, 2001, (a) for the Company as a whole and, (b) for each of the Company's subsidiaries or divisions involved in the AG drug business, if any.
4. For each AG drug on the list of AG drugs provided by the FTC, state the (a) proprietary/trade name of the AG, if any; (b) proprietary/trade name of the brand-name drug for which the NDA authorizes the marketing of the AG; (c) active ingredient; (d) dosage form; (e) NDA number of the brand-name drug that authorizes the marketing of the AG (5 digits, no letter); (f) dosage strength; (g) 14-digit GPI (Medi-Span=s Generic Product Identifier); (h) the AG=s 9-digit National Drug Code (NDC) number for each strength (labeler and product code separated by a hyphen); (i) name of the firm/business entity associated with each NDC labeler code; (j) date of launch for each NDC number; (k) date of discontinuance for each NDC number, if any; and (l) date of the first public announcement of the marketing or intended marketing of the AG.
5. Submit a list of the Company's orally administered prescription AG drug products of any capsule or tablet form that were launched after Jan. 1, 2001, but are not on the FTC=s list of AG drugs (if any), and provide the information requested in Item 4.
6. *Sales of AG drugs, by NDC.* For each AG drug addressed in Items 4 and 5, for sales in the United States from Jan. 1, 2001-March 31, 2007, state the (a) applicable month and year; (b) the drug identifying information described in the second paragraph of Instruction (D); (c) the AG=s 11-digit NDC number (including labeler, product, and package size codes separated by hyphens); (d) package size; (e) package type; total sales to all customers, net of discounts, rebates, promotions, returns and chargebacks, in (f) units (as represented by the NDC=s package size code), and in (g) dollars.
7. *Total sales of AG drugs.* For each AG drug addressed in Items 4 and 5, for sales in the United States from Jan. 1, 2001-March 31, 2007, state the (a) applicable month and year; (b) the drug identifying information described in the second paragraph of Instruction (D); (c) the Company's total sales attributable to all strengths and package sizes of the dosage form under consideration, net of discounts, rebates, promotions, returns and chargebacks, in dollars; and (d) the total sales in prescriptions.
8. *Prices of AG drugs: WAC and AWP.* For each AG drug addressed in Items 4 and 5, for sales the United States from Jan. 1, 2001-March 31, 2007, state the (a) applicable month and year; (b) the drug identifying information described in the second paragraph of Instruction (D); (c) the AG=s 11-digit NDC number (including labeler,

product, and package size codes separated by hyphens); (d) package size; (e) package type; (f) wholesale acquisition cost ("WAC," *see* 42 U.S.C. § 1395w-3a(b)(6)(B)); and (g) the average wholesale price ("AWP").

9. *Prices of AG drugs: AMP.* For each AG drug addressed in Items 4 and 5, for the period from Jan. 1, 2001-March 31, 2007, state the (a) applicable quarter and year; (b) the drug identifying information described in the second paragraph of Instruction (D); (c) the AG=s 9-digit NDC number (including labeler and product codes separated by a hyphen); and (d) the average manufacturer price ("AMP") as defined by, and reported to, the Centers for Medicare and Medicaid Services (CMS).
10. Submit all documents that were prepared by or for any officer(s) or director(s) of the Company and/or, if applicable, the marketing entity, or that are in the files of any current or prior Company (and/or marketing entity) senior vice president (or equivalent position) with product line responsibility (during all or part of the period from Jan. 1, 2002-April 3, 2006) for an AG drug addressed in Items 4 and 5 (or, in the case of unincorporated entities, individuals exercising similar functions), as follows. (a) For each AG drug addressed in Items 4 and 5, submit planning, decisional, or strategy documents prepared from January 1, 2002 to April 3, 2006, including studies, surveys, analyses, and reports (both internal and external), that evaluated, considered, or analyzed (but did not merely refer to) the marketing or possible marketing of an AG or AGs (as a response to current or future generic competition, or for other reasons), including but not limited to whether or not to license or otherwise market a brand-name drug product as an AG drug product; reasons for marketing an AG and/or refraining from marketing an AG; the timing of AG launch relative to a 180-day exclusivity period; the marketing of an AG during 180-day exclusivity; the marketing of an AG in the context of paragraph IV certifications and settlements of litigation; the marketing of AGs upon expiration of patents or marketing exclusivities claiming a brand-name drug product or its use; and the profitability or other benefits of marketing an AG drug. (b) With respect to AGs in general, submit documents as described in (a) of this Item.
11. For the AG drugs addressed in Items 4 and 5: (a) If the Company and the brand-name company entered into an agreement that licensed or otherwise authorized the marketing of the identified drug product as an AG, submit the agreement. (b) Submit copies of any public announcements, e.g., press release(s), of the planned marketing or launch of each AG.
12. Submit planning, decisional, or strategy documents dated Jan. 1, 2006-April 29, 2007 that discuss the effect(s) or possible effect(s) of the enactment of Section 6003 of the Deficit Reduction Act of 2005, P.L. 109-171,[383] on the marketing of AGs after Jan. 1, 2007.

By direction of the Commission.

Deborah Platt Majoras
Chairman

SEAL
Date of Order: December 10, 2007

Appendix A. General Instructions

A. Organization of Responses and Due Dates of Parts

The Company's Special Report must be filed by March 19, 2008.

B. Responses to Questions

The Special Report should be entered into the Excel spreadsheets provided with this Order whenever possible. The FTC has entered the question numbers and the information that must be provided in the header row of each column. To efficiently enter the requested information, companies may wish to electronically "copy and paste" drug identifying or other information that must be entered on more than one row or worksheet. When it is not possible to enter the required answer or information into the applicable worksheet, or no worksheet has been provided, restate the Item and provide the required answer or information. If any question cannot be answered fully, give the information that is available and explain in detail in what respects and why the answer is incomplete.

All responses to Items 1-2 and 4-5 should be submitted to the FTC in both paper and in electronic form (as Excel, Word, or WordPerfect documents) on machine-readable CDs or DVDs.

C. Definitions

The following definitions apply to all Items:

(1) "Active ingredient" means a drug=s nonproprietary established name, including the established names for all active ingredients, as defined at 21 C.F.R. § 299.4 and used in the Orange Book.[384]

(2) "ANDA" means Abbreviated New Drug Application, as set forth in 21 U.S.C. § 355(j).

(3) "ANDA-generic drug" means a drug marketed or sought to be marketed pursuant to an approved ANDA and usually sold under the established name of the active ingredient(s).

(4) "Authorized generic ("AG") drug" means any drug sold, licensed or marketed under an NDA approved by the FDA under 21 U.S.C. § 355(c); and marketed, sold or distributed (directly or indirectly) without using the listed drug's brand-name and with a different NDC product number or labeler number (or both).[385]

(5) "Brand-name" drug means an innovator drug product marketed pursuant to an approved NDA under a proprietary, trademark-protected name.

(6) "Capsule" means all dosage forms of capsules as set forth in Appendix C of the Orange Book, including capsule; capsule, delayed release (DR); capsule, delayed release pellets (DRP); and capsule, extended release (XR).

(7) "Company" means Company A, its domestic and foreign parents, predecessors, divisions, subsidiaries, affiliates, partnerships and joint ventures, and all directors, officers, employees, agents and representatives of the foregoing. The terms "subsidiary", "affiliate" and "joint venture" refer to any person in which there is partial (50 percent or more) or total ownership or control between the company and any other person. As used in this definition, the term "person" includes the company

and means any natural person, corporate entity, partnership, association, joint venture, government entity, or trust.

(8) "Documents" means all computer files and written, recorded, and graphic materials of every kind in the possession, custody or control of the Company.

(9) "ANDA" means a New Drug Application, as set forth in 21 U.S.C. § 355(b) and approved under 21 U.S.C. § 355(c).

(10) "Tablet" means all dosage forms of tablets as set forth in Appendix C of the Orange Book, including tablet; tablet, chewable (C); tablet, coated particles (CP); tablet, delayed release (DR); tablet, delayed release, orally disintegrating (DR OD); tablet, extended release (XR); tablet, orally disintegrating (OD).

D. Data Submissions

Unless modified by agreement in writing with the staff of the Federal Trade Commission, all numerical data submitted in response to Items 6-9 must be submitted in a spreadsheet format both on paper and on machine-readable CDs or DVDs. The Commission will accept database and spreadsheet data in the following formats: MS Excel, MS Access, tab-delimited or fixed width text files. All financial information required to be submitted by this Order should be in whole dollar amounts. For Items 6-9, the applicable month (quarter) and year requested refers to each month and year for which the Company provides the information called for by the given Item. If the information is not kept in the form requested, the Company is encouraged to contact the Commission representative to discuss alternative formats in which the information may be provided.

To identify the drug for which data is being provided in response to Items 6-9, state on the applicable row or page the (b)(1) proprietary/trade name of the AG, if any; (b)(2) proprietary/trade name of the brand-name drug for which the NDA authorizes the marketing of the AG; (b)(3) active ingredient; (b)(4) dosage form; (b)(5) NDA number (5 digits, no letter) of the brand-name drug that authorizes the marketing of the AG; and the (b)(6) dosage strength (except for Item 7). See the Excel spreadsheets provided by the FTC, which should be used to provide this data whenever possible.

E. Document Submissions

This Special Order covers documents in the Company's possession, custody or control, wherever the documents are located. However, unless or until the Commission notifies Company otherwise in writing, the Commission will not seek to enforce the Special Order to compel the production of documents that were located outside the United States at the time Company received the Special Order. In order to expedite the receipt of documents reflecting the views of all recipients of Special Orders, the Commission requests your cooperation in producing any such documents on a voluntary basis by the date specified in this Special Order.

Provide two paper copies of each document. Group the documents by drug product. For each document, indicate the name of the person from whose files the document came and whether the document was generated within the Company or externally; if generated externally, provide the name of the source of the document. All documentary responses should be Bates-stamped.

F. Responsibilities of Company Officials

The Special Report is required to be subscribed and sworn to by an official of the Company who has prepared or supervised the preparation of the Special Report from books, records, documents, correspondence, and other data and material in the Company's possession. Each subscriber to the Special Report is to give his or her full name, title, and contact information in a notarized certification at the end of the Special Report, as set forth in Appendix B.

G. Questions

Any questions you have relating to the scope or meaning of this Order, or suggestions for possible modifications thereto, should be directed to Karen A. Goldman, Federal Trade Commission, Office of General Counsel, 600 Pennsylvania Ave., N.W., Washington, DC 20580, (202) 326-2574, kgoldman@ftc.gov.

H. Submission of Report

The Special Report must be Bates-stamped.

You are advised that penalties may be imposed under applicable provisions of federal law for failure to file Special Reports or for filing false reports.

Two copies of the Special Report required by this Order should be submitted to the attention of Karen A. Goldman, Federal Trade Commission, Room H-503, 600 Pennsylvania Ave., NW, Washington, DC 20580 by 5:00 PM on the dates specified herein.

Instructions for Specific Items

1-3. Self-explanatory.

4. The FTC has provided a list of AG drugs marketed by the Company during the relevant time frame that must be addressed in the Company's Special Report. The list is limited to AGs that were first launched in the United States after Jan. 1, 2001. A blank list will be provided if the FTC is not aware of any AGs. Using the Excel spreadsheet containing this list, enter the information requested in Item 4. Enter the specific dosage form, e.g., capsule DR, capsule XR, tablet DR, or tablet XR. Enter each strength for each dosage form on a different row. When entering the 14-digit GPI, separate the two-digit fields with dashes.

   The response to Item 4(h) should include all of the Company's 9-digit NDC numbers used in the marketing, sale, or distribution of the AG in the United States. However, do not include NDC numbers that cover repackaged or relabeled drug products (such as those for use in institutions) that were previously sold under one of the aforementioned NDCs. If the NDCs associated with the AG have changed, provide all NDC numbers that have been used. If there are multiple NDC numbers for a given strength, each should be entered on a different row.

5. Add to the Excel spreadsheet containing the FTC=s list of AGs any other AGs that fit the specified criteria but were not on FTC=s list. Follow the instructions for Item 4 for entering the requested information on these AGs.

6. Item 6 requests monthly net sales data for AGs for all 11-digit NDCs arising from the 9-digit NDCs provided in response to Item 4(h) and Item 5, i.e., including all package size codes for those NDCs.
7. The responses to Item 7 represents combined sales from all strengths and NDC numbers.
8. Item 8 requests monthly WAC and AWP for all 11-digit NDCs arising from the 9-digit NDCs provided in response to Items 4(h) and 5.
9. Item 9 requests the quarterly AMP (*see* 42 U.S.C. § 1396r-8(k)(1)), for all 9-digit NDCs provided in response to Items 4(h) and 5.
10. When responding to Item 10(b), do not duplicate documents provided in response to Item 10(a).
11. For press releases, the source of the document need not be provided.
12. Self-explanatory.

Appendix B. Certification

This Special Report, together with any and all appendices and attachments thereto, was prepared and assembled under my supervision in accordance with instructions issued by the Federal Trade Commission in its Special Orders for the Authorized Generic Drug Study. Subject to the recognition that, where so indicated, reasonable estimates have been made because books and records do not provide the required information, the information is, to the best of my knowledge, true, correct, and complete. Where copies rather than original documents have been submitted, the copies are true, correct, and complete.

____

Type or Print Name and Title

____

Type or Print Company Name and Address

____

Type or Print Phone Number and E-Mail Address

____

(Signature)

Subscribed and sworn to before me at the City of __________________, *State of* ______________________, *this day of* ____________, *20* ___.

____

(Notary Public)

My Commission Expires: __________________

APPENDIX G. LIST OF AUTHORIZED GENERIC DRUGS IN STUDY

BRAND NAME	ACTIVE INGREDIENT	DOSAGE FORM	NDA#
Accupril	quinapril hydrochloride	tablets	19885
Accuretic	hydrochlorothiazide; quinapril hydrochloride	tablets	20125
Actigall	ursodiol	capsules	19594
Agrylin	anagrelide	capsules	20333
Aldactazide	hydrochlorothiazide; spironolactone	tablets	12616
Aldactone	spironolactone	tablets	12151
Allegra	fexofenadine hydrochloride	tablets	20872
Amaryl	glimepiride	tablets	20496
Ambien	zolpidem tartrate	tablets	19908
Amoxil	amoxicillin	capsules	62216
Amoxil	amoxicillin	tablets	50754
Amoxil	amoxicillin	tablets, chewable	50761
Arava	leflunomide	tablets	20905
Augmentin	amoxicillin; clavulanate potassium	tablets	50564, 50720
Augmentin	amoxicillin; clavulanate potassium	tablets, chewable	50726
Azulfidine Entabs	sulfasalazine	tablets, delayed release	7073
Biaxin	clarithromycin	tablets	50662
Carnitor	levocarnitine	tablets	18948
Ceftin	cefuroxime axetil	tablets	50605
Celexa	citalopram hydrobromide	tablets	20822
Cipro	ciprofloxacin hydrochloride	tablets	19537
Cleocin HCl	clindamycin hydrochloride	capsules	50162
Colazal	balsalazide	capsules	20610
Colestid	colestipol hydrochloride	tablets	20222
Cyclessa	desogestrel; ethinyl estradiol	tablets	21090
Cytotec	misoprostol	tablets	19268
Daypro	oxaprozin	tablets	18841
Declomycin	demeclocycline hydrochloride	tablets	50261
Desogen	desogestrel; ethinyl estradiol	tablets	20071
Diamox	acetazolamide	capsules, extended release	12945
Diflucan	fluconazole	tablets	19949
DITROPAN XL	oxybutynin chloride	tablets, extended release	20897
Dostinex	cabergoline	tablets	20664
Estrostep Fe	ethinyl estradiol; norethindrone acetate	tablets	20130
Flexeril	cyclobenzaprine hydrochloride	tablets	17821
Flumadine	rimantadine hydrochloride	tablets	19649

BRAND NAME	ACTIVE INGREDIENT	DOSAGE FORM	NDA#
Fosamax	alendronate sodium	tablets	20560
Glucophage XR	metformin hydrochloride	tablets, extended release	21202
Glucotrol XL	glipizide	tablets	20329
Glucovance	glyburide; metformin hydrochloride	tablets	21178
Imitrex	sumatriptan	tablets	20132
Inspra	eplerenone	tablets	21437
K-Dur	potassium chloride	tablets, extended release	19439
Lamictal CD	lamotrigine	tablets, chewable	20764
Lamisil	terbinafine hydrochloride	tablets	20539
Limbitrol	amitriptyline hydrochloride; chlordiazepoxide hydrochloride	tablets	16949
Lotensin	benazepril hydrochloride	tablets	19851
Lotensin HCT	benazepril hydrochloride; hydrochlorothiazide	tablets	20033
Lotrel	amlodipine besylate; benazepril hydrochloride	capsules	20364
Macrobid	nitrofurantoin; nitrofuran-toin, macrocrystalline	capsules	20064
Macrodantin	nitrofurantoin, macrocrystalline	capsules	16620
Marinol	dronabinol	capsule	18651
Mestinon	pyridostigmine bromide	tablets	9829
Micro-K	potassium chloride	capsules, extended release	18238
Microzide	hydrochlorothiazide	capsules	20504
Mobic	meloxicam	tablets	20938
Monodox	doxycycline	capsules	50641
Monopril	fosinopril sodium	tablets	19915
MS Contin	morphine sulfate	tablets, extended release	19516
Myambutol	ethambutol hydrochloride	tablets	16320
Neurontin	gabapentin	capsules	20235
Neurontin	gabapentin	tablets	20882
Nolvadex	tamoxifen citrate	tablets	17970
Nor-QD	norethindrone	tablets	17060
Norvasc	amlodipine besylate	tablets	19787
OMNICEF	cefdinir	capsules	50739
Ortho Micronor	norethindrone	tablets	16954
Ortho Tri-Cyclen	ethinyl estradiol; norgestimate	tablets	19697

Appendix G. (Continued)

BRAND NAME	ACTIVE INGREDIENT	DOSAGE FORM	NDA#
Ortho-Cyclen	ethinyl estradiol; norgestimate	tablets	19653
Ortho-Novum 7/7/7	ethinyl estradiol; norethindrone	tablets	18985
Ovcon 35	ethinyl estradiol; norethindrone	tablets	17716
Oxandrin	oxandrolone	tablets	13718
OxyContin	oxycodone	tablets, extended release	20553
Pamine	methscopolamine bromide	tablets	8848
Parlodel	bromocriptine	capsules	17962
Paxil	paroxetine hydrochloride	tablets	20031
Paxil CR	paroxetine hydrochloride	tablets, extended release	20936
Plendil	felodipine	tablets, extended release	19834
Pletal	cilostazol	tablets	20863
Ponstel	mefenamic acid	capsules	15034
Pravachol	pravastatin sodium	tablets	19898
Prilosec	omeprazole	capsules, delayed release	19810
Proscar	finasteride	tablets	20180
Protonix	pantoprazole sodium	tablets, delayed release	20987
Purinethol	mercaptopurine	tablets	9053
Razadyne	galantamine hydrobromide	tablets	21169
Razadyne ER	galantamine hydrobromide	capsule, extended release	21615
Rebetol	ribavirin	capsules	20903
Remeron SolTab	mirtazapine	tablets, orally disintegrating	21208
Restoril	temazepam	capsules	18163
Retrovir	zidovudine	tablets	20518
Risperdal	risperidone	tablets	20272
Ritalin SR	methylphenidate hydrochloride	tablets	18029
Robinul	glycopyrolate	tablets	12827
Salagen Tablets	pilocarpine hydrochloride	tablets	20237
Seasonale	ethinyl estradiol; levonorgestrel	tablets	21544
Sonata	zaleplon	capsules	20859
Sporanox	itraconazole	capsules	20083
Tambocor	flecainide acetate	tablets	18830

BRAND NAME	ACTIVE INGREDIENT	DOSAGE FORM	NDA#
Tiazac	diltiazam hydrochloride	capsules, extended release	20401
Tofranil-PM	imipramine pamoate	capsules	17090
Toprol-XL	metoprolol succinate	tablets, extended release	19962
Tri-Norinyl	ethinyl estradiol; norethindrone	tablets	18977
Ultracet	acetaminophen; tramadol hydrochloride	tablets	21123
Uniretic	hydrochlorothiazide; moexipril hydrochloride	tablets	20729
Unithroid	levothyroxine sodium	tablets	21210
Univasc	moexipril hydrochloride	tablets	20312
Urocit-K	potassium citrate	tablets	19071
Verelan PM	verapamil hydrochloride	capsules, extended release	20943
Wellbutrin SR	bupropion hydrochloride	tablets, extended release	20358
Xanax XR	alprazolam	tablets	21434
Yasmin	drospirenone, ethinyl estradiol	tablets	21098
Zaroxolyn	metolazone	tablets	17386
Zithromax	azithromycin	tablets	50711, 50730, 50784
Zocor	simvastatin	tablets	19766
Zofran	ondansetron hydrochloride	tablets	20103
Zofran ODT	ondansetron hydrochloride	tablets, orally disintegrating	20781
Zoloft	sertraline hydrochloride	tablets	19839
Zyban	bupropion hydrochloride	tablets, extended release	20711

Appendix H. Methods

I. General

A. Definition of Authorized Generic Drug

For purposes of the study, "authorized generic ("AG") drug" means any drug sold, licensed or marketed under a New Drug Application ("NDA") approved by the FDA under 21 U.S.C. § 355(c) and marketed, sold or distributed (directly or indirectly) without using the listed drug's brand-name and with a different National Drug Code ("NDC") product number or labeler number (or both).[386]

Typically, the name of an AG is the nonproprietary established name of its active ingredients,[387] but in some cases a trade name different from the brand-name of the listed drug is used.

B. Timing and Dates

All chronological information is reported by calendar year.

C. Reporting by Drug

In Chapters 2 and 7, data are presented by drug (NDA), rather than by strength; a drug is counted as having only one AG, one first patent challenge, and one entry by 180-day exclusivity even if these conditions occur for multiple strengths. Also, a drug is counted as having an AG if at least one strength had an AG, as having a first patent challenge if one strength had a challenge, and as having entry by 180-day exclusivity if such entry occurs for one strength. In addition, chronological information about AGs, patent challenges, and 180-day exclusivity is generally presented in terms of the timing of the first such event for each drug. For example, Figure 2-1 reports AG launches by the year of the first launch of any strength. Counting by drug is consistent with the perception that decisions about whether to launch an AG or bring a patent challenge are usually made on a drug basis,[388] presumably because the economic incentives for such decisions arise from the overall sales of the drug.

Chronological information on AGs, patent challenges, and exclusivities is also presented by drug. This captures the overall trends in a way that is compatible with company counts and analysis of sales levels by drug. The overall trends observed when reporting by drug are very similar to those obtained by strength.

An exception to reporting by drug is in Figure 4-1 of Chapter 4, which shows the timing of the launch of AGs relative to the launch of bioequivalent ANDA-generic versions of the same brand-name drug. Unlike other timing information in the report that is presented by year, Figure 4-1 considers very small differences in the timing of launch of the AG and the ANDA-generic (in the order of days or weeks), as well as larger differences. Generally, companies launch all strengths of an AG at the same time, but sometimes launch times differ, especially when the launch times of first ANDA-generics of different strengths are different. Thus, to ensure that both small and large differences in launch timing for each strength were observed and appropriately weighted in the results, Figure 4-1 reports launch timing by strength.

D. Dosage Forms Included in the Study

AGs and other drugs included in the study were limited to tablet and capsule dosage forms in Appendix C of the FDA publication, the "Orange Book."[389] This limitation facilitates the economic analysis because certain dosage forms, such as injectables, are sold primarily outside the retail channels included in National Prescription Audit ("NPA") sales data from IMS Health.[390]

E. Inflation Adjustment

All sales were deflated to December 2008 dollars using the monthly producer price index series for finished goods.[391]

II. Identification of AGs, their NDA-holders, and Distributors

A. Sources of Information

We developed a list of AGs that meet the above definition based on information from the following sources. (1) *FDA National Drug Code (NDC) database, cumulative and current (online) Directory.*[392] The NDC database was used because it provides information on two numerical codes that are key aspects of the definition of an AG, the product and labeler numbers. Thus, we searched the FDA's historical NDC database and current online information for NDAs with some NDC numbers for which the tradename was an active ingredient or other name different from that of the brand-name drug, and the "product code" or "labeler code" was different from those of the brand-name drug.[393] NDC information was also used to identify the distributors of AGs when other sources identified the AG but did not provide the name of the distributor. (2) *Companies sent the Special Orders.* Companies were asked to identify AGs marketed pursuant to their NDAs and AGs distributed pursuant to other companies' NDAs. (3) *The FDA's List of Authorized Generic Drugs.*[394] After it became available, we included AGs from the FDA's List of Authorized Generic Drugs. Because the *List* does not include information on the distributor of the AG, and its launch and discontinuance dates are often unknown or approximate, we used other sources for this information. (4) *RED BOOK.*[395] The RED BOOK includes AGs but does not identify them as such; it was used primarily to confirm information from other sources on AGs and their distributors. In addition, since the RED BOOK provides prices of marketed drugs, it was used to confirm that drugs identified on the basis of NDCs or pre-launch information had entered the market. (5) *Internet Information.* AGs were identified from a variety of internet sources, such as press releases, Securities and Exchange Commission (SEC) reports, and pharmacy benefit manager lists of new generic drugs.

B. Time of Launch of AGs Included in the Study

The list included AGs first launched between January 1, 2001 and December 31, 2008. Launch dates were obtained from company submissions, press releases, and other sources. To cover all AGs that launched into markets without established AG sales during that period, the list also included a few AGs that had been marketed during the 1990s, discontinued, and then relaunched between 2001–08 after a period off the market.[396] AGs that were first launched before the study period and re-launched between 2001–08 by a different distributor without a period off the market were not included in the list, unless the change in distributor had competitive implications.[397] The list of AGs in the Illinois Formulary was a primary source regarding AGs launched before the study period.[398]

III. Companies Included in the Study

A. Companies That Received Special Orders

Most companies included in the study[399] were sent Special Orders. Companies received Special Orders if, based on information available at the time the Orders were prepared in 2007, the company (or a predecessor or subsidiary)[400] held an NDA or ANDA, at any time after 2001, for a drug included in the study, or was a licensee regarding an application for such a drug.[401] Companies that held NDAs or ANDAs for drugs included in the study were identified using the Orange Book.[402]

Generally, companies with rights in relevant NDAs were sent Brand-Name (or Authorized Generic) Special Orders, and companies with rights in relevant ANDAs were sent Generic Special Orders.[403] Because some companies had rights in both relevant NDAs and ANDAs, they were sent Special Orders for both brand-name and generic companies.

1. Brand-Name Company Special Orders

Companies received Brand-name Special Orders if they held the NDA for (i) the brand-name version of an AG included in the study or (ii) a brand-name drug that first faced generic competition after January 1, 2001, for which at least one ANDA with a paragraph IV certification was filed; or (iii) a brand-name drug for which at least one ANDA with a paragraph IV certification was filed after January 1, 2001, and generic entry had not yet occurred.

2. Generic Company Special Orders

Companies received Generic Special Orders if they held an ANDA for (i) a bioequivalent generic version of an AG included the study; or (ii) a bioequivalent generic version of a brand-name drug that first faced generic competition after January 1, 2001, for which at least one ANDA with a paragraph IV certification was filed.[404]

3. Authorized Generic Company Orders

Two companies received AG Special Orders because they distributed an AG included in the study, but did not hold any NDA or ANDA described in (1) or (2) above.

4. Licenses and Assignments of NDAs and ANDAs

In addition, some companies that did not hold the relevant NDAs or ANDAs received Special Orders based on apparent licenses regarding the brand-name and generic drugs approved under the FDA applications described above.[405] Licenses were inferred from comparisons of the company name listed for a drug (NDA or ANDA) in the Orange Book, cumulative NDC database, and RED BOOK. For example, a licensee relationship would be inferred when a company listed in the RED BOOK as the manufacturer of a drug differed from the NDA or ANDA-holder listed in the Orange Book (and was there was no successor or subsidiary relationship between the companies).[406] In such cases, the NDC database typically contained NDCs for both companies, with the application holder having the earlier record. Internet sources such as press releases and SEC reports were used to confirm the nature of the relationship and to identify additional licensees.

Companies that appeared to be licensees of the NDAs described above received Brand-name Special Orders; licensees of the ANDAs described above received Generic Special Orders. Inclusion of such licensee companies ensured that companies that sold a brand-name or ANDA-generic drug but did not hold the relevant NDA or ANDA were included in the study.

Orange Book-RED BOOK-NDC database comparisons sometimes led to the identification of earlier application holders when the company presently listed as the NDA or ANDA-holder in the Orange Book had acquired the application by assignment (there was no predecessor or subsidiary relationship between the companies). The assignor often had discontinued NDCs in the cumulative NDC database. Internet sources were used to confirm likely assignments.

B. Companies That Did Not Receive Special Orders

A few companies were included in the study but did not receive Orders because they related to AGs that were identified after the Special Orders were prepared in 2007-8, or because their relationship to AGs identified before the Orders were prepared was learned thereafter.

Methods Related to Chapter 2

IV. Company Information

A. Categorization of Companies as Brand-Name, Generic, or Authorized Generic

Generally, companies were categorized in the text or figures of Chapter 2 as brand-name, generic, or authorized generic companies based on the type of Special Order that they received.

Companies that received both Brand-Name and Generic Special Orders because they held both NDAs and ANDAs may operate primarily as brand-name or generic companies, or have a mixture of both businesses. Thus, Figures 2-2 and 2-3 refer to "NDA-holding" companies rather than brand-name companies, to avoid referring to companies with primarily generic businesses as brand-name companies because they held a few NDAs.

B. Updating of Company Names

The companies identified in figures in Chapter 2, and in Appendix C are companies that were sent Special Orders and other companies that were not sent Orders but were subsequently identified as related to AGs. The company names listed are those of parent and successor pharmaceutical companies relating to AGs or other drugs included in the study. Grouping companies under the largest and most recent organizational unit with a pharmaceutical business focuses the information presented on recent, rather than historical, aspects of the industry.[407]

1. Brand-Name Company Names

(a) *Mergers*. Whether a merger took place before or after AG launch, the predecessor company no longer exists or exists as a subsidiary, so the companies shown in Figures 2-2 through 2-4 are successor/parent companies.[408] In each figure the AGs at issue are included in the counts of any successor/parent pharmaceutical company.

(b) *Assignments of NDAs*. When an NDA was assigned to another company, the AG is included in the count of the NDA-holder at the time of launch (or its successor or parent) in Figures 2-2 through 2-4. Thus, when an NDA was transferred before launch, the AG is included in the count of the assignee;[409] for transfers after launch, AGs are included in the count of the assignor.

2. Generic Company Names

Generally, the naming conventions discussed above for brand-name companies also apply to generic companies shown in Figures 2-5 and 2-6; AG, contract, settlement agreement, and exclusivity counts were attributed to successor/parent pharmaceutical companies. In Figure 2-5, counts were attributed to assignees for agreements assigned before AG launch, and to assignors when transferred after launch. However, because multiple generics (ANDAs and AGs) can compete in regard to one drug, attribution of counts to a single successor/parent company can sometimes obscure differences in generic practices relating to AGs and paragraph IV certifications. Accordingly, counts for two large generic companies that were independent for most of the study period, Ivax and Andrx, were presented separately from those of the two companies that acquired them (respectively, Teva and Watson).[410]

C. Licensees of NDAs

Companies that distributed brand-name drugs pursuant to licenses with holders of NDAs relating to AGs are not shown in Figures 2-2 and 2-4; the AG is attributed to the holder of the relevant NDA even when the brand was sold by another company. Figure 2-3, however, about in-house distribution of AGs, includes such licensees (rather than the NDA-holder, to avoid double-counting) when the licensee distributed the brand and its generic subsidiary distributed the AG.[411]

D. Counts of 180-Day Exclusivities by Company

The number of exclusivities held by the seven companies in Figure 2-6 (59) is high relative to the total number of exclusivities for all companies shown in Figure 2-7 (66) because the latter figure reports only one exclusivity per drug, but multiple companies may hold exclusivities for a given drug, as a result of shared exclusivity on the same strength, or different companies holding exclusivities on different strengths.[412]

V. Chronological Trends in Authorized Generic Drugs

A. AGs' Relationship to 180-Day Exclusivity Periods

Information on 180-day exclusivity periods was obtained from historic Orange Book records, the FDA's letters approving relevant ANDA-generic drugs, company information, and other sources. Information on whether an exclusivity period lacked an AG because a settlement agreement prohibited its marketing was obtained from agreements submitted by companies pursuant to the Special Orders or filed with the FTC pursuant to the Medicare Prescription Drug, Improvement, and Modernization Act of 2003 ("MMA").[413]

1. Determination by Drug

The relationship between exclusivity periods and AGs was analyzed by drug. For Figure 2-7, a drug (NDA) was counted as having generic entry by exclusivity if a generic had exclusivity for any strength, and as having an AG during exclusivity if an AG was marketed at any time during an exclusivity period for any strength of the drug. Similarly, for Figure 2-8, an AG was counted as having been marketed during exclusivity if at any time it was marketed during an exclusivity period for any strength of a drug.

2. Time of 180-Day Exclusivity and AG Launch

Analysis of trends in the relationship between 180-day exclusivities and AGs involves reporting the dates of two distinct events – the onset of exclusivity and the launch of an AG. The choice of which date to use in graphing the results depends on which condition – exclusivity or AG – is present in all the results being presented. Figure 2-7, which analyzes the competitive conditions of exclusivity periods, reports on exclusivity periods with and without AGs. Accordingly, it reports trends in the competitive conditions of exclusivity periods according to the year an exclusivity began, which is usually, but not always, the year of any AG launch. For exclusivities with AGs, the year the exclusivity began is that of the first exclusivity strength with an AG;[414] for exclusivities without AGs, it is that of the first exclusivity. The start date of exclusivity was calculated as 180 days before the end date listed in the Orange Book.[415]

By contrast, Figure 2-8 examines the relative abundance of AGs marketed during exclusivity and apart from exclusivity. It includes AGs launched after the conclusion of exclusivity and AGs for drugs for which there was no exclusivity period.[416] Because Figure 2-8 reports information about AGs regardless of whether there was exclusivity, it provides the information according to the year of AG launch. For AGs marketed apart from exclusivity, the date is that of the first launch of any strength; for AGs marketed during exclusivity, the date is that of the first launch of any strength marketed during exclusivity.[417]

Accordingly, yearly counts of exclusivities with AGs in Figure 2-7 and AGs marketed during exclusivity in Figure 2-8 may differ slightly because the former is reported on the basis of the date of exclusivity, and the latter on the basis of the date of AG launch.

3. AG Entry by Pre-Entry Brand Sales

Figure 2-9 depicts the propensity of AG introductions for drugs with various levels of pre-entry brand sales,[418] measured as the annualized expenditures on the brand drug in the three months prior to first generic entry, broken down by whether first generic entry was by 180-day exclusivity or not. A drug is classified as having an AG if an AG was introduced for any strength of the drug. Similarly, if a first-filer on any strength received an exclusivity period, the drug is classified as having had an exclusivity period.

In order to be able to calculate the pre-generic entry brand sales based on the three months prior to generic entry, it was necessary to only consider drugs with first generic entry starting in the fourth month after the first date for which sales data was available. Consequently, this graph is based on data for drugs with first generic entry starting in April of 2003, unlike other tabulations in this chapter that do not require the pre-entry sales, and can thus start earlier.

B. AG Launch by Highest Patent Certification in ANDAs

To determine the highest patent certification in ANDAs for each drug for which an AG was marketed, we used the FDA's application database to identify all ANDAs filed with respect to the NDA under which the AG is approved.[419] This information was graphed according to the year the AG was launched (2001–2008), not the year of certification, which generally would have been much earlier.

Methods Related to Chapter 7

VI. Trends in ANDA Filings and Patent Certifications

To analyze trends in ANDA filings (Figures 7-1 and 7-2), we obtained information on ANDAs from the FDA's application database, the Center-wide Oracle-based Management Information System (COMIS).[420] Unlike other analyses in Chapters 2 and 7, the analysis of trends in ANDA filings from 2000–2007 included ANDAs for drugs that were not otherwise included in the study, including dosage forms that are not capsules or tablets. Thus, for Figure 7-1 we determined the numbers of ANDAs filed per year based on the filing ("clock") dates of all dosage forms of ANDAs filed during that period.

We also used the FDA's application database to examine trends in PIII and PIV patent certifications from 2000–2007 (Figure 7-2). Although a patent certification must be made with respect to every patent listed in the Orange Book, the application database lists only the highest certification made. Thus, if an ANDA contains a Paragraph IV certification for any patent, the database shows a Paragraph IV certification even if the applicant also made Paragraph II (the patent is expired) or Paragraph III certifications for other patents.

VII. Drugs Subject to a First Patent Challenge

To examine trends in drugs subject to a first patent challenge (Figure 7-3), the dates of the first patent challenge for a given drug (i.e., for a particular dosage form and NDA) were determined for all tablet and capsule forms of drugs for which the first challenge occurred from 2003 through 2008. We used the FDA's Paragraph IV Patent Certifications website[421] for challenges from March 2, 2004, through the end of 2008 and the FDA's application database for those between January 1, 2003, and March 2, 2004.[422] When using the FDA's application database, which lacked certification dates, we estimated the date of the first PIV certification by assuming that the date of filing was the same as the date of certification, unless the FDA's Paragraph IV website showed a later certification date. Thus, we identified all drugs for which the first ANDA with a PIV certification was filed between January 1, 2003, and March 2, 2004, and excluded the three drugs for which the FDA's Paragraph IV Patent Certifications website showed a later date for the first PIV certification.

Similar to other analyses, the dates of first patent challenge are presented by drug (NDA), rather than by strength. This is consistent with the observation that in most cases, the same patents are listed for each strength of a drug, and most ANDAs include all strengths of a drug. When the first PIV certifications for different strengths were made on different dates, as occasionally occurs, the earliest date was used. The use of a single PIV certification date for a drug simplifies the determination of the sales level of a drug at the time of patent challenge, by ensuring that the sales of a single year are used.[423]

VIII. Drugs Subject to a First Paragraph III Certification

To evaluate the extent to which generic companies chose to make PIII rather than PIV certifications and wait until patent expiration to enter the market, we examined trends in "first PIII certifications" for drugs for which the first PIII was between 2003 and 2007 (Table 7-3). We define "first PIII" drugs as those for which the highest certification in all ANDAs was a PIII. Thus, if an ANDA with a first PIII is amended to include a PIV certification, or if a prior or subsequent ANDA for the same drug includes a PIV certification, the drug is categorized as a first PIV rather than a first PIII. In essence, the first PIII and first PIV drugs represent the population of patent-protected drugs that generic companies viewed as available for patent challenge.[424]

The year of the "first PIII certification" for a given drug (i.e., for a particular dosage form and NDA) was estimated from ANDA filing dates in the FDA's application database.[425] Using the database, we identified all ANDAs filed from 2003–2007 for which the highest certification was a PIII certification. Based on the established name, dosage form, and strengths, we determined the reference-listed drug for each ANDA, and excluded those for which the drug was listed on the FDA's Paragraph IV Patent Certification website as of February 7, 2011. We excluded from the remaining ANDAs those for drugs for which an earlier-filed ANDA made a PIII certification, and thus determined, for each brand-name drug not subject to a PIV certification, the year of filing of the first ANDA with a PIII certification.

IX. Sales Levels of Drugs Subject to a First Paragraph III or IV Certification

To assess the financial incentives underlying decisions to attempt to enter the market before patent expiration by making a PIV certification, or to make a PIII certification and wait to enter after patent expiration (Tables 7-1, 7-2, 7-4; Figure 7-4), we determined the sales level of brand-name drugs subject to first PIII or PIV certifications. The sales level used was that of the year of the first PIII or PIV certification, according to IMS Health NPA data.

For ten drugs for which the first PIV certification was in the same year as NDA approval, with less than a full year's sales for that year, we annualized the sales based on sales from NDA approval to the end of the year.[426] Annualization based on the first year's sales is consistent with the limited sales data that must have been available to the generic companies at the time of PIV certification, as well as the analysis of drugs for which a full year of sales was available for the year of the first PIV certification. No first PIII certifications occurred in the same year as NDA approval, so annualization was not necessary for first PIII drugs.

X. New Chemical Entities–Shared Exclusivity

Drugs with New Chemical Entity ("NCE") exclusivity[427] were used to examine the frequency of patent challenges under circumstances likely to result in shared 180-day exclusivity (Figure 7-5, Table 7-5).

A. Percentage of NCEs that Received a First-Day PIV Certification

To ensure that each NCE analyzed was approved a full 4 years (or 4.5 years, for those with pediatric exclusivity) before the first day an ANDA with a PIV could be filed, only the first-approved NDA for each NCE was included in the analysis.[428] Accordingly, each NCE analyzed was at the same stage in its life cycle with respect to sales, public awareness, and other factors that could affect a decision to challenge a patent.

For the first-approved NDA for each NCE approved from 1998–2004, we determined the first date on which an ANDA with a paragraph IV certification could be filed, including any pediatric exclusivity, and the date of the first PIV certification, if any, as described *supra* in Section VII.[429] Using the cumulative Orange Book database, we excluded from the analysis NDAs that were not available for patent challenge or for which a patent challenge would not advance entry, including those that lacked listed patents on the first day on which a patent could be challenged, or lacked patent protection after the expiration of regulatory exclusivity (e.g., after the expiration of NCE exclusivity or Orphan Drug Exclusivity). The remaining NCEs were used to determine the number and percentage for which an ANDA with a paragraph IV certification had been filed on the first possible day (Figure 7-5).

B. Number of ANDAs Filed on the First Possible Day

We used information from the FDA's application databases to determine the number of ANDAs filed on the first possible day.[430] Only NCEs with first-day ANDAs were included in calculations of the mean number of first-day ANDAs per NCE (Table 7-5), so that the results reflect the likely number of competitors during any 180-day exclusivity with respect to NCEs that received a first-day patent challenge. Similarly, although companies occasionally submitted multiple first-day ANDAs for the same drug (e.g., for different strengths), we counted only one ANDA per company to ensure that the count reflects the likely number of competitors during 180-day exclusivity. However, because the FDA may not deem all such filings as "substantially complete" or approvable, or a company may withdraw an application or decide not to market an approved ANDA product (e.g., because of a merger of two filers), these numbers should be considered only estimates of the number of companies that will compete during exclusivity.

APPENDIX I. TECHNICAL DATA APPENDIX

This appendix describes the sources of data used in the analysis of Chapters 3 and 6 and details the criteria used to construct the data sample. Additionally, it summarizes characteristics of the sample, and discusses how the analysis was tailored to account for some of these characteristics.

I. Data Sources

The data for this Report were acquired from several sources. The retail and wholesale price, expenditure, and quantity data were licensed from IMS Health, Inc. Authorized generic products and their distributors were identified based on information produced by pharmaceutical companies pursuant to the Commission's information requests ("Special Orders"), press releases, and information provided by the FDA.[431] The following sections describe, in detail, the data obtained from each of these sources and how they have been combined for use in the Report.

A. IMS Health Inc.

The FTC purchased a license from IMS Health for information representing nationally aggregated, monthly sales information for each non-injectable prescription medication distributed in the United States over the period from January 2003 through December 2008. This information included: (1) the National Sales Perspective (NSP) Survey, which represents wholesale level quantity and dollar sales[432] information for products purchased by retail and non-retail pharmacies; and (2) the National Prescription Audit (NPA) Survey, which represents retail quantity and dollar sales information for prescriptions dispensed primarily at retail pharmacies. All sales information in both sets of data is reported in nationally aggregated form within channels, and for the analysis presented here, the data have been aggregated across channels.

In addition to monthly sales information, both surveys provided detailed information about each product. This information included the 11-digit National Drug Code (NDC), strength, dosage form, therapeutic class, manufacturer and name of the active ingredient(s) in a single dose. IMS also provided the date the product was first recorded as having sales (dates as early as 1950 are reported), whether the medication was sold over-the-counter or as a prescription, and whether the manufacturer of the product is a generic or a brand-name manufacturer.[433] Taken together, the data provide information on each product at the 11-digit NDC level of specificity, broken down by pharmacy channel. A product is defined in the analysis as an active ingredient(s)-dosage form-strength-therapeutic class-manufacturer combination.[434]

The sample of products analyzed was limited to tablet and capsule dosage forms of prescription products that first faced generic competition during the period 4/2003–12/2008.[435] All products that are not oral solids, including syrups, ointments, and liquids of any kind, were excluded. Over-the-counter medications and vitamins were also excluded because they often are sold in channels that IMS does not survey. All decongestants were excluded because the set of active ingredients included in decongestant combinations was very large and often changed over time, making it difficult to track a product from year to year. In addition, products that represented outliers based on extreme values in both the quantity and revenue data have been excluded.[436] Tables at the end of this appendix list the set of products included in the sample (Table I-3), the dosage form mapping used (Table I-4), the list of suppliers counted as repackagers (Table I-5), and the lists of decongestant (Table I-6) and vitamin (Table I-7) therapeutic classes excluded.

Products were defined as beginning to face generic competition during the period on the basis of the manufacturer, brand status, and sales information provided by IMS. The manufacturer and brand status information were used to classify each product into one of two types: brand and generic. A product was treated as facing generic competition if at least one generic manufacturer (including the AG distributor) of the product had positive sales prior to the end of the sample. The product was treated as having begun to face generic competition during the sample period if it faced generic competition during the period and all generic manufacturers had zero sales prior to April 2003. The date of generic entry was defined as the first date on which a manufacturer other than the brand was observed with positive sales.[437] Exclusivity periods were limited to no more than 6 months time, and the non-exclusivity period was limited to the first three years after generic entry.[438]

Company and FDA information were used to classify generic products as either ANDA-generics or authorized generics. The number of generic manufacturers producing each product was defined as the count of manufacturers observed with positive sales during the month. The indicator of whether the molecule faced an AG competitor was similarly defined by whether the AG manufacturer had positive sales during the month. The manufacturer count included the AG manufacturer but excluded firms that were determined likely to be repackagers.[439] Repackagers purchase supplies from manufacturers and distribute them in some alternate form of packaging, such as blister packs.[440]

B. FDA and Company Data

Sales information from IMS was supplemented with data collected from the FDA and the product manufacturers. These sources were used to identify whether a firm issued an authorized generic and the name of the AG marketer when applicable. They were also used to determine details about relevant Hatch-Waxman related legal actions associated with each product, including whether the product faced a Paragraph IV challenge and the end date of exclusivity periods associated with Paragraph IV challenges.

AGs were identified using information produced by pharmaceutical companies pursuant to the Special Orders and information provided by the FDA.[441] The Special Orders requested the proprietary/trade name of the AG, the proprietary name of the brand-name drug for which the NDA authorizes the marketing of the AG, the active ingredient, the dosage form, the NDA number of the brand-name drug that authorizes the marketing of the AG, and the strength of the AG. This information was collected from both the generic and brand-name manufacturers. In addition, brand-name manufacturers were requested to provide the name of the entity associated with each NDC labeler code, enabling identification of the AG distributor.

The most relevant Hatch-Waxman related information was whether the product faced a Paragraph IV patent challenge and whether a generic manufacturer was granted exclusivity related to a Paragraph IV challenge. A list of drugs facing Paragraph IV challenges was downloaded from the FDA website.[442] For each drug associated with a 180-day exclusivity period, the date that generic exclusivity ended was determined from information provided by the FDA. A month was treated as part of the exclusivity period if the 28th day of the month occurred prior to the exclusivity end date.[443]

This information was supplemented with settlement data from the company responses to the Special Orders. The Special Orders requested all firms to identify whether the marketing of an AG occurred pursuant to a litigation settlement agreement. The Special Orders asked brand-name firms whether the firm had entered a litigation settlement agreement not to market the AG or to delay doing so. Settlement information received from the Special Orders was confirmed and verified using information collected by the FTC pursuant to the Medicare Modernization Act. The data were coded to distinguish whether the settlement licensed the AG distribution rights to the litigant, or whether the terms of the settlement restricted the distribution of an AG.

C. Bureau of Labor Statistics

All dollar values for expenditures and prices were normalized to be in December 2008 dollars using the monthly Producer Price Index (PPI) for finished goods (WPSSOP3000) over the period of our data (January 2003 through December 2008). These data were obtained from the Bureau of Labor Statistics.[444]

II. Properties of the Data

As detailed above, this Report considers a very wide range of drugs, from pain killers to anti-cholesterol drugs to antibiotics. The benefit of this approach is that the analysis can be informed by a large sample size. A potential danger is that the analysis could produce misleading results by comparing apples to oranges. This section describes the heterogeneity observed in the sample and the steps that were taken to tailor the analysis accordingly.

A. Sample Characteristics

Table I-1 presents product-level information describing the variables used to construct the regression samples. More than 60% of the products in the sample face a Paragraph IV certification. However, less than 40% of all products, and 63% of products facing a Paragraph IV certification, were observed with an exclusivity period. AGs were observed for roughly half of the products in the sample, with half distributed through a licensee and half through a subsidiary of the brand-name firm.

Settlements between brand-name and ANDA-generic firms can be important determinants of whether an AG is observed for a product. Table I-1 reports that 14% of products in the sample are involved in a settlement involving an AG. Nearly two-thirds of these settlements named the litigant as the AG distributor, whereas the rest restricted the ability of the brand to issue an AG.

B. Heterogeneity of Products Based on Market Size

The regression analyses in Chapters 3 and 6 often include product-characteristic controls in an attempt to control for the non-random determinants of the competitive environment, such as the presence of an AG. The importance of controlling for the determinants of the competitive environment can be seen in Figure I-1, which plots the pre-entry retail sales of the brand-name product against the relative frequencies of Paragraph IV challenges, AG entry, and the maximum number of generic competitors observed for that product in any month in our sample.

This figure shows that all three of these competition measures are generally increasing in pre-entry retail dollar sales. The horizontal axis measures retail sales of the brand-name product just prior to generic entry, grouped in deciles. So, for example, the first point on the Paragraph IV line shows that about 20% of the smallest 10% of products faced Paragraph IV challenges. The frequency of Paragraph IV challenges increases as the pre-entry brand sales grow (moving to the right on the graph), with over 90% of the largest 10% of products getting challenged. The presence of AG competitors follows a similar pattern. Less than ten percent of products in the lowest sales deciles have an AG competitor, but nearly 90% of the products in the highest sales decile have an AG competitor. The third statistic counts the maximum number of manufacturers observed for each product (measured on the vertical axis to the right) over the entire sample. Figure I-1 shows that products with larger pre-entry brand sales tend to attract more generic competitors. The average number of generic competitors in the lowest sales deciles is slightly more than three per product, but products in the highest sales decile have an average of over nine generic competitors per product by the end of the sample period.

Table I-1. Hatch-Waxman Act and Authorized Generic Statistics

Variable	Obs.	Mean
Hatch-Waxman and Authorized Generic Information		
Paragraph IV	312	0.625
Exclusivity	312	0.394
Authorized Generic	312	0.535
AG is Distributed by a Licensee	312	0.272
AG is Distributed by a Subsidiary	312	0.263
Settlements Involving an AG		
Settlements Involving an AG	312	0.138
Litigant Named the AG Distributor	312	0.087
Settlement Terms Require no AG	312	0.051

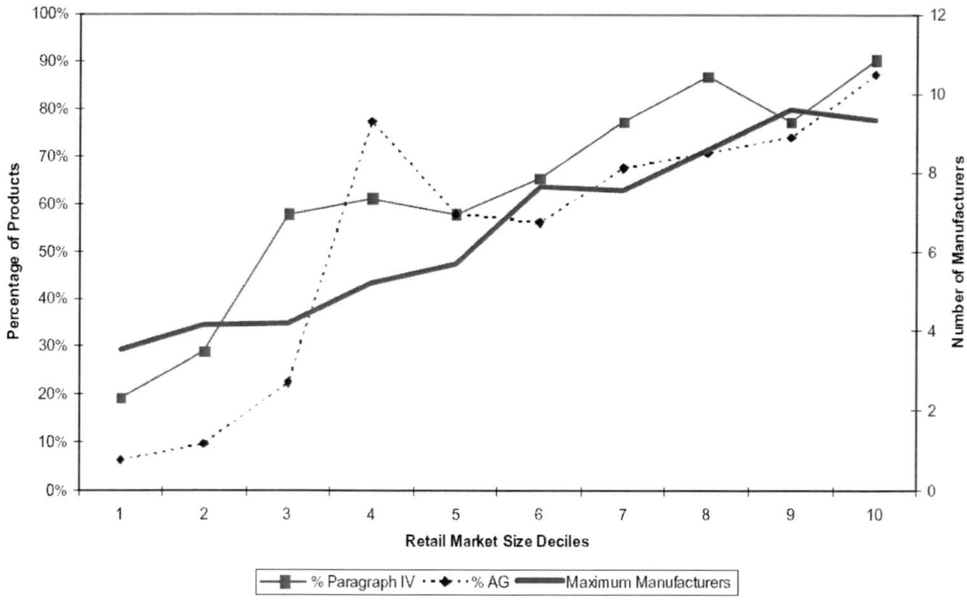

Figure I-1. The Influence of Market Size.

Figure I-1 demonstrates that products facing competition from an AG are potentially different from other types of drugs with respect to the size of the market, and thus, potentially, the attractiveness of generic entry. As noted in Chapter 3, the regression analysis includes product characteristic controls to help control for these influences. The product characteristics used include the dosage form of the product, therapeutic class indicator variables, and the month since generic entry began. Table I-2 presents the relative frequencies of dosage forms and therapeutic class characteristics observed in the sample. The vast majority of products are immediate release tablets (67.9%) or capsules (11.5%). However, extended-release tablets and capsules represent a non-trivial fraction of the sample, accounting together for nearly 15% of products.

C. Controlling for Product Heterogeneity with Product Characteristic Effects

The therapeutic class indicators utilized in the analysis were provided by the data vendor, IMS Health. The classes were used to group products treating similar conditions together.[445] The regression analysis uses therapeutic class indicators to help control for potentially unobserved differences, between products with and without AGs, that are constant across the condition treated. The drugs in the sample are classified into 31 different therapeutic classes. Of these 31 therapeutic classes, 15 contain drugs that are observed with an exclusivity period. Over half of the products in the sample belong to the three largest classes, Vascular Agents, Psychotherapeutics, and Neurological Disorders. In contrast, each of the 12 smallest classes includes less than 1% of the products.

Although a therapeutic class may contain a small fraction of the products in the sample, it could represent a large fraction of dollars sold.[446] For example, the contraceptives therapeutic class includes among the fewest products of all therapeutic classes in the sample, but in terms of dollars sold, contraceptives are among the largest therapeutic classes. The size of the class, as measured in terms of dollars sold, is an important determinant of the competitive environment. This relationship can be seen in Figure I-2 which plots a market-size metric,[447] the proportion of products observed with an AG, and the proportion of products facing a Paragraph IV challenge for the therapeutic classes observed in the sample of 312 products. The figure sorts the therapeutic classes by the proportion of Paragraph IV challenges, showing those with the smallest fraction of Paragraph IV challenges on the left and those with the highest fraction of Paragraph IV challenges on the right.

Table I-2. Product Characteristics Summary Statistics

Variable	Obs.	Mean	Std. Dev.
Dosage Form			
Tablet	312	0.679	0.467
Capsule	312	0.115	0.320
Chewable	312	0.006	0.080
Orally Disintegrating	312	0.038	0.193
Extended Release Capsule	312	0.035	0.185
Extended Release Tablet	312	0.112	0.316
Sustained-Release Tablet	312	0.013	0.113
Therapeutic Class			
Allergy/Cold Preps*	312	0.013	0.113
Amebacide/Antibacterial Agent	312	0.006	0.080
Analgesics*	312	0.035	0.185
Anti-arthritics	312	0.013	0.113
Anti-Fungal Agents*	312	0.019	0.138
Anti-hyperlipidemic Agent*	312	0.032	0.176
Anti-Infectives Systemic*	312	0.074	0.262
Anti-nauseant*	312	0.016	0.126
Antineoplastic Agents	312	0.003	0.057

Table I-2. (Continued)

Variable	Obs.	Mean	Std. Dev.
Therapeutic Class			
Anti-Obesity	312	0.003	0.057
Anti-viral*	312	0.035	0.185
Cardiac Agents	312	0.010	0.098
Contraceptives	312	0.003	0.057
Dermatologicals	312	0.003	0.057
Diabetes Therapy*	312	0.054	0.227
Diuretics & Aquaretics	312	0.010	0.098
Gastrointestinal*	312	0.022	0.148
Genitourinary*	312	0.019	0.138
Hemostatic Modifiers	312	0.013	0.113
Hormones*	312	0.026	0.158
Miscellaneous Preps	312	0.003	0.057
Musculoskeletal*	312	0.035	0.185
Neurological Disorders*	312	0.131	0.338
Ophthalmic Preparations	312	0.003	0.057
Parasympathetics	312	0.003	0.057
Psychotherapeutics*	312	0.163	0.370
Sedatives & Hypnotics	312	0.022	0.148
Smoking Deterrents	312	0.003	0.057
Thyroid Therapy	312	0.013	0.113
Tuberculosis Therapy	312	0.003	0.057
Vascular Agents*	312	0.208	0.407

*At least one drug in the therapeutic class is observed during exclusivity.

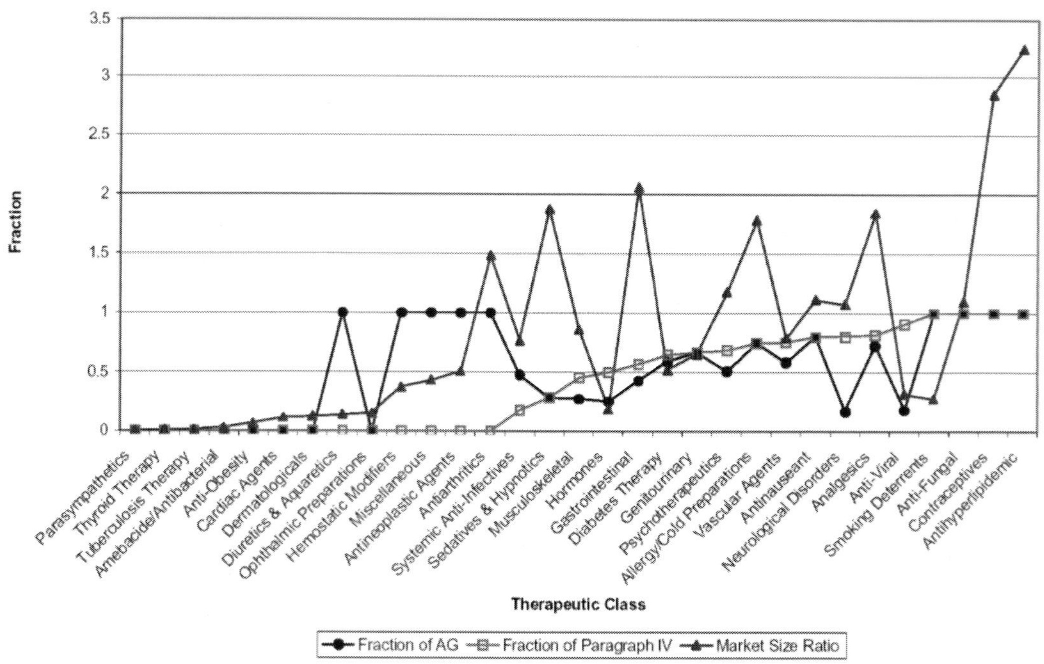

Figure I-2. Therapeutic Class, Hatch-Waxman Act and Authorized Generics.

Figure I-2 suggests that the therapeutic class indicators help to explain much of the relationship between Paragraph IV challenges, AG competition and market size. The therapeutic classes with very few Paragraph IV challenges, such as the Parasympathetics, located on the left of the graph, are small products in terms of pre-entry sales. These small products are also unlikely to be observed with AG competition. In contrast, the therapeutic categories with a high percentage of products facing Paragraph IV challenges, located on the far right of the graph, are typically very large products in terms of pre-entry sales. These categories always face Paragraph IV challenges, are very likely to face AG competition, and include some of the largest products in the sample. However, the therapeutic classes in the middle of the graph can fall anywhere in the distribution of pre-entry sales. In this way, the therapeutic classes appear to be able to control for conditions that explain Paragraph IV entry and AG competition that are not entirely explained by market size.[448]

III. Detailed Lists Describing the Sample

Table I-3. Products Used in the Analysis by Therapeutic Class

Allergy/Cold Preps
Cetirizine, 10mg Tablet
Fexofenadine, 180mg, 30mg, 60mg Tablets
Amebacide/Antibacterial Agent
Metronidazole, 375mg Capsule
Metronidazole, 750mg Extended-Release Tablet
Analgesics
Acetaminophen/Propoxyphene, 100-500mg Tablet
Acetaminophen/Tramadol, 37.5-325mg Tablet
Hydrocodone/Ibuprofen, 7.5-200mg Tablet
Ibuprofen/Oxycodone, 5-400mg Tablet
Oxycodone, 10mg, 20mg, 40mg, 80mg Extended-Release Tablets
Sumatriptan, 100mg, 25mg, 50mg Tablets
Antiarthritics
Leflunomide, 10mg, 20mg Tablets
Meloxicam, 15mg, 7.5mg Tablets
Anti-Fungal Agents
Fluconazole, 100mg, 150mg, 200mg, 50mg Tablets
Itraconazole, 100mg Capsule
Terbinafine, 250mg Tablet
Antihyperlipidemic Agent
Colestipol, 1000mg Tablet
Pravastatin, 10mg, 20mg, 40mg, 80mg Tablets
Simvastatin, 10mg, 20mg, 40mg, 5mg, 80mg Tablets
Anti-Infectives Systemic
Amoxicillin/Clavulanic Acid, 250-125mg Tablet
Azithromycin, 250mg, 500mg, 600mg Tablets
Cefdinir, 300mg Capsule
Cefpodoxime Proxetil, 100mg, 200mg Tablets

Table I-3. (Continued)

Anti-Infectives Systemic
Cefprozil, 250mg, 500mg Tablets
Ciprofloxacin, 1000mg, 500mg Extended-Release Tablets
Ciprofloxacin, 100mg, 250mg, 500mg, 750mg Tablets
Clarithromycin, 500mg Extended-Release Tablet
Clarithromycin, 250mg, 500mg Tablets
Demeclocycline, 150mg, 300mg Tablets
Ofloxacin, 200mg, 300mg, 400mg Tablets
Antinauseant
Granisetron, 1mg Tablet
Ondansetron, 4mg, 8mg Orally Disintegrating/Ecteric Coateds
Ondansetron, 4mg, 8mg Tablets
Antineoplastic Agents
Mercaptopurine, 50mg Tablet
Anti-Obesity
Benzphetamine, 50mg Tablet
Antiviral
Didanosine, 200mg, 250mg, 400mg Extended-Release Capsules
Famciclovir, 125mg, 250mg, 500mg Tablets
Ganciclovir, 250mg, 500mg Capsules
Ribavirin, 200mg Capsule
Zidovudine, 100mg Capsule
Zidovudine, 300mg Tablet
Cardiac Agents
Midodrine, 10mg, 2.5mg, 5mg Tablets
Contraceptives
Drospirenone/Ethinylestradiol, 3-0.03mg Tablet
Dermatologicals
Tretinoin, 10mg Capsule
Diabetes Therapy
Acarbose, 100mg, 25mg, 50mg Tablets
Glimepiride, 1mg, 2mg, 4mg Tablets
Glipizide, 10mg, 2.5mg, 5mg Extended-Release Tablets
Glipizide/Metformin, 2.5-250mg, 2.5-500mg, 5-500mg Tablets
Glyburide/Metformin, 1.25-250mg, 2.5-500mg, 5-500mg Tablets
Metformin, 500mg, 750mg Extended-Release Tablets
Diuretics and Aquaretics
Metolazone, 10mg, 2.5mg, 5mg Tablets
Gastrointestinal
Balsalazide, 750mg Capsule
Glycopyrrolate, 1mg, 2mg Tablets
Omeprazole, 10mg, 40mg Extended-Release Capsules
Pantoprazole, 20mg, 40mg Orally Disintegrating/Ecteric Coateds

Genitourinary
Butabarbital/Hyoscyamine/Phenazopyridine, 150-0.3-15mg Tablet
Finasteride, 5mg Tablet
Flavoxate, 100mg Tablet
Oxybutynin, 10mg, 15mg, 5mg Extended-Release Tablets
Hemostatic Modifiers
Anagrelide, 0.5mg, 1mg Capsules
Cilostazol, 100mg, 50mg Tablets
Hormones
Desmopressin, 0.1mg, 0.2mg Tablets
Estrogenic Sub,Conjugated, 0.45mg Tablet
Hydrocortisone, 5mg Tablet
Methylprednisolone, 16mg, 32mg Tablets
Oxandrolone, 10mg, 2.5mg Tablets
Miscellaneous Preps
Cabergoline, 0.5mg Tablet
Musculoskeletal
Alendronate, 10mg, 35mg, 40mg, 5mg, 70mg Tablets
Cyclobenzaprine, 5mg Tablet
Dantrolene, 100mg, 25mg, 50mg Capsules
Etidronic Acid, 200mg, 400mg Tablets
Neurological Disorder
Clonazepam, 0.125mg, 0.25mg, 0.5mg, 1mg, 2mg Orally Disintegrating/Ecteric Coateds
Divalproex, 125mg, 250mg, 500mg Tablets
Gabapentin, 100mg, 300mg, 400mg Capsules
Gabapentin, 600mg, 800mg Tablets
Galantamine, 16mg, 24mg, 8mg Extended-Release Capsules
Galantamine, 12mg, 4mg, 8mg Tablets
Lamotrigine, 25mg, 5mg Chewables
Lamotrigine, 100mg, 150mg, 200mg, 25mg Tablets
Levetiracetam, 250mg, 500mg, 750mg Tablets
Oxcarbazepine, 150mg, 300mg, 600mg Tablets
Ropinirole, 0.25mg, 0.5mg, 1mg, 2mg, 3mg, 4mg, 5mg Tablets
Zonisamide, 100mg, 25mg, 50mg Capsules
Ophthalmic Preparations
Acetazolamide, 500mg Extended-Release Capsule
Parasympathetics
Bethanechol, 5mg Tablet
Psychotherapeutics
Alprazolam, 0.5mg, 1mg, 2mg, 3mg Extended-Release Tablets
Bupropion, 300mg Extended-Release Tablet
Bupropion, 100mg, 150mg, 200mg Sustained-release Tablets
Citalopram, 10mg, 20mg, 40mg Tablets
Dexmethylphenidate, 10mg, 2.5mg, 5mg Tablets
Lithium, 300mg Extended-Release Tablet
Methamphetamine, 5mg Tablet
Mirtazapine, 15mg, 30mg, 45mg Orally Disintegrating/Ecteric Coateds

Table I-3. (Continued)

Psychotherapeutics
Mirtazapine, 45mg Tablet
Nefazodone, 100mg, 150mg, 200mg, 250mg, 50mg Tablets
Paroxetine, 12.5mg, 25mg, 37.5mg Extended-Release Tablets
Paroxetine, 10mg, 20mg, 30mg, 40mg Tablets
Protriptyline, 10mg, 5mg Tablets
Risperidone, 0.25mg, 0.5mg, 1mg, 2mg, 3mg, 4mg Tablets
Sertraline, 100mg, 25mg, 50mg Tablets
Tranylcypromine, 10mg Tablet
Trimipramine, 25mg, 50mg Capsules
Venlafaxine, 100mg, 25mg, 37.5mg, 50mg, 75mg Tablets
Sedatives and Hypnotics
Methylphenobarbital, 100mg, 32mg, 50mg Tablets
Zaleplon, 10mg, 5mg Capsules
Zolpidem, 10mg, 5mg Tablets
Smoking Deterrents
Bupropion, 150mg Sustained-release Tablet
Thyroid Therapy
Thyroid Gland, 15mg, 240mg, 300mg, 90mg Tablets
Tuberculosis Therapy
Isoniazid/Rifampin, 300-150mg Capsule
Vascular Agents
Amlodipine, 10mg, 2.5mg, 5mg Tablets
Amlodipine/Benazepril, 10-20mg, 2.5-10mg, 5-10mg, 5-20mg Capsules
Benazepril, 10mg, 20mg, 40mg, 5mg Tablets
Benazepril/Hydrochlorothiazide, 10-12.5mg, 20-12.5mg, 20-25mg, 5-6.25mg Tablets
Bendroflumethiazide/Nadolol, 40-5mg, 80-5mg Tablets
Carvedilol, 12.5mg, 25mg, 3.125mg, 6.25mg Tablets
Diltiazem, 360mg, 420mg Extended-Release Capsules
Eplerenone, 25mg, 50mg Tablets
Felodipine, 10mg, 2.5mg, 5mg Extended-Release Tablets
Fosinopril, 10mg, 20mg, 40mg Tablets
Fosinopril/Hydrochlorothiazide, 10-12.5mg, 20-12.5mg Tablets
Hydrochlorothiazide/Metoprolol, 100-25mg, 100-50mg, 50-25mg Tablets
Hydrochlorothiazide/Moexipril, 15-12.5mg, 15-25mg, 7.5-12.5mg Tablets
Hydrochlorothiazide/Quinapril, 10-12.5mg, 20-12.5mg, 20-25mg Tablets
Isradipine, 2.5mg, 5mg Capsules
Metoprolol, 100mg, 200mg, 25mg, 50mg Extended-Release Tablets
Moexipril, 15mg, 7.5mg Tablets
Nimodipine, 30mg Capsule
Nisoldipine, 20mg, 30mg, 40mg Extended-Release Tablets
Quinapril, 10mg, 20mg, 40mg, 5mg Tablets
Ramipril, 1.25mg, 10mg, 2.5mg, 5mg Capsules

Table I-4. Mapping from IMS Data to Dosage Form

Three-Lettered Code (as provided by IMS)	Analysis Dosage Form
ABA Tablets Uncoat Regular Ordinary Tablet	Tablet
ACA Tablets Coated Regular Ordinary Tablet	Tablet
AAA Capsules Regular Ordinary	Capsule
AAE Capsules Regular Soluble	Capsule
AAF Capsules Regular Sprinkle	Capsule
ABC Tablets Uncoat Regular Chewable	Chewable
ACC Tablets Coat Regular Chewable	Chewable
ABD Tablets Uncoat Regular	Buccal/Sublingual
BBD Tab Uncoat Long Acting Buccal/Sub-Lingual	Buccal/Sublingual
AGD Lozenge Reg Buccal/Sub-Lingual	Buccal/Sublingual
ABE Tablets Uncoat Regular Sol	Orally Disintegrating/ Ecteric Coated
ABZ Tablets Uncoat Regular Other	Orally Disintegrating/ Ecteric Coated
ACZ Tab Coated Regular Other	Orally Disintegrating/ Ecteric Coated
BAA Capsules Long Acting Ordinary	Extended-Release Capsule
BAZ Capsules Long Acting Other	Extended-Release Capsule
AAZ Capsules Regular Other	Extended-Release Capsule
BBA Tablets Uncoat Long Acting Ordinary	Extended-Release Tablet
BBE Tablets Uncoat Long Acting Solution	Extended-Release Tablet
BBZ Tablets Uncoat Long Acting Other	Extended-Release Tablet
BCA Tablets Coated Long Acting Ordinary	Extended-Release Tablet
BCZ Tablets Coated Long Acting Other	Extended-Release Tablet
AGA Lozenge Regular Ordinary Lozenge	Lozenge
RB Mouth Throat Lozenges Lozenge	Lozenge
BGA Lozenge Long Acting Ordinary	Extended-Release Lozenge
BDA Granulate Long Acting Ordinary	Extended-Release Granule
Doseform=Tablet/Capsule	Other

Table I-5. Firms Counted as Repackagers

Allscripts Pharmaceuticals
Altura Pharmaceuticals
American Generic
American Health Packager
American Pharmaceuticals
American Pref Pharmaceuticals
American Regent
American Therapeutical
American Urologic
AQ Pharmaceuticals
Blenheim Pharmacal
Blu Pharmaceuticals
Bryant Ranch Pre-packager
DHS
Dispensexpress

Table I-5. (Continued)

Dispensing Solution
Dr.X
GSMS
Keltman Pharmaceuticals
Major Pharmaceuticals
Marlex Pharmaceuticals
Mckesson Packaging Services
Nucare Pharmaceuticals
Palmetto Pharmaceuticals
PD-RX Pharmaceuticals
Pharma Medical
Pharma Pac
Pharmpak
Physicians Total Care
Physician Partner
Physician Therapeutics
Prepak Systems
Quality Care Pharmaceuticals
Repackager
Rxpak Division
Southwood Pharmaceuticals
St Marys Mpp
Stat Rx
UDL Laboratories
Vibranta

Table I-6. List of USC5 Decongestant Therapeutic Classes Excluded

14310 Anti-histamine/Decongestant
14330 Anti-histamine/Decongestant/Analgesic
14390 Comb W/O Expectorant,Other
14510 Expectorant/Decongestant
14560 Expectorant/Decongestant/Analgesic
34380 Narcotic Cough/Expectorant
34510 Non-Narcotic Cough/Decongestant
34520 Non-Narcotic Cough/Anti-histamine
34540 Non-Narcotic Cough/Decongestant/Anti-histamine
34560 Non-Narcotic Cough/Anti-histamine/Analgesic
34570 Non-Narcotic Cough/Decongestant/Anti-histamine/Anal
34590 Non-Narcotic Cough Comb W/O Expectorant,Other
34610 Non-Narcotic Cough/Decongestant/Expectorant
34650 Non-Narcotic Cough/Decongestant/Analgesic/Expectorant
34680 Non-Narcotic Cough/Expectorant

Table I-7. List of USC5 Vitamin Therapeutic Classes Excluded

11420 Vitamin K & Related, Oral
32200 Lipotropics
37340 Emollients & Protectives
43100 Enzymes, Local/Topical
48111 Ferrous, Iron Alone
48112 Ferrous, Iron Combination
48120 Liver
48130 Vitamin B12
48190 Hematinics, Other
60500 Calcium Supplements
60600 Complete Food Supplement
60700 Nutrients & Supplements
73000 Tonics
76110 Multivitamin Prenatal
76121 Multivitamin-Pediatric Chewable W/Fluoride
76122 Multivitamin-Pediatric Drops W/Fluoride
76123 Multivitamin-Pediatric Liquid W/Fluoride
76131 Multivitamin-Pediatric Chew without Fluoride
76132 Multivitamin-Pediatric Drops without Fluoride
76133 Multivitamin-Pediatric Liq without Fluoride
76140 Multivitamin General
76212 B-Complex, Plain, Oral
76222 B-Complex, W/C, Oral
76230 B-Complex, Other Combination
76310 Ascorbic Acid
76320 Vitamin A
76330 Vitamin A & D
76340 Vitamin D
76350 Niacin
76380 Vitamin E
76390 Vitamins,Other
84210 Natural Medicine Other, Herbals
84220 Natural Medicine Other, Nutritn
84230 Natural Medicine Other, Topical

APPENDIX J. AUTHORIZED GENERICS AND THE MEDICAID REBATE PROGRAM

I. Background

A. The Medicaid Rebate Program: An Overview

In 1990, Congress established the Medicaid Drug Rebate Program.[449] That program required drug manufacturers that want to participate in the Medicaid program to agree to rebate to the state a portion of the price of each drug provided to Medicaid beneficiaries, in accordance with the terms of a standard national rebate agreement.[450]

The 1990 legislation set out a rebate formula for both brand and generic drugs. A brand manufacturer was required to rebate an amount equal to the product of the total number of units of each dosage form and strength paid for under the Medicaid state plan times the *greater* of (i) either a flat rebate amount (currently 15.1% of the average manufacturer price ("AMP")) and (ii) the difference between the *AMP* and the *best price* ("BP") for the drug. Additionally, brand manufacturers had to pay a supplemental rebate for drugs that exceeded a stated percentage increase in the cost of living index. The rebate for generic drugs was set at 11% of AMP, and there was no supplementary inflation-based rebate.

Over time a number of issues in applying the formulas surfaced. One of these issues concerned the treatment of authorized generics – in particular, whether brand companies had to include AGs in their calculations of AMP and best price for the corresponding brand drug. Some generic companies contended that the original Medicaid rebate legislation had created a loophole for AGs and that AGs should be included in the calculations.[451] Congress addressed the issue in the Deficit Reduction Act of 2005 (the "DRA").[452]

B. The DRA and the Treatment of Authorized Generics

Section 6003 of the DRA specifically requires brand manufacturers to include authorized generic sales in their calculations of both the AMP and best price when they report these prices for covered outpatient drugs to the Secretary.[453] The DRA also required CMS to promulgate regulations detailing precisely how the AMP was to be calculated. The effective date of the law was January 1, 2007.

On December 22, 2006, CMS published proposed regulations, including rules on the inclusion of AG prices in the calculation of AMP and best price.[454] The proposed rule would have required the brand manufacturer to factor into its calculation of the AMP and Best Price for a given drug all the sales of the corresponding AG, even if the AG were manufactured or marketed by a different company.[455]

This drew significant adverse comments. Among other things, commenters argued that the rule as proposed would require brand companies (the NDA holders) to obtain pricing data from other companies marketing the AG, which could raise antitrust concerns.[456] Accordingly, the proposal was revised when the Final Rule was promulgated on July 17, 2007. The Final Rule does not contemplate a "blended"AMP, *i.e.*, an AMP that reflects the price of AGs, other than in narrow circumstances. Moreover, the Final Rule does not require the NDA holder to factor in the AG sales of a secondary manufacturer in calculating "best price"; it, does, however, have to factor in the *transfer price* of the AG to the secondary manufacturer.[457] Thus, the final rule resulted in potentially greater rebate liability to the brand companies that offered AGs than did the proposed rule because the difference between the AMP (which would not, in most cases, include the lower AG prices) and the best price (which would include what were expected to be low transfer prices for the AG) would typically be greater.[458]

C. This Study and the Impact of the DRA

Some commenters predicted that the DRA changes would significantly increase brand companies' Medicaid rebates, and that this likely would result in a substantial decrease in AGs.[459] Some documents obtained from the companies offered similar projections.[460] Indeed, one comment asserted that the DRA provisions would so greatly discourage the marketing of AGs that this study, to the extent that it would be based on historical data, would not be useful.[461]

These concerns appear overstated. As discussed in Chapter 2, although the number of AG launches fell off in 2007–2008 from the high levels observed in 2003–2006, substantial numbers of AGs continue to be introduced. The DRA clearly did not bring a halt to the introduction of AGs.[462]

In order to help examine this issue further, the Commission's Special Orders required the brand-name companies and the specialized AG companies to produce "planning, decisional or strategy documents . . . that discuss the effect(s) or possible effect(s) of the enactment of Section 6003 of the Deficit Reduction Act of 2005, P.L. 109-171 on the marketing of AGs after Jan. 1, 2007."[463] The documents that were submitted, combined with the data regarding the number of AG launches, suggest that the DRA changes have not fundamentally undermined AG marketing. The analysis, however, necessarily bears a caveat: the timing of the DRA changes in relationship to this study may have shaped and limited the response to the Commission's information request in ways that understate the changes' effects.[464]

II. Company Documents Analyzing the DRA's Impact on AG Marketing

Although limited,[465] the documents that were produced show that for most drugs the companies expected their Medicaid rebates to increase because of the DRA changes, but that the amount of the expected increase was expected to vary significantly from drug to drug.[466] They indicate that for any given drug, the expected financial impact of the DRA changes depended on a variety of factors including the percentage of sales attributable to Medicaid[467] and the timing of the AG launch.[468] Assessing the documents, however, is difficult because most antedate issuance of the final version of the regulations and consequently could understate the DRA changes' effect.[469]

Adding further complexity, the documents suggest that focusing narrowly on just the "best price" calculation and its Medicaid rebate effects may be insufficient: other regulatory changes and effects may also be relevant. For example, the documents of several companies observed that enactment of the Part D Medicare program would substantially decrease the companies' exposure to additional Medicaid rebates for certain classes of drugs used by the elderly.[470] This might reduce the impact of changes in the "best price" calculation. On the other hand, the documents of one company in particular focused on the severe financial impact the DRA changes would have on the prices that it could charge for oral contraceptive drugs under the Section 340B Program.[471] Because the Medicaid rebate is also a reference point for 340B ceiling prices, a higher Medicaid rebate can also translate into a significantly lower ceiling price for drugs sold to 340B institutions.[472]

With regard to operational effects, the documents show that some companies *considered* whether to drop anticipated launches of new AGs or to discontinue marketing particular AGs because of the expected negative impact of the DRA changes on profitability. In only a few instances, however, do documents suggest that companies ultimately *decided* against launching or in favor of terminating AGs because of the DRA changes.

In only one case do the documents record a decision not to launch an AG largely because of the DRA.[473] In that case the company viewed the percentage of the drug's sales to Medicaid recipients as high (23%) and expected high levels of generic competition.[474] Essentially the added Medicaid rebates turned the marginal financials for the AG launch into significant losses under all reasonable scenarios, and the company decided not to proceed with the launch.

The documents also reveal two companies that decided to discontinue marketing a total of three AGs largely because of the DRA. One company decided to stop marketing two AGs (both in the same therapeutic category) when the AGs had not been profitable for the past two years and the expected impact of the DRA changes on the amount of Medicaid rebates was expected to be significant.[475] The other case was similar: the brand company and its AG distributor agreed to terminate their contract for the AG several days prior to the effective date of the DRA final rule when the AG had been only marginally profitable in any event and the additional Medicaid rebate liability would have made future marketing unprofitable.[476] It thus appears that the prospect of increased Medicaid rebates may have tipped the balance against AG marketing on some already-marginal drugs.

At the same time, documents produced by several companies suggest that the larger Medicaid rebates would not lead to diminished AG marketing efforts. In many cases the AG was profitable, and would continue to be so notwithstanding the larger Medicaid rebates. Thus, even in some cases where the additional rebates were expected to be substantial, AG marketing was not discontinued.[477] Furthermore, in some instances other considerations may also have shaped reactions. The documents of one company, for example, show that despite expected losses on sales of certain AGs because of the DRA changes, customer expectations and other strategic considerations impelled it to continue introducing AGs.[478]

In short, the documents do not indicate that brand companies viewed the DRA changes as sounding a death knell for their AG programs, or that those changes caused the companies to abandon AG marketing or even to revise their AG strategies in a fundamental way. Instead, the companies analyzed the impact of the DRA changes on particular drugs, but ultimately decided to make relatively few changes with respect to introducing new AGs or terminating those already in the market. As noted above, however, this analysis is based largely on documents that predated issuance of the final rule, and hence, could understate the financial impact of the DRA changes and the brand companies' response.

APPENDIX K. PATENT CHALLENGES: IMPACT ON GENERIC ENTRY AND BRAND EXCLUSIVITY

The length of brand exclusivity – the period when generics are not available, from NDA approval to generic entry – depends on both the length of patent protection obtained by a brand-name company and the extent to which patent challenges reduce the protected period. The following figures, which are based on the set of drugs for which generic entry took place via 180-day exclusivity from 2001–2008,[479] suggest that both factors contributed to variations in the length of brand exclusivity.

As shown in Figure K-1, the length of patent protection obtained by brand-name companies increased from 2001–2008: the period between NDA approval and expiration of the last-to-expire patent gradually rose by about 3–4 years.

At the same time, generic companies sought to reduce the period of brand exclusivity by challenging patents. As shown in Figure K-2, the number of years by which patent challenges reduced the period of patent protection varied. On average, generic entry first occurred about four years before expiration of the last patent in 2001. This average rose to about 8–10 years before expiration from 2003–2005 but then fell back to about seven and one-half years during 2006–2008.

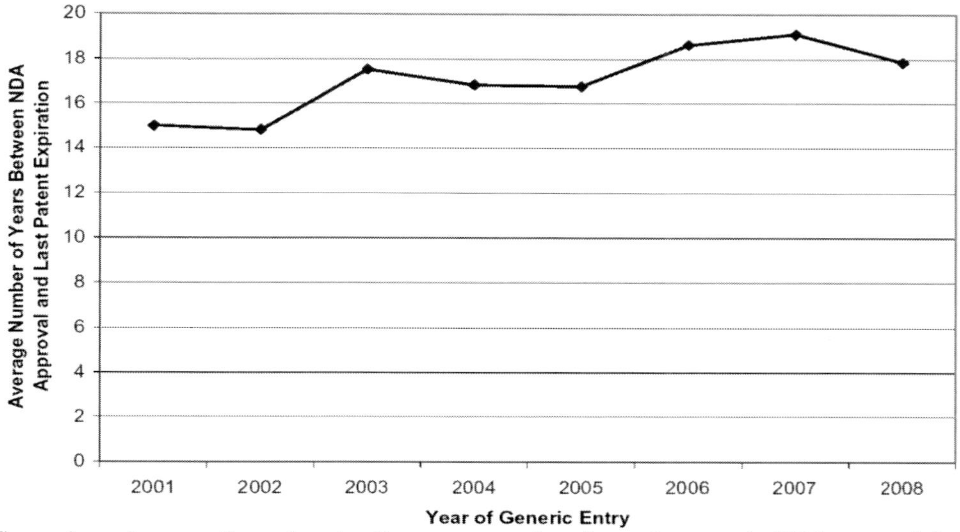

The figure shows, by year of generic entry, the average number of years between the NDA approval date and the last patent expiration date for 66 brand-name drugs that experienced generic entry by 180-day exclusivity from 2001–2008. The drugs are limited to tablet and capsule dosage forms. See supra Appendix H, Section I.D.

Figure K-1. Years of Brand Patent Protection.

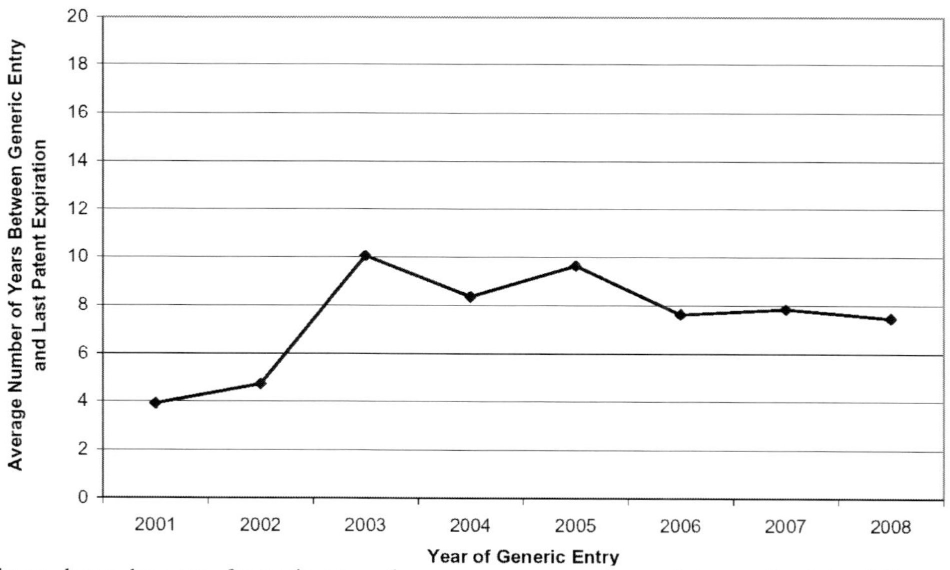

The figure shows, by year of generic entry, the average number of years between the date of first generic entry and the last patent expiration date for 66 brand-name drugs that experienced generic entry by 180-day exclusivity from 2001–2008. The drugs are limited to tablet and capsule dosage forms. See supra Appendix H, Section I.D.

Figure K-2. Years Generic Entered Before Brand Patent Expiration.

The length of brand exclusivity equals the maximum length of a brand's patent protection minus the extent to which patent challenges reduce the period of protection. As shown in Figure K-3, brands' exclusivity went from a high of 11 years in 2001 to a low of 7–8 years in 2003–2005, and then rose to 10–11 years from 2006–2008. Although the change in length of exclusivity is not statistically significant, the increase in brand exclusivity in 2006–2008 appears to arise from both an increase in the maximum period of patent protection and a decrease in the effect of patent challenges.

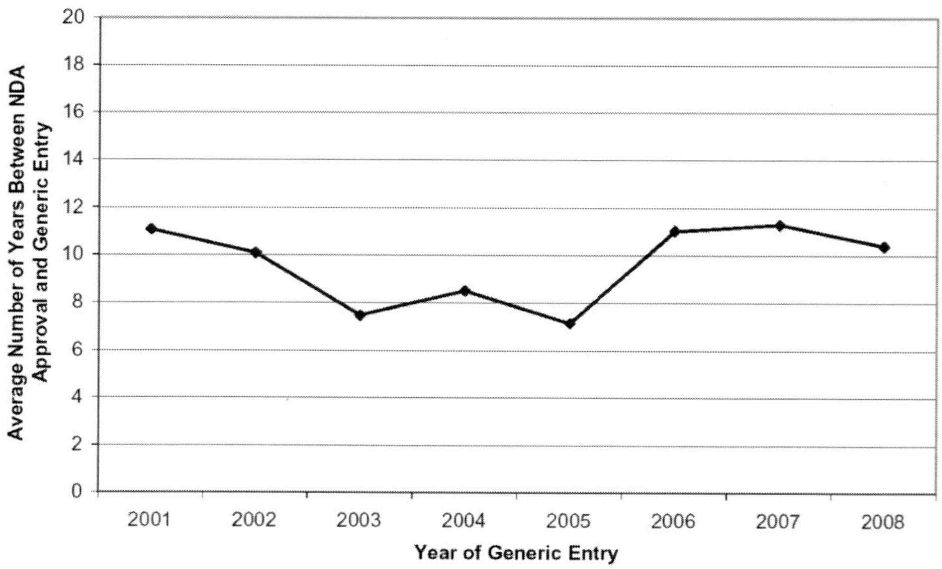

The figure shows, by year of generic entry, the average number of years between the NDA approval date and the first generic launch date for 66 brand-name drugs that experienced generic entry by 180-day exclusivity from 2001–2008. The drugs are limited to tablet and capsule dosage forms. See supra Appendix H, Section I.D.

Figure K-3. Years of Brand Exclusivity.

Appendix L. Technical Modeling Appendix

The discussion throughout Chapters 3 and 6 refers to regression models that relate competition variables (such as the presence of an AG) to measures of specific market outcomes, such as generic prices and first-filer revenues. This appendix presents the details of those regression models. The appendix begins with a detailed presentation of the models used within the exclusivity period. The models estimated outside of exclusivity are modifications of these initial models, and the discussion of them simply highlights the changes.

I. Models Applied During the 180-Day Exclusivity Period

The regression models employed to analyze the impact of AGs go beyond a simple comparison of means between markets with and without an AG. The models statistically control for other factors that may vary across markets, and which may be correlated with the introduction of an AG using regression analysis. This section provides a detailed description of the chosen specification, the variables included in the model, and how the estimation results are used to calculate the statistics of interest that are presented in the Report. The discussion begins with the pricing models.

A. Generic Price Model

Using both the retail and wholesale data, the regression pricing models estimate the relationship between the relative prices of all generic products, competition variables, and product characteristic controls. Of primary interest is the relationship between the dependent variables and the AG. The presence of an AG is represented by an indicator variable that interacts with the total number of generic manufacturers of the product in the particular month.[480] The model also includes indicator variables representing the product characteristic controls listed in Table I-2 and indicator variables for the number of months since generic entry. As described in Chapter 3, all models estimate standard errors that are clustered around the molecule of the product. Identical models are estimated weighting each observation (product-month) by the pre-entry sales of the brand-name product.[481] The estimation equation for the full control pricing model was

$$(\frac{p}{p_{b_0}})_{mdft} = \alpha + \beta_1 ag_{mdft} + \beta_2 man2_{mdft} + \beta_3 man3_{mdft} + \beta_4 man4_{mdft}$$
$$+ \beta_5 (ag \cdot man2)_{mdft} + \beta_6 (ag \cdot man3)_{mdft} + \beta_7 (ag \cdot man4)_{mdft} + \delta_t + \delta_{year} + \delta_{df} + \delta_{tc} + \varepsilon_{mdft}$$

where,

Variables

p: monthly price of the product (various prices are used depending on the analysis[482])
p_{b0}: Pre-entry price of the brand-name product (three-month average)
ag: An indicator of whether an AG has positive sales during the month
man2-man4: Dummy variable indicators representing the count of generic manufacturers 2-4
and,

Estimated Coefficients

α : Regression constant
β_1 -β_7 : Competition variable coefficients
δ_t : Vector of five month-since-entry indicator variables (month 0 is excluded[483])

δ_{df} : Vector of six dosage form indicator variables (tablets are excluded)
δ_{year}: Vector of five calendar year indicator variables (year 2008 is excluded)
δ_{tc} :Vector of fourteen therapeutic class indicator variables (analgesics are excluded)
ε : Error term.

The left-hand side of the equation is the relative price for each product (where the subscript *mdft* refers to the molecule, dosage-form-strength, and month-since-entry). For the analysis reported in Tables 3-1 and 3-2, this price was constructed by taking the total dollars spent on all generic products (including the AG) during the month and dividing by the total extended units consumed during the month. The pre-entry average brand price, p_{b0}, was constructed to be the total expenditures on the brand over the three months prior to generic entry divided by the total extended units of the brand sold over the same period.

The right-hand side of the equation includes the competition and product characteristic variables. The competition variables include an indicator for whether an AG is present (ag), indicators for the total number of manufacturers in the market (man2-man4), and interactions of the AG with the total number of manufacturers. The product characteristic variables control for the months since generic entry, the dosage form, and the therapeutic class. The indicator for whether an AG is present is set to equal one if the AG manufacturer has positive sales during the month, and zero otherwise. Similarly, the manufacturer count and product characteristic indicators equal one if the market conditions are true, and zero otherwise. For example, man2 is equal to one if the market has exactly two generic manufacturers, and is zero otherwise. Similarly, the capsule indicator is set to one if the product is a capsule, and is zero otherwise. The estimation equation for the models with "no controls" is identical to the model above, but excludes the product characteristic controls represented by the vectors δ_t, δ_{df}, δ_{year}, and δ_{tc}.

The competition variable coefficient estimates from the regressions were used to estimate the AG effect on price. For the exclusivity analysis in Chapter 3, the estimated AG price effect represents the percentage change due to adding an AG to an ANDA-Only market. The percentage price change was evaluated at the constant using the following equation:[484]

$$\%\Delta P = \frac{P^*_{+AG} - P^*_{ANDA}}{P^*_{ANDA}} = (\beta_1 + \beta_2 + \beta_5)/\alpha,$$

In the above equation, P* represents the predicted relative price from the regression. This price was predicted for markets with an AG and two manufacturers (P^*_{+AG}), and for markets without an AG and only one manufacturer (P^*_{ANDA}). The percentage change in price was calculated as the percentage difference in the predicted price of a market with two manufacturers and an AG and a market with one manufacturer and no AG. The percentage was evaluated at the predicted price of the market with one manufacturer and no AG.

B. Revenue Models

The modeling approach employed for the revenue analysis is very similar to that used in the pricing equation. However, the revenue model predicts the relative revenues at the firm level, for the first-filer ANDA-generics and brand-name firms (both on the brand-name product only, and on the brand-name product combined with the AG), rather than market averages. As in the pricing models, all specifications include indicator variables for each observed count of manufacturers, and these manufacturer count variables are also interacted with the AG indicator to allow the impact of the AG to vary depending on the number of competitors. The model with full controls also includes indicator variables representing product characteristics. However, the revenue estimation equations vary slightly across entities (i.e., the brand-name product, the brand-name firm, and the ANDA-generic firm). For example, there are no first-filer revenues in months where only an AG is on the market, and thus no "AG-Only" term is estimated in the generic revenue model.

1. First-Filer Generic Firm Revenues

The equation for the "full control" revenue model for ANDA-generic firms is presented below:

$$\frac{R_g}{R_{b_0}} = \alpha + \beta_1 man2 + \beta_2 man3 + \beta_3 man4$$

$$+ \beta_4(ag \cdot man2) + \beta_5(ag \cdot man3) + \beta_6(ag \cdot man4) + \delta_t + \delta_{year} + \delta_{df} + \delta_{tc} + \varepsilon$$

where,[485]

Variables

R_g: Contemporaneous generic revenues in market
R_0: Pre-entry brand revenues (three-month average)
ag: Indicator of whether an AG has positive sales during the month
man2-man4: Dummy variable indicators representing the count of generic manufacturers 2-4
ε: Error term

and,

Estimated Coefficients

α: Regression constantβ_1-β_7: Competition variable coefficients
δ_t: Five month-since-entry indicator variables (month 3 is excluded)
δ_{year}: Five calendar year indicator variables (year 2008 is excluded)
δ_{df}: Six dosage form indicator variables (tablets are excluded)
δ_{tc}: Fourteen therapeutic class indicator variables (Analgesics are excluded).

The left-hand side of the equation represents the ANDA-generic firms' relative revenues for each product. Relative revenues were constructed by dividing contemporaneous market revenues for first-filer generic firms, R_g, by pre-entry brand revenue.[486] All of the other variables are defined exactly as in the pricing equation. The AG effect was calculated analogously to the effect in the pricing model, considering the effect of adding an AG to an ANDA-Only market.

The first-filer revenue effect of introducing an AG to an ANDA-Only market was calculated using the following equation:[487]

$$\%\Delta R_{FF} = \frac{Rg^*_{+AG} - Rg^*_{ANDA}}{Rg^*_{ANDA}} = (\beta_1 + \beta_4) / \alpha$$

The same naming conventions used for the pricing regressions were also used for the revenue equation. R* represents the predicted revenues from the regression. The predicted revenue for markets with one ANDA and an AG is represented by Rg^*_{+AG}, whereas the predicted revenue for a market with one ANDA manufacturer but no AG is represented by Rg^*_{ANDA}. The above equation calculates the predicted revenue change from adding an AG to an ANDA-Only market.

2. Brand-Name Firm Revenues

The brand-name product revenue and the brand-name firm (brand-name product + AG) revenue equations are analogous to the first-filer equation, and appear identical to each other. They are represented below:

$$\frac{R_b}{R_0} = \alpha + \beta_1 ag + \beta_2 man2 + \beta_3 man3 + \beta_4 man4$$
$$+ \beta_5 ag \cdot man2 + \beta_6 ag \cdot man3 + \beta_7 ag \cdot man4 + \delta_t + \delta_{year} + \delta_{df} + \delta_{tc} + \varepsilon$$

The above equation regresses relative brand revenues against product characteristic controls and a set of competition variables that are very similar to those in the first-filer revenue equation. The relative brand-name product revenues are constructed by dividing the contemporaneous brand-name product revenues by the pre-entry brand revenues. Similarly, the relative brand-name firm revenues are constructed by dividing the brand-name firm revenues, which include the revenues from the AG product, by the pre-entry brand revenues. The primary difference between the first-filer equation and the brand equation is the AG-only term included in the brand equation. The brand-name product and the brand-name firm are sometimes observed facing an AG competitor without an ANDA competitor. This coefficient identifies the revenue for those markets with only an AG competitor.

The effect of an AG on brand revenues is given below:

$$\%\Delta R_{brand} = \frac{Rb^*_{+AG} - Rb^*_{+ANDA}}{Rb^*_{+ANDA}} = (\beta_1 + \beta_2 + \beta_5) / \alpha$$

The predicted percentage change in brand revenues is the predicted revenues for markets with an AG and an ANDA less the predicted revenues for markets with only an ANDA divided by the predicted revenues for markets with only an ANDA.

II. Models Employed Outside of a 180-Day Exclusivity Period

The potential for many manufacturers to sell a product outside an exclusivity period necessitates several modifications to the regression analysis detailed above. The main modification is that more indicator variables are included in the regression to account for greater numbers of manufacturers. Separate manufacturer indicators are included for up to ten manufacturers, and a single indicator is included for all drugs with greater than ten manufacturers. The models also include a single indicator variable representing the effect of the AG on the variable of interest (either relative prices or relative revenues). The effect of the AG is estimated solely through the AG indicator.[488] The models also track data on the product for a longer period (typically 30–36 months). Consequently, the models outside of exclusivity include a larger set of month indicators corresponding to this longer period. For the products without an exclusivity period, month indicators are interacted with whether the product faced a Paragraph IV challenge.

The AG effects are also calculated somewhat differently outside of exclusivity by treating an AG as replacing an ANDA-generic manufacturer, rather than adding to the number of firms. During exclusivity, entry by an AG clearly adds an additional manufacturer, because the number of ANDA-generic manufacturers does not decrease to compensate for this entry. However, outside of exclusivity, ANDA-generic manufacturers that observe the presence of an AG may adjust their entry decisions accordingly. Consequently, the analysis outside exclusivity treats AG entry as displacing an ANDA-generic.[489] For example, the analysis outside of exclusivity addresses the question: "do markets with five ANDA-generics behave differently than markets with four ANDA-generics and an AG?" In contrast, the analysis during exclusivity addresses the question "do markets with an ANDA-generic and no AG behave differently than markets with an ANDA-generic and an AG?" Using the notation from above, the price effect of an AG outside of exclusivity is calculated using estimates from the model as:

$$\%\Delta P = \frac{P^*_{+AG} - P^*_{ANDA}}{P^*_{ANDA}} = \beta_1 / \alpha .$$

The price at which these effects are measured can be especially important outside of exclusivity because average prices with ten manufacturers can be much lower than average prices with two manufacturers. In exclusivity, markets were relatively homogeneous, so these effects were evaluated at the average price for a market with only one ANDA competitor, which happened to be estimated by the intercept term, α. Outside of exclusivity, the average number of manufacturers is five, so this is used as the excluded category in the set of manufacturer count indicators. Consequently, the intercept term reflects prices in markets with five manufacturers, which is where the effect is evaluated. The other omitted categories are psycho-therapeutic tablets and the first month of non-exclusivity. These categories represent the largest categories, in terms of the number of products, observations, and pre-entry brand sales, in the sample.

End Notes

[1] The Federal Trade Commission conducted this study at the request of Senators Grassley, Leahy, and Rockefeller, as well as at the request of Representative Waxman, all of whom asked the Commission to examine the competitive effects of authorized generic drugs. *See* Letter from Senators Charles Grassley, Patrick Leahy, and John Rockefeller to Deborah Platt Majoras, Chairman, Fed. Trade Comm'n (May 9, 2005) (*infra* Appendix A); Letter from Hon. Henry A. Waxman, U.S. House of Representatives, to Deborah Platt Majoras, Chairman, Fed. Trade Comm'n (Sept. 13, 2005) (*infra* Appendix B). Then-Commissioner Leibowitz also requested the FTC to study "the competitive implications of authorized generics." Jon Leibowitz, Commissioner, Fed. Trade Comm'n, Health Care and the FTC: The Agency as Prosecutor and Policy Wonk, Remarks at the Antitrust in HealthCare Conference 9–10 (May 12, 2005), http://www.ftc.gov/speeches/leibowitz/050512healthcare. pdf.

[2] 21 U.S.C. § 355(j)(5)(b)(iv) (2010). Exclusivity now may be "shared" by two or more applicants filing on the same day. *See* 21 U.S.C. § 355(j)(5)(B)(iv)(I)–(II)(bb) (2010).

[3] *See* Teva Pharm. Indus. Ltd. v. Crawford, 410 F.3d 51, 54 (D.C. Cir. 2005).

[4] FED. TRADE COMM'N, AUTHORIZED GENERICS: AN INTERIM REPORT ("Interim Report") (2009), http://www.ftc. gov/os/2009/06/P062105authorizedgenericsreport.pdf.

[5] *Id.*, Executive Summary, at 2.

[6] *Id.*

[7] For instance, for a drug with brand sales of $130 million, a generic that does not anticipate AG competition will expect a patent challenge to be profitable if it has at least a 4 percent chance of winning; with AG competition, that generic would need at least a 10 percent chance of winning to expect a patent challenge to be profitable. Under this mode of analysis, the AG might discourage a challenge only if the generic thinks the chance of winning is between 4 and 10 percent, i.e., when the challenge is unlikely to be successful. For larger drugs, the presence of an AG is critical to the patent-challenge decision only when the expected likelihood of success is even less than 10 percent.

[8] An absence of documents is not necessarily determinative: generic companies simply might not have recorded the reasons for a decision to refrain from filing a patent challenge. In reaching its conclusions, the Commission considered all the evidence before it; no single category, including the documents provided by generic firms, was dispositive.

[9] While the Report finds that AGs have infrequently been launched for drugs in markets with less than $50 million of annual brand sales, generic documents discussing assumptions about AG competition do not draw distinctions based on market size. The documentary evidence regarding this point, however, is limited.

[10] "Paragraph IV" generic drug applications, filed with the Food and Drug Administration pursuant to 21 U.S.C. § 355(j)(2)(A)(vii)(IV), certify that a patent is invalid or will not be infringed by the generic drug and begin the process of generic entry via patent challenge.

[11] New chemical entities are drugs for which the active ingredient has not received previous FDA approval. For new chemical entities, the first day that applications with Paragraph IV certifications are allowed is four years after approval of the brand-name drug. This is a specific, known day, on which filers will expect to share exclusivity.

[12] FTC staff estimates that "pay-for-delay" arrangements, overall, cost American consumers $3.5 billion per year. FED. TRADE COMM'N, PAY-FOR-DELAY: HOW DRUG COMPANY PAY-OFFS COST CONSUMERS BILLIONS 8–10 (2010), http://www.ftc.gov/os/2010/01/100112 payfordelayrpt.pdf.

[13] *See, e.g.*, CONG. BUDGET OFFICE, HOW INCREASED COMPETITION FROM GENERIC DRUGS HAS AFFECTED PRICES AND RETURNS IN THE PHARMACEUTICAL INDUSTRY 31 (1998), http://www.cbo.gov/ftpdocs/6xx/ doc655/pharm.pdf. "No AG" agreements also deny consumers the benefit of price discounts from AG competition during the 180-day exclusivity period.

[14] Of the 39 agreements from FY 2004 to FY 2010, 24 were made between FY 2004 and FY 2009 (an average of four per year), while 15 were made in FY 2010. The 15 agreements in FY 2010 in which brand-name firms agreed not to introduce an AG were nearly 60% of the 26 agreements that year containing payments to a first-filer generic and a restriction on that firm's ability to market its product.

[15] Authorized generic drugs (often referred to in this Report as "AGs") are drugs that are approved as brand-name drugs but are marketed as generic drugs. AGs do not bear the brand-name or trademark of the brand-name drug or manufacturer, but the brand-name and AG products are chemically identical.

[16] *See* Letter from Senators Charles Grassley, Patrick Leahy, and John Rockefeller to Deborah Platt Majoras, Chairman, Fed. Trade Comm'n (May 9, 2005) (*infra* Appendix A).

[17] Drug Price Competition and Patent Term Restoration (Hatch-Waxman) Act of 1984, Pub. L. No. 98417, 98 Stat. 1585 (1984) (codified in scattered sections of 15, 21, 28 & 35 U.S.C.).

[18] *See* Letter from Hon. Henry A. Waxman, U.S. House of Representatives, to Deborah Platt Majoras, Chairman, Fed. Trade Comm'n (Sept. 13, 2005) (*infra* Appendix B). Then-Commissioner Leibowitz also requested the

FTC to study "the competitive implications of authorized generics." Jon Leibowitz, Commissioner, Fed. Trade Comm'n, Health Care and the FTC: The Agency as Prosecutor and Policy Wonk, Remarks at the Antitrust in HealthCare Conference 9–10 (May 12, 2005), http://www.ftc.gov/speeches/leibowitz/ 050512healthcare.pdf.

[19] *See infra* Chapter 2.

[20] *See* Andrx Citizen Petition, FDA Docket No. 2004P-0563/CP1 (Dec. 27, 2004), http://www.fda.gov/ohrms/dockets/dockets/04p0563/04p-0563-cp0000-01-vol1.pdf (urging the FDA to "inform McNeil Specialty Pharmaceuticals that any authorized version of Concerta® that is introduced and marketed as a 'generic' drug before or during the initial product launch of the first ANDA-approved version will be regarded as misbranded and subject to regulatory action"); Teva Citizen Petition, FDA Docket No. 2004P-0261/CP1 (June 10, 2004), http:// www.fda.gov/ohrms/dockets/dailys/04/June04/061004/04p-0261-cp00001-toc.htm (urging the FDA to "prevent Pfizer Inc. from marketing a generic version of its Accupril® (quinapril) drug products until after the expiration of Teva's 180-day exclusivity period for generic quinapril products"); Mylan Citizen Petition, FDA Docket No. 2004P-0075/CP1 (Feb. 18, 2004), http://www.fda.gov/ohrms/dockets/dailys/04/feb04/021804/04p-0075-cp00001-vol1.pdf (urging the FDA "to prohibit the marketing and distribution of [AGs] until the expiration of any 180-day generic drug exclusivity to which an ANDA applicant is entitled"); *see also* Apotex Comment in Support of Mylan Citizen Petition, FDA Docket No. 2004P-0075/EMC1 (Mar. 24, 2004), http://www.fda.gov/ohrms/dockets/dailys/04/ apr04/040204/04P-0075-emc00001.pdf.

[21] *See, e.g.*, Mylan Pharm., Inc. v. FDA, No. Civ.A. 104CV242, 2005 WL 2411674 (N.D. W. Va. Sept. 29, 2005), *aff'd*, 454 F.3d 270 (4th Cir. 2006); Teva Pharm., Indus., Ltd. v. FDA, 355 F. Supp. 2d 111 (D.D.C. 2004), *aff'd*, Teva Pharm. Indus. Ltd. v. Crawford, 410 F.3d 51 (D.C. Cir. 2005); *see also* SmithKline Beecham Corp. v. Apotex Corp., 383 F. Supp. 2d 686 (E.D. Pa. 2004).

[22] FED. TRADE COMM'N, AUTHORIZED GENERICS: AN INTERIM REPORT ("Interim Report") (2009), http://www.ftc.gov/os/2009/06/P062105authorizedgenericsreport.pdf.

[23] *See* 21 U.S.C. § 355(b), (c) (2010).

[24] *See* 21 U.S.C. § 355(j) (2010). Generic drugs approved through the filing of an ANDA will be referred to as "ANDA-generic" drugs when necessary to distinguish them from AGs.

[25] Under 21 U.S.C. § 355(j)(2)(A)(vii)(IV), a generic manufacturer certifies that each relevant patent is "invalid or will not be infringed by the manufacture, use, or sale of the new [ANDA] drug for which the application is submitted."

[26] OFFICE OF GENERIC DRUGS, U.S. FOOD & DRUG ADMIN., APPROVED DRUG PRODUCTS WITH THERAPEUTIC EQUIVALENCE EVALUATIONS ("Orange Book") (31st ed. 2011), *available at* http://www.accessdata.fda.gov/scripts/cder/ob/default.cfm.

[27] Unless otherwise specifically noted, all references in this Report to exclusivity or an exclusivity period are to 180-day exclusivity. Exclusivity now may be "shared" by two or more applicants filing on the same day. *See* 21 U.S.C. § 355(j)(5)(B)(iv)(I)–(II)(bb) (2010).

[28] *See, e.g.*, Richard G. Frank, *The Ongoing Regulation of Generic Drugs*, 357 NEW ENG. J. MED. 1993, 1993 (2007), *available at* http://www.nejm.org/doi/pdf/10.1056/NEJMp078193.

[29] *See* PHARM. RESEARCH AND MFRS. OF AM. ("PhRMA"), PHARMACEUTICAL INDUSTRY PROFILE (2010), http://www.phrma.org/sites/default/files/159/profile_2010_final.pdf (citing IMS Health data); *see also* GENERIC PHARM. ASS'N, 2010 ANNUAL REPORT 17 (2010), http://www.gphaonline.org/sites/default/files/Annual%20Report%202010.pdf (also citing IMS Health data).

[30] *See* CONG. BUDGET OFFICE, HOW INCREASED COMPETITION FROM GENERIC DRUGS HAS AFFECTED PRICES AND RETURNS IN THE PHARMACEUTICAL INDUSTRY 27 (1998), http:// www.cbo.gov/ftpdocs/6xx/doc655/pharm.pdf.

[31] Public Comment from the GPhA to the Fed. Trade Comm'n 2 (June 27, 2006), http://www.ftc.gov/os/comments/genericdrugstudy3/062806gpha.pdf.

[32] *See* Teva Pharm. Indus. Ltd. v. Crawford, 410 F.3d 51, 54 (D.C. Cir. 2005).

[33] *See, e.g.*, Fair Prescription Drug Competition Act, S. 373, 112th Cong. (2011); H.R. 741, 112th Cong. (2011).

[34] In recent years, the Commission has undertaken two other major empirical studies to address competition policy issues affecting the pharmaceutical industry. *See* fed. TRADE COMM'N, PHARMACY BENEFIT MANAGERS: OWNERSHIP OF MAIL-ORDER PHARMACIES (2005), www.ftc.gov/reports/pharmbenefit05/050906pharmbenefitrpt.pdf; FED. TRADE COMM'N, GENERIC DRUG ENTRY PRIOR TO PATENT EXPIRATION (2002), www.ftc.gov/os/2002/07/ genericdrugstudy.pdf. This Report draws upon the knowledge and experience accumulated in conducting these earlier studies.

[35] IMS CONSULTING, IMS HEALTH, ASSESSMENT OF AUTHORIZED GENERICS IN THE U.S. (2006)(written for PhRMA), http://replay.web.archive.org/20061009134405/http://www. phrma.org/files/IMS%20Authorized%20Generics%20Report_6-22-06.pdf. *See infra* Chapter 3.

[36] Aidan Hollis & Bryan A. Liang, *An Assessment of the Effect of Authorized Generics on Consumer Prices*, 10 J. BIOLAW & BUS. 10, 16 (2007) (written for GPhA) (an earlier version of this paper was made available by GPhA in July 2006, *available at* http://www. gphaonline.org/sites/default/files/GPhA_AG_Study.pdf). *See infra* Chapter 3.

[37] Ernst R. Berndt, Richard Mortimer & Andrew Parece, *Do Authorized Generic Drugs Deter Paragraph IV Certifications? Recent Evidence* (2007) (working paper written for PhRMA), http://www.analysisgroup.com/uploadedFiles/Publishing/Articles/PhRMA_Authorized_Generic_Entry .pdf; *see also* Ernst R. Berndt et al., *Authorized Generic Drugs, Price Competition, and Consumers' Welfare,* 26 HEALTH AFF. 790 (2007), *available at* http://content.healthaffairs.org/cgi/reprint/26/3/790.pdf. *See infra* Chapter 7, Section II.B.

[38] HOWREY LLP, THE SHORT-TERM AND LONG-TERM COMPETITIVE IMPACT OF AUTHORIZED GENERICS (2009) (written for PhRMA), http://www.ftc.gov/os/comments/genericdrugs tudy3/091028pharmresearch.pdf.

[39] OMB approval was obtained pursuant to requirements of the Paperwork Reduction Act, 44 U.S.C. §§ 3501-21 (2007). *See* Agency Information Collection Activities; Comment Request, 72 Fed. Reg. 25,304 (FTC May 4, 2007); Agency Information Collection Activities; Comment Request, 71 Fed. Reg. 16,779 (FTC Apr. 4, 2006).

[40] 15 U.S.C. § 46(b) (2010).

[41] Special Orders list the information that each company must provide to the FTC.

[42] Brand-name companies were included in the study if they marketed an AG or had a brand-name drug subject to a Paragraph IV certification that was included in the study. *See infra* note 31.

[43] These are companies that marketed ANDA-generic versions of brand-name drugs subject to a Paragraph IV certification, ANDA-generic drugs bioequivalent to an AG, or an AG not based on the company's or parent company's NDA. Thus, the generic companies included ANDA-generic subsidiaries of brand-name companies, but not subsidiaries that market only AGs on behalf of the parent.

[44] *See infra* Appendix G. The final count of 119 relevant AGs treats different dosage forms as separate AGs. Injectables and solutions were excluded to provide a more uniform data set.

[45] In general the Special Orders sought information on (i) AGs launched after January 1, 2001 and all drugs related to them, *i.e.*, brand-name versions of AG drugs and all bioequivalent generic drugs; (ii) brand-name drugs that first faced generic competition after January 1, 2001, for which at least one ANDA with a Paragraph IV certification was filed, and all bioequivalent generic drugs; and (iii) brand-name drugs for which at least one ANDA with a Paragraph IV certification was filed after January 1, 2001, but for which generic entry had not yet occurred. There was substantial overlap between the first two categories.

[46] The time periods covered by the Report's analyses vary due to the availability of information from diverse sources. *See infra* Appendix H.

[47] *See infra* Appendix D, ¶ 27, at D-6 (Brand-Name Drug Company Special Order covering the period from January 1, 2002 through April 3, 2006); *see also infra* Appendix F, ¶ 10, at F-3 (Authorized Generic Drug Company Special Order requesting similar information from companies that marketed AGs, but not ANDA-generic drugs).

[48] *See infra* Appendix E,. ¶¶ 18-19, at E-4, E-5 (Generic Drug Company Special Order covering the period from January 1, 2003, through April 3, 2006).

[49] This data set, which is the basis for much of the Report, includes all tablet and capsule dosage forms ("oral solids") of AGs that were first marketed between 2001 and 2008. Other dosage forms, such as injectables or solutions, were excluded to provide a more uniform data set. Counts reflect the number of NDAs (individual brand-name drugs) rather than the number of strengths ("products"), avoiding multiple counts for drugs with more than one strength. AGs were identified from information provided by the FDA, company responses to the Special Orders, and other sources. The time periods covered by the Report's analyses vary due to the availability of information from diverse sources. *See infra* Appendix H for more information on the definition and identification of AGs, criteria for inclusion in the study, and how they were counted. *See infra* Appendix G for a list of all AGs covered by the study.

[50] *See infra* Figures 2-7 and 2-8, and accompanying discussion.

[51] *See, e.g., See, e.g.,* JOHN R. THOMAS, CONG. RESEARCH SERV., AUTHORIZED GENERIC PHARMACEUTICALS: EFFECTS ON INNOVATION 8–9 (2008); Letter from William K. Hubbard, FDA, to Stuart A. Williams, Mylan Pharmaceuticals Inc. and James N. Czaban, Heller Ehrman, Re: Docket Nos. 2004P-0075/CP1 & 2004P-0261/CP1, at n.9 (July 2, 2004), http://www.fda.gov/ohrms/DOCKETS/dailys/04/july04/070704/04p-0075-pdn0001. pdf (listing authorized generic drugs launched as long ago as 1992); Kurt R. Karst, *Authorized Generics—Historical Overview and Current Issues,* REG. AFF. FOCUS, Mar. 2005.

[52] During the 1990s, AGs were not marketed during 180-day exclusivity, because there were almost no exclusivity periods as a result of the requirement that the first generic applicant defend successfully against a brand-name company's patent infringement lawsuit. When this requirement was eliminated, exclusivities began to increase, and the opportunity for marketing during the valuable exclusivity period grew. *See* FED. TRADE COMM'N, GENERIC DRUG ENTRY PRIOR TO PATENT EXPIRATION 57–58 (July 2002), http://www.ftc.gov/os/2002/07/genericdrugstudy.pdf (citing Mova v. Shalala, 955 F. Supp. 128 (D.D.C. 1997), *aff'd,* 140 F. 3d 1060 (D.C. Cir. 1998)). There were no awards of exclusivity from 1992–1997. For tablet and capsule prescription drugs, one exclusivity was awarded in 1998, two in 1999, and one in 2000. *See* Figure 2-7 for data on exclusivities and AGs from 2001–2008.

[53] *See infra* Chapter 4, Sections I, II.

[54] *See, e.g.,* Sandra Levy, *Why Authorized Generics are Making a Comeback,* DRUG TOPICS, Nov. 3, 2003, *available at* http://drugtopics.modernmedicine.com/drugtopics/article/ articleDetail.jsp?id=111159; Robert P.

Rezick & James B. Kobak, *Permission Granted*, PHARMACEUTICAL EXECUTIVE, May 2004. All seven AGs launched in 2001 were marketed by generic subsidiaries. In 2002, three were marketed by contract and four by subsidiaries. In 2003, 15 were marketed by contract (including four settlements), and four by subsidiaries.

[55] See, e.g., Leila Abboud, *Drug Makers Use New Tactic to Ding Generic-Drug Firms,* WALL ST. J., Jan. 27, 2004, at B1; Lewis Krauskopf, *Generic Drug Companies Fighting Threat from Big Brands,* THE RECORD, Aug. 22, 2004.

[56] *See* Letter from William K. Hubbard, FDA, *supra* note 3; *supra* Chapter 1, notes 7, 18, and accompanying text.

[57] Deficit Reduction Act of 2005 ("DRA"), Pub. L. No. 109-171, § 6003, 120 Stat. 4, 60–61 (2006) (codified as amended at 42 U.S.C. § 1396r-8).

[58] Details regarding the DRA requirements and information derived from the Special Orders regarding the DRA's likely effects are presented in Appendix J. However, subsequent changes in the DRA implementing regulations, which occurred after the cut-off date for document production, may limit the utility of the information produced.

[59] *See* BUREAU OF COMPETITION, FED. TRADE COMM'N, AGREEMENTS FILED WITH THE FEDERAL TRADE COMMISSION UNDER THE MEDICARE PRESCRIPTION DRUG, IMPROVEMENT, AND MODERNIZATION ACT OF 2003: OVERVIEW OF AGREEMENTS FILED IN FY 2010 (2011), http://www.ftc.gov/os/2011/05/1105 mmaagreements.pdf.

[60] *See infra* Chapter 4, Section III.A. (AG launch usually simultaneous with ANDA-generic entry); FED. TRADE COMM'N, PAY-FOR-DELAY: HOW DRUG COMPANY PAY-OFFS COST CONSUMERS BILLIONS 5 (2010), http://www.ftc.gov/os/2010/01/100112payfordelayrpt.pdf.

[61] *See infra* Chapter 8.

[62] Also, a "No AG" agreement for one drug prohibited the launch of an AG for part of 2007, and no AG was launched thereafter. For a few other drugs, "No AG" agreements prohibited the launch of AGs only during exclusivity or for some strengths, but because an AG version of the drug was launched, the AG count in Figure 2-1 was unaffected.

[63] This issue is explored in Chapter 3, Section III.B.3.

[64] These were companies that had rights to the NDA for a brand-name drug that was included in the study because it was related to an AG, a paragraph IV certification, or first generic entry (with or without exclusivity) within specific time frames. The group of 55 companies that received the FTC's Special Order for brand-name companies, and four other companies that were identified later, included most major brand-name companies. *See infra* Appendix C. A few companies generally regarded as generic companies received both brand and generic Special Orders, because in addition to their ANDA-generic business they held a few NDAs that were the basis for marketing AGs. *See infra* Appendix H for more information on the criteria for inclusion of drugs and companies in the study.

[65] *See, e.g., infra* Chapter 5, text accompanying note 17.

[66] *See infra* text accompanying note 28 (agreements usually provide for AG launch upon ANDA-generic entry or the date of expected ANDA-generic launch); Chapter 4, Section III.A (AG launch usually occurs at ANDA-generic entry).

[67] *See infra* Chapter 3, Section III.C.2; Chapter 4, Section I.A. Brand strategies to address the loss of revenue at generic entry by promoting sales of a new patent-protected drug at the expense of a product for which generic entry has occurred (a "product hop") could be less effective or even incompatible with an AG, e.g., if the brand discontinues the NDA for the product experiencing generic entry.

[68] *See, e.g.,* FED. TRADE COMM'N & U.S. DEP'T OF JUSTICE, IMPROVING HEALTH CARE: A DOSE OF COMPETITION ch. 7, at 20 (2003), http://www.ftc.gov/reports/healthcare/040723health carerpt.pdf (discussing promotion and advertising of brand-name drugs to physicians and consumers, and noting the absence of such efforts with regard to generic products); FED. TRADE COMM'N, PHARMACY BENEFIT MANAGERS: OWNERSHIP OF MAIL ORDER PHARMACIES 6–7, 44–46 (2005), http://www.ftc.gov/reports/pharmbenefit05/050906pharmbenefitrpt. pdf (discussing competition for placement of brand-name but not generic drugs on PBM formularies); Haiden A. Huskamp et al., *Generic Entry, Reformulations and Promotion of SSRIs in the US,* 26 PHARMACOECONOMICS 603, 604, 606 (2008) (reviewing literature showing that brand-name drug promotional efforts decline significantly upon generic entry).

[69] *See, e.g.,* Company Document ("CD"), July 2004 (generic drugs are a "Commodity business; Highly competitive and price-driven; . . . Minimal focus on marketing"); CD, Dec. 8, 2004 (identifying "Competitive Pricing" first in a list of "Key Success Factors for Gx Manufacturers" in marketing to wholesalers and retailers).

[70] *See, e.g.,* CD, Dec. 8, 2004 (identifying "Broad portfolio" among "Key Success Factors"); CD, Mar. 31, 2005 (noting "[s]ome customer preference for larger ANDA portfolios"); CD, July 2004 (top generic firms provide "Product Quality & Consistency of Supply . . . lapses in supply [ruin relationship with customer] . . . Self-manufacturing is seen as a major advantage").

[71] The business model for the brand subsidiaries varied. From 2001–2008, the period covered by Figure 2-3, Greenstone, a subsidiary of Pfizer, was the primary example of a brand subsidiary with a generic portfolio limited to AGs of the parent's brand-name drugs. Beginning in 2009, however, Greenstone expanded its portfolio to include ANDA-generics and AGs for which the applications are held by other companies. *See,*

e.g., Lisa Lucarelli Chandler & Harry Dutt Samaroo, *Pfizer and the Greenstone Brand: A Sustainable Competitive Advantage?,* 10 J. MED. MARKETING 155, 157, 161 (2009), *available at* http://mmj.sagepub.com/content/10/2/155 ("The Greenstone subsidiary has morphed from a unit that marketed only Pfizer legacy products to a full line generic company" as a result of agreements with Aurobindo Ltd. and Claris Lifesciences Ltd. to market a variety of their generic products); Greenstone LLC, Press Release, Greenstone Selected as Eisai Partner to Launch Authorized Generic of Aricept® (Donepezil Hcl) Tablets (Sept. 8, 2010), http://www.greenstonellc.com/press-release-1.aspx. Other brand subsidiaries listed in Figure 2-3 also offered ANDA-generic or AG versions of other companies' brand-name drugs. Sandoz, a subsidiary of Novartis, and Roxane, a subsidiary of Boehringer Ingelheim, are examples.

[72] These include Watson, Teva, Barr, Mallinckrodt, and K-V Pharma. AGs marketed in-house represented a small fraction of the generic business of these companies, the bulk of which was ANDA-generic drugs, but also included AGs arising from agreements with brand-name companies. Although Barr merged with Teva and became Teva's subsidiary, Barr is treated as a separate company for purposes of this study because the merger did not become effective until December 23, 2008, close to the end of the period covered by the study. For more information on the study's treatment of companies that merged, *see infra* Appendix H.

[73] This addresses AGs marketed between January 1, 2001 and December 31, 2008. *See infra* Appendix H, Section II. The first number differs from the number of AG agreements identified *infra* in Chapter 8, which includes agreements that provide for the marketing of AGs in the future.

[74] A settlement in which the brand-name firm designates the first-filer to be the authorized generic (or grants the first-filer an exclusive license) does not undermine a generic's incentives to challenge patents because the AG neither competes against the first-filer's product nor reduces the first-filer's revenues. Such agreements are one form of a settlement in which the brand agrees to refrain from offering a competing AG. *See infra* Chapter 8.

[75] Exclusive supply and distribution agreements that authorize the marketing of an AG by the first-filer can raise competitive concerns. They are effectively "No AG" agreements, because, although the AG is marketed, there is no competing ANDA-generic. *See infra* Chapter 8.

[76] *See infra* Chapter 4, note 40 and accompanying text.

[77] Watson and Par are examples. As noted above, a generic licensee may be a subsidiary of another brand-name firm. *See supra* note 23.

[78] The specialized AG marketer is Prasco. Another AG marketer, Heritage Pharmaceuticals, did not expressly state that it specialized in AGs but had no ANDA-generic drugs with a paragraph IV certification or first generic entry (with or without exclusivity) within the study's time frames.

[79] *See, e.g.,* CD, May 18, 2004.

[80] *See, e.g.,* Agreement, 2007 ("[Generic Co.] acknowledges and agrees that during the Term, it shall not . . . file an ANDA . . . with the FDA or manufacture, market, sell or distribute any Competing Equivalent Product."); Agreement, 2006 (similar).

[81] *See, e.g.,* Agreement, 2007 (generic may manufacture and market an ANDA-generic product after the exclusivity period but is required to pay the same profit split on its ANDA-generic product as on the AG). Some settlement agreements also call for a profit split on ANDA-generic products. *See* Settlement Agreement, 2005 (marketing of ANDA-generic version); *id.* (royalty of 5% of net sales of the ANDA-generic); Settlement Agreement, 2005 (option to market ANDA-generic instead of AG); *id.* (requiring the generic to pay 20% of its profits on the ANDA-generic product). This Report cites all agreements arising from settlements or patent litigation, including settlements, licenses and supply and distribution agreements, as settlement agreements.

[82] *See infra* Chapter 4, note 46; *cf.* Settlement Agreement, 2001 ("Buyer may discount . . .Generic Products or sell . . . Generic Products at a loss or without compensation . . . after negotiation of terms acceptable to [brand] to compensate [brand] for any loss of Net Profit distribution . . . incurred by [brand] as a result of such actions by Buyer").

[83] *See, e.g.,* Agreement, 2004 ("'Transfer Price' means an amount equal to Manufacturer's Direct Cost for the Product."); Agreement, 2003 ("Delivery Price" is equal to the "Seller's Cost of Goods for the manufacture and supply of such Product"); Agreement, 2004 ("[generic co.] shall pay to [brand-name co.] a transfer price equal to [brand-name co.]'s actual cost of Product").

[84] *See infra* Chapter 4, Section III.B.

[85] The inverse relationship between exclusivities and AGs could also arise from brand-name company preferences; as discussed above, some brand-name companies will not contract with generic firms that have filed an ANDA or made a Paragraph IV certification for a bioequivalent product. *See supra* text accompanying note 31.

[86] Generic companies may tap the high revenues available during 180-day exclusivity by marketing AGs. The top four companies for marketing AGs by contract (Figure 2-6) sold about one-third of such AGs during 180-day exclusivity, about the same fraction as for AGs overall (Figure 2-8). Generic company documents discussing plans to market AGs highlighted their value during 180-day exclusivity. *See generally* CD, Jan. 15, 2006 ("Strategic Rationale" for entering into an agreement to market two AGs: "Accelerates path to profitability . . . by accessing profit share during exclusivity period . . . ."); CD, May 6, 2005 (favorable AG opportunities include "Paragraph IV exclusivities (key value drivers)").

[87] Data regarding recent trends in the timing of generic entry and the length of brand-name firm exclusivity are presented in Appendix K.

[88] For example, the Prescription Access Litigation Project has argued that "the intent [of marketing an AG] is not to foster true competition but merely to sabotage the ability of the ANDA filer to take advantage of the 180-day exclusivity period provided for by Hatch Waxman." Public Comment from the Prescription Access Litig. Project et al. to the Fed. Trade Comm'n 4 (June 5, 2006), http://www.ftc.gov/os/comments/genericdrugstudy3/060605pal.pdf. Similarly, the Generic Pharmaceutical Association ("GPhA") stated, "Authorized generics occur when a brand company introduces or licenses a 'generic' version of its product to compete with the true generic during the 180-day exclusivity period, awarded to the first generic manufacturer to challenge the patent." Public Comment from the GPhA to the Fed. Trade Comm'n 1 n.2 (June 27, 2006), http://www.ftc.gov/os/ comments/genericdrugstudy3/062806gpha.pdf.

[89] *See supra* note 4 and accompanying text.

[90] Although subject to fluctuation from year to year, the number of exclusivity periods generally has grown during the period analyzed; whereas nineteen exclusivity periods started in 2001–2003, twenty-nine began in 2006–2008. *See* Figure 2-7.

[91] Most "No AG" agreements do not restrict launch of an AG after the expiration of 180-day exclusivity, although the restrictions have lasted longer on some products with low sales. *See infra* Chapter 8, Figure 8-3.

[92] AGs marketed outside or without exclusivity included those launched after conclusion of an exclusivity period as well as AGs for drugs for which there was no exclusivity period. (Also, in one instance the first-filer marketed, and discontinued, an AG before its 180-day exclusivity period began.) This calculation excludes AGs launched during exclusivity that the brand continued to market after the exclusivity period expired. Nor does it include drugs for which first generic entry occurred prior to January 1, 2001.

[93] AGs "[n]ot marketed during an exclusivity period" include four AGs that were marketed by the ANDA-generic that was the first-filer for the relevant drug. These AGs, like others marketed apart from exclusivity, likely would not have created a disincentive for patent challenges; indeed, they contributed to the first-filers' revenues. A fifth first-filer AG was marketed during a 180-day exclusivity period shared by two competitors, which, under the circumstances, likely would have anticipated a third competitor during the exclusivity period.

[94] Figure 2-9 examines the rate of AG launch by pre-entry market size for drugs for which first generic entry occurred during the April 2003–December 2008 period analyzed. Because the purpose of that figure is to examine whether 180-day exclusivity affects the propensity to launch an AG, the appropriate comparison is between first generic entry with and without exclusivity at similar sales levels. Launches of AGs into mature markets are not included because the decision whether to launch an AG into a mature market involves consideration of an additional factor, the ability to gain share in a market with established generic competitors. By contrast, other figures in this chapter include AGs launched into mature markets as well as those launched at first generic entry because the analyses are intended to show the circumstances of launch of all AGs.

[95] First generic entry may occur without 180-day exclusivity because no ANDA included a Paragraph IV certification, e.g., all generic applicants may have certified to the FDA that they would wait for patent expiration before entering. Moreover, even when an ANDA included a Paragraph IV certification, entry occurs without exclusivity under a number of circumstances, e.g., if the first-filer loses the infringement litigation and obtains FDA approval of its ANDA after patent expiration; launches its ANDA-generic product more than 180-days after exclusivity was triggered by a court decision; or relinquishes or forfeits its exclusivity. *See, e.g.,* David E. Korn, Erika Lietzan & Shaw W. Scott, *A New History and Discussion of 180-Day Exclusivity,* 64 FOOD & DRUG L.J. 335 (2009); Shashank Upadhye, GENERIC PHARMACEUTICAL PATENT AND FDA LAW ch. 13, 14 (2010).

[96] *See infra* Chapter 4, Section I.A.

[97] A Paragraph I certification requires an ANDA applicant to state that "patent information has not been filed," while a Paragraph II certification requires an applicant to state that "such patent has expired." 21 U.S.C. §§ 355(j)(2)(A)(vii)(I), (II). Certification under Paragraph III identifies the date on which the patent will expire, 21 U.S.C. § 355(j)(2)(A)(vii)(III), and indicates that the applicant is seeking ANDA approval only after patent expiration.

Twelve AGs were "old antibiotics" that originally were approved under 21 U.S.C. § 357, and thus were exempt from the Hatch-Waxman patent listing, patent certification, and 180-day exclusivity provisions of 21 U.S.C. § 355. Although no patent certifications could have been made for these drugs, the FDA database lists them among ANDAs with Paragraph I filings. Eleven of the 12 were marketed from 2001–2006. Even if the 11 "old antibiotics" were excluded from the analysis of those years, about half of the AGs from 2001–2006 (40 out of 81) arose from NDAs of drugs for which there was no patent challenge.

[98] One possibility is that they could reflect a decline in the prevalence of drugs that were not subject to patent challenges, rather than a shift in the reasons for AG launch. *See* Chapter 7, Section II; *see also* AARON GAL & NIKHIL R. CHARI, BERNSTEIN RESEARCH, THE LONG VIEW: U.S. GENERIC PHARMACEUTICALS -A BOTTOM-UP MODEL OF THE U.S. COMMODITY GENERICS MARKET IN 2009, at 3, 7, 13, 14 (by dollar or prescription volume, Paragraph IV drugs increased in prevalence from 2004 through 2008 and comprised the bulk of generic market entry beginning in 2006). Another possibility is that the drop in AGs marketed apart from

exclusivity and Paragraph IV certifications could have arisen from decisions not to market less profitable AGs as a result of implementation of the Deficit Reduction Act in 2007. *See infra* Appendix J.

[99] FED. TRADE COMM'N, AUTHORIZED GENERICS: AN INTERIM REPORT ("Interim Report") (2009), http://www.ftc.gov/os/2009/06/P062105authorizedgenericsreport.pdf.

[100] The analysis performed in this chapter allows for careful consideration of the statistical properties of the estimates. The analysis of price effects, for instance, often yields estimated effects that would not be unlikely to have been observed even if the true effect was zero, in which case the estimated effects are characterized as not statistically different from zero or "statistically insignificant." Just how unlikely the estimated effect would be if the true effect actually was zero is often referred to as the level of significance. For instance, if the significance level associated with an estimated effect is 10%, that would generally be considered weaker evidence that the observed data was inconsistent with a true average effect of zero than if the significance level is 5%.

[101] IMS CONSULTING, IMS HEALTH, ASSESSMENT OF AUTHORIZED GENERICS IN THE U.S. (2006) (written for the Pharm. Research and Mfrs. of Am. ("PhRMA")), http://replay.web. archive.org/20061009134405/http://www.phrma.org/files/IMS%20Authorized%20Generics%20Report_6-22-06.pdf ("the IMS Study").

[102] *Id.* at 9–11.

[103] Aidan Hollis & Bryan A. Liang, *An Assessment of the Effect of Authorized Generics on Consumer Prices,* 10 J. BIOLAW & BUS. 10, 20–21 (2007) (written for the Generic Pharm. Ass'n ("GPhA")) (an earlier version of this article was made available by GPhA in July 2006, *available at* http://www.gphaonline.org/sites/default/files/GPhA_AG_Study.pdf) ("Hollis and Liang").

[104] *Id.* at 11–12.

[105] *Id.* at 14.

[106] For example, the authors contend that minor drugs such as Ganciclovir should not be weighted as heavily as major drugs such as Fluoxetine. *Id.* at14.

[107] PHRMA, HOWREY LLP & CAPANALYSIS, AUTHORIZED GENERICS BENEFIT CONSUMERS BY REDUCING PRICES: A REPLY TO HOLLIS & LIANG (2007), http://www.howrey.com/files/ News/29b5c3ee-6dd3-480f-9c42-c2dd170f7e94/Presentation/NewsAttachment/0e5f5d06-0649-453a-8784-efe59844cea1/ Authorized%20 Generics%20Benefit%20Report.pdf.

[108] *Id.* at 6–8.

[109] HOWREY LLP, THE SHORT-TERM AND LONG-TERM COMPETITIVE IMPACT OF AUTHORIZED GENERICS 14–15 (2009) (written for PhRMA), http://www.ftc.gov/os/comments/generic drug study3/091028pharmresearch.pdf.

[110] Estimating the impact on consumers in pharmaceutical markets is indeed a very difficult task, due not only to the prevalence of private health insurance, but also government programs. The Centers for Medicare and Medicaid Services estimate that in 2007, consumers' out-of-pocket payments accounted for 21% of expenditures on pharmaceuticals; private health insurance paid for 44%; and public funds covered the remaining 35%. *See National Health Expenditure Data: Historical*, CTRS. FOR MEDICARE AND MEDICAID SERVS., http://www.cms.gov/NationalHealthExpendData/02_NationalHealthAccountsHistorical.asp. The extent to which a given retail price increase is passed on to each of these types of payers depends on contracts between retail pharmacies and pharmacy benefit managers; contracts between pharmacy benefit managers and health insurance plan sponsors; provisions of health benefit plans; and Medicare and Medicaid regulations. Untangling this web of dependencies is beyond the scope of this Report.

[111] A detailed description of these sources and how they were processed is provided in Appendix I.

[112] The full reference for data that will be referred to as retail or NPA data is: IMS Health, IMS National Prescription Audit Plus 7™, Years 2003 to 2008, Data Extracted January 2009. The channels included in our National Prescription Audit data are Chain Stores, Food Stores, Independents, Long-Term Care, and Mail Service. The full reference for data that will be referred to as wholesale or NSP data is: IMS Health, IMS National Sales Perspectives™, January 2003 to December 2008, Retail and Non-Retail Channels, Data Extracted February 2009. The channels included in our National Sales Perspectives data are: Chain Stores, Clinics, Federal Facilities, Food Stores, HMOs, Home Health Care, Independents, Long-Term Care, Mail Service, Misc-Other, Misc-Prisons, Misc-Universities, and Non-Federal Hospitals. The analysis presented here aggregates all sales across channels.

[113] The monthly Producer Price Index (PPI) for finished goods (WPSSOP3000) over the period of our data (January 2003 through December 2008) is obtained from the Bureau of Labor Statistics. *See Producer Price Indexes*, BUREAU OF LABOR STATISTICS, http://www.bls.gov/ ppi/data.htm.

[114] Throughout this chapter and Chapter 6, the term "product" refers to a full specification of active ingredient(s), dosage form, and strength. The term "molecule" refers to the set of active ingredients that are included in a single tablet or capsule. The definition of a "product" using IMS data, for purposes of this chapter and Chapter 6, differs from the definition of a "drug" used elsewhere in this Report in describing data from the FDA. FDA drug information is provided at the NDA and ANDA level, whereas IMS product information is provided at the level of the molecule-dosage-form-strength-therapeutic class.

[115] Sales of a generic or AG product prior to the end of an FDA-granted exclusivity period are treated as occurring during an exclusivity period.

[116] The analysis in this chapter compares prices and expenditures before and shortly after first generic entry. In order to ensure availability of at least three months' data prior to generic entry, the analysis is limited to products with first generic entry no earlier than April 2003. Chapters 3 and 6 do not cover introductions of AGs that occurred from 2003 through 2008 if another generic entered prior to April of 2003. As such, this should be seen as an analysis of the impact of AGs on recently genericized markets.

[117] For instance, among products with 180-day exclusivity, the average market size for products with an AG was more than twice that when no AG was launched ($381 million versus $178 million). The difference was even more pronounced for products that were not subject to a Paragraph IV challenge. As was the case for Figure 2-9, market size is calculated throughout this chapter as the annualized retail sales of the brand-name product based on the three months prior to generic entry, measured in December 2008 dollars.

[118] The endogeneity of the decision to issue an AG was also addressed by using instrumental variables regression analysis. These regressions used either market size, brand-name firm identity, or both to predict whether an AG would be launched, and then estimated the impact of the predicted presence of an AG on prices. The results of this analysis did not differ substantively from the results reported here.

[119] In addition, AG competitors might replace potentially more aggressive ANDA-generic competitors outside of the 180-day exclusivity period. In this way, consumers could face higher prices for generic products outside of exclusivity. Chapter 6 explores this issue.

[120] Other competitive environments are possible due to legal provisions that allow for shared exclusivity; settlement arrangements between brand-name and ANDA-generic firms; or other market anomalies. For example, the third most commonly observed competitive arrangement during exclusivity is an AG-only market, but this is a distant third. Generally, such arrangements can be explained by settlements between brand-name and ANDA-generic firms or short-run supply problems for the ANDA-generic firm. Our econometric specifications account for the possibility that atypical competitive environments could generate atypical market outcomes by including in the price regressions an indicator variable for these markets. The coefficient on this indicator variable is rarely statistically significant.

[121] Of the 40 molecules observed during exclusivity, only seven (16.7%) have at least one strength or dosage form that faces an AG competitor and one that does not. For the typical molecule in the sample, either all or none of the strengths face AG competition.

[122] Because the sample is limited to oral solid dosage forms, the extended units are equivalent to molecule-strength-dosage-form combinations. In other words, the analysis is done at the 9-digitNational Drug Code level.

[123] For both the retail and wholesale analysis, the monthly generic market price for a product is calculated as the total sales dollars of *all* generic products divided by the extended units sold by *all* generic manufacturers. For example, in markets that have both an ANDA and an AG in the market, this calculation represents the sum of the total sales dollars from the ANDA and the AG divided by the total extended units sold by the ANDA and the AG. Consequently, in markets with more than one manufacturer the generic price is a weighted average of all generic manufacturer prices.

[124] To be more precise, let G be the average price of a generic product in the current month, and B the average price of the brand-name product in the three months prior to generic entry. The generic relative price would be calculated as G/B. The generic discount off the pre-entry brand price, as discussed in the Interim Report, *supra* note 1, is 1-G/B.

[125] *See infra* Appendix L for details regarding the exact specification of the model.

[126] These prices are plotted for one month only, so that all data points reflect markets that have had the same amount of time to adjust to generic entry. Month four data reflect conditions after the markets have had some time to adjust to generic entry, but before the end of exclusivity was imminent. Corresponding graphs for other months are not substantially different.

[127] The manufacturers are included in the regression by a set of indicator variables that describe the competitive environment. For example, all of the models include dummy variable indicators (variables that take the value of one if true and zero if false) representing each possible number of manufacturers, whether an AG is present, and interactions between the two. The dependent variable is the generic relative price. Logarithmic transformations of the relative price result in nearly identical AG effects in all pricing models. *See infra* Appendix L for a more detailed description of the model employed and its assumptions.

[128] Similarly, controlling for other product attributes, such as dosage form and the months since entry, can help control for factors that could be related to the presence of an AG and price. For example, a consumer may be more reluctant to switch to generic forms of a product with an extended release formula, and producing generic versions of extended-release drugs may be relatively more costly than for typical drugs, making those products both less attractive as AG markets and likely to experience higher relative generic prices. Controlling for the number of months since entry can take separate account of any market dynamics associated with a product's life cycle, such as the decline of advertising's influence over time.

[129] The Interim Report, *supra* note 1, estimated the difference in the discounts between markets with an AG and markets without an AG. In order to convert the differences from that report to a percentage change in the generic price as reported here, they would need to be divided by the average price of the generic. For example, the Interim Report found that the unweighted average difference between retail discounts in ANDA+AG and

ANDA-Only markets was -4.2%. Dividing that by the ANDA-Only Mean Relative Price of 0.86 from the unweighted analysis in Table 3-1 would yield -4.8%, which is very close to what is reported here, given that the standard error of the estimated effect is reported in Table 3-1 to be 2.8%. The Interim Report also estimated the difference to be -4.3% when taking a weighted average (and dropping clopidogrel from the analysis, as was done here), which is similar to the analysis in column (iii) of Table 3-1. Dividing that -4.3% difference by the weighted average generic price of 0.9 yields a percentage change in the discount of about -4.8%, which is also quite close to the -4.2% reported in column (iii).

[130] "Clustering" standard errors is a statistical technique to account for the fact that some observations may essentially be co-determined. For instance, if a company sells both 100mg and 200mg tablets of the same drug, there is no reason to expect the 200mg tablets to be exactly twice as expensive as the 100mg tablets. However, it is entirely possible that the company would want to price a 200mg tablet somewhat higher than a 100mg tablet. If so, the prices of these products should not be treated as independent observations. Similarly, it may not be reasonable to assume that the price of the 200mg tablet in one month is independent of the price of the 200mg tablet in the preceding month. Although clustering the standard errors assumes that observations of different clusters are independent, the clustering allows calculation of standard errors that account for correlation between observations within the same cluster. Thus, a decision to cluster by molecule allows the model to determine the correlation between observations of the same molecule but with different months, strengths, and dosage forms. However, observations from different molecules are assumed to be independent from each other.

[131] A 95% Confidence interval indicates that if the data generating process were repeated many times, and the estimations were performed on each instance of the data generating process, roughly 95% of the confidence intervals would contain the true average AG effect. The 95% confidence intervals for these AG effects can be calculated using the estimated AG effect and their standard errors, where the interval is (Estimated AG Effect)±1.96×(Standard Error). As a rule of thumb, similar confidence intervals can be calculated for all such effects by doubling the standard error and adding and subtracting that from the estimated effect.

[132] Clustering the standard errors has a big impact on the estimated standard errors. If the regression in column (i) is performed without clustering, the estimated effect does not change (-3.8%), but the estimated standard error drops from 2.8% to 0.7%, which would imply a 95% confidence interval of [5.2%, -2.4%]. Incorrectly treating all the observations as if they were independent would cause the statistical significance of the analysis to be greatly overstated.

[133] Although the estimated effects of AG competition are larger using wholesale prices rather than retail prices, this is partially explained by the fact that the base wholesale prices are lower. Averaged across all drugs in the sample, the pre-entry brand wholesale prices are on average 10% lower than pre-entry brand retail prices. Furthermore, larger discounts off these brand prices are observed in the wholesale data. The base ANDA-Only mean relative prices, off of which these AG effects are taken, are lower at the wholesale level.

[134] The results are remarkably stable with regard to model specification: they are nearly identical in sign and magnitude whether the model includes no product characteristics or a full set of indicators. identifying the product of interest.

[135] Another way to address this question would be to compare generic prices in markets with one ANDA competitor and one AG to generic prices in markets with only two ANDA competitors. Unfortunately, the number of observations of the latter type of market condition was insufficient to allow for meaningful statistical analysis.

[136] A word of caution with respect to the measurement of brand prices and revenues in this chapter and Chapter 6 is warranted. Rebates paid by brand-name companies are not included in our data. Rebates can be substantially scaled back upon generic entry, and the impact of such practices will not be reflected in the brand prices or revenues reported here. This may cause the levels of both brand prices and revenues following generic entry to be understated in our data. Since this impact would be present regardless of whether an AG is launched, we have no reason to believe it biases our estimate of AG impacts on either brand prices or revenues.

[137] These prices are for the same set of products used in the generic product analysis during exclusivity. All of the products considered eventually face an FDA-granted exclusivity period. Price changes are measured relative to the month of generic entry.

[138] The model that produces these percentage changes regresses the logarithm of brand price against product fixed-effects and time dummy variables. The models are estimated separately for the sample with and without an AG. Both series plotted in Figure 3-3 represent the coefficient estimates on the month-since-entry dummy variables. Dummy variable coefficients in log-linear models are approximations of the average percent change.

[139] In contrast, the average retail relative prices for brand-name products were slightly higher than the pre-entry brand prices.

[140] This result may be surprising in light of economic research dating back to Frank and Salkever (1997), which shows that brands generally raise their prices upon generic entry. *See* Richard G. Frank & David S. Salkever, *Generic Entry and the Pricing of Pharmaceuticals*, 6 J. ECON. & MGMT. STRATEGY 75 (1997). However, this new finding only appears in the context of 180-day exclusivity periods, and we know of no published study that restricts attention to brand pricing during 180-day exclusivity periods. A report submitted to the FTC by

Howrey LLP on behalf of PhRMA, *supra* note 9, at 23, also found brand that wholesale prices dropped following generic entry in markets with an AG.

141 *See infra* Chapter 8.

142 The price effects reported in Table 3-6 are the predicted results from a regression model that includes the full set of controls employed in Tables 3-1 and 3-2.

143 Technically, issuing an AG could be profit-maximizing if the costs of issuing an AG were lower than not issuing an AG. This seems unlikely.

144 Our measure of wholesale expenditures is the total dollars reported in the IMS National Sales Perspective (NSP) database, which is the total amount paid by pharmacies.

145 The wholesale data include wholesaler margins, which may differ on the products that pass through wholesalers. This could bias the results if the proportions of products going through wholesalers are systematically different for products with and without AG sales. However, we have no reason to believe that is the case.

146 Profits are obviously preferable to revenues as a metric for estimating AG competition effects. Although profits cannot be estimated directly, Chapter 6 uses revenue estimates in a break-even simulation that considers firm costs in an effort to address the impact of AG competition on the profitability of generic entry through patent challenges.

147 Differences in the sample sizes reported in Tables 3-2 and 3-7 reflect the fact that some of the products considered in the price analysis do not have an ANDA firm present in the market and therefore would not be included in the analysis of AG effects on ANDA revenues. These products represent "AG Only" markets, discussed earlier.

148 Table 3-7 reports results from four model specifications that are very similar to those used in developing Tables 3-1 and 3-2. The regression models control for how the number of manufacturers and their type affect the variable of interest, which in this case is the relative expenditures on the first-filer generic (rather than the relative market price). The specifications differ with respect to what variables are included in a way that is exactly analogous to those presented in Tables 3-1 and 3-2. In contrast to the pricing model, the revenue model focuses on those revenues generated by a subset of generic firms, specifically, ANDA-generic firms, rather than considering overall market revenues. (The pricing model considered the effect of AG competition on a weighted average of all generic prices, including the AG price, rather than the prices of ANDA-generic firms.)

149 A note of caution is appropriate in interpreting these results: a failure to control for unobserved characteristics relevant to the decision to market an AG is virtually certain to bias the estimates of changes in brand expenditures. The point has particular relevance here. In the pricing context, unobserved market characteristics that influence the decision to launch an AG may or may not be correlated with generic pricing. However, market characteristics that explain the decision to launch an AG almost certainly are strongly correlated with the amount of revenue that the brand expects to lose when facing generic competition.

150 Here, all AGs are treated as if they are marketed by a subsidiary of the brand-name company. Sometimes the brand-name firm will license the rights to distribute an AG to an independent marketer, in which case, the brand-name firm will not receive all of the revenue associated with sales of the AG. The brand-name firm, however, typically receives both a transfer price and a share of any profits – usually a large share, unless a patent litigation settlement is involved. *See supra* Chapter 2, Section I.B.2.b.ii; *infra* Chapter 4, Section III.B; Company Document, Oct. 12, 2004 (stating that the share of profits awarded to generic firms in AG marketing arrangements had fallen to 10 percent or less).

151 All of the estimates are imprecisely estimated, and neither model that controls for product characteristics can reject the hypothesis that introducing an AG has no effect on brand-name firm revenues.

152 Public Comment from the Generic Pharm. Ass'n ("GPhA") to the Fed. Trade Comm'n 3 (June 27, 2006), http://www.ftc.gov/os/comments/genericdrugstudy3/062806gpha.pdf.

153 Public Comment from Gilbert's LLP to the Fed. Trade Comm'n 1–2 (June 5, 2006), http:// www.ftc.gov/os/ comments/genericdrugstudy3/060605gilberts.pdf (contending that "the ultimate goal of brand name companies in launching authorized generics is to neutralize the legislative scheme intended by Congress to nurture a vigorous generic industry").

154 *See* Henry Grabowski, *Competition between Generic and Branded Drugs*, *in* PHARMACEUTICAL INNOVATION: INCENTIVES, COMPETITION, AND COST-BENEFIT ANALYSIS IN INTERNATIONAL PERSPECTIVE 153, 154–58 (Frank A. Sloan & Chee-Ruey Hsieh eds., 2007) (generic share increased from 19% in 1984 to 51% in 2002).

155 *See* PHARM. RESEARCH AND MFRS. OF AM. ("PHRMA"), PHARMACEUTICAL INDUSTRY PROFILE (2010), http://www.phrma.org/sites/default/files/159/profile_2010_final.pdf (citing IMS Health data); *see also* GPHA, 2010 ANNUAL REPORT 23 (2010), http://www.gpha online.org/sites/default/files/GPhA%202010%20Annual%20Report.pdf (also citing IMS Health data); Company Document ("CD"), Oct. 10, 2007 ("Generic revenue & Rx penetration is at an all time high and continues to out pace branded product growth.").

156 *See, e.g.*, Tracy L. Regan, *Generic Entry, Price Competition, and Market Segmentation in the Prescription Drug Market,* 26 INT'L J. INDUS. ORG. 930, 939–940 (2008) (reporting brand share six months after entry of approximately 40 percent, based on generic entries from 1998–2001); *see also* Grabowski, *supra* note 3, at 158–59 (citing Atanu Saha et al., *Generic Competition in the U.S. Pharmaceutical Industry*, 13 INT'L J. ECON. BUS. 15 (2006)) (finding brand share six months after entry of about 60 percent, based on generic entry in the

1990s); CD, May 25, 2006 (showing brand market share at 26 weeks of approximately 70 percent, based on 1991–1993 CBO data).

[157] *See, e.g.*, CD, May 25, 2006 (in 2005, brand share 26 weeks after entry was less than 20 percent, based on IMS data); CD, Mar. 31, 2006 (indicating that a single generic product sold during 180-day exclusivity can be expected to erode branded share by "about 80% in the first few months"); CD, Sept. 27, 2004 ("Accelerating Rate of Generic Penetration . . . 80% conversion within 4–6 weeks, compared to 60% within 6–8 months just a few years ago"); *see also* Murray Aitken, Ernst R. Berndt & David M. Cutler, *Prescription Drug Spending Trends in the United States: Looking Beyond the Turning Point*, 28 HEALTH AFF. w151, w155 (2009) ("[I]n 2002 branded products retained 28 percent of their prescription volume twelve months after patent expiry. In 2007 that figure dropped to 14 percent."). The Commission's Interim Report found that during the sixth month of exclusivity, brand share of retail quantities dispensed averaged under thirty percent in markets without AGs and approximately sixteen percent in markets where AGs were present. FED. TRADE COMM'N, AUTHORIZED GENERICS: AN INTERIM REPORT ("Interim Report") ch. 1, at 15–16 (2009), http://www.ftc.gov/os/2009/06/P062105authorizedgenericsreport.pdf.

[158] *See, e.g.*, MEDCO, 2009 DRUG TREND REPORT 22 (2009), http://medco.mediaroom.com/ file.php/177/2009+DRUG+TREND+REPORT.pdf (reporting that 30 days after generic entry, Fosamax lost 84 percent of its market share at retail).

[159] *See, e.g.*, CD, 2006 (denoted "DRAFT") ("launch [subsidiary's] generic products to maximize post-LOE return and provide [parent] a competitive generic offering").

[160] CD, June 28, 2004 (the brand's AG subsidiary is the "[c]ornerstone of US LOE strategy to leverage [the brand's] strengths and capture value post-LOE").

[161] CD, undated.

[162] *See, e.g.* CD, Nov. 2004 ("[p]rovides high margin to [branded firm] during exclusivity period . . . [a]bility to launch on day one of competitors 180 day exclusivity provides greatest dollar return"); CD, undated (illustrating greater AG revenue potential during 180-day exclusivity period than with no exclusivity).

[163] CD, Dec. 1, 2006.

[164] CD, Nov. 11, 2005; *see also* CD, Sept. 15, 2005 (without 180-day exclusivity, "economic potential is minimal").

[165] *See, e.g.*, CD, Nov. 4, 2004 (forecast of brand and AG sales, gross margin, royalties, and business unit contribution with different numbers of generics and with no AG, simultaneous launch, and early launch); CD, Sept. 8, 2005 (best- and worst-case forecasts of sales, share, and margin).

[166] *See, e.g.*, CD, May 5, 2004 ("Key Success Factors" for AG include "Assessment of . . . sales cannibalization; Accurate forecasting of the financial return"); CD, June 7, 2003 (forecast methodology based on recent market share and price erosion); CD, 2005–2006 (sales forecasts with best- and worst-case assumptions regarding sales, share, and erosion); CD, undated (forecasts of profits and profit share used in selecting AG distributor). These forecasts are evidence that brand-name companies are looking at AGs as a revenue opportunity.

[167] *See, e.g.*, CD, undated ("Financials: Proj[ected] vs. actual: Branded share erosion; Share captured by the authorized generic; Price erosion; [Brand Firm] Sales / BUC").

[168] *See, e.g.*, CD, Mar. 31, 2006 (launching an AG simultaneously with third party entry "[d]elivers incremental revenue which otherwise would be lost to the generic challenger"); CD, 2005 (AGs generate "*incremental* volume and profits"); CD, Mar. 22, 2005 (launching AG would result in "incremental net trade sales and net income"). Indeed, many brand-name firms' documents suggest that if the supply of ANDA-generic products is sufficient to satisfy demand, marketing an AG will not accelerate erosion of brand sales. *See, e.g.*, CD, 2005 (AG can be used to "[r]ealize a share of the generic market, without cannibalizing the Rx tail"); CD, July 2003 (analysis of previous AGs indicated that "Authorized Generics Do Not Negatively Impact Brand Share"); CD, Feb. 8, 2002 ("the substitution of brand to generic on this product will occur at the same rate irrespective of [an AG] launch or not"); CD, Nov. 2004 (stating that when an AG is launched in response to generic entry, there is "[n]o acceleration of brand erosion" because there is "no incentive for customer to accelerate substitution"). This is consistent with firm analyses finding that so long as one generic substitute is available, presence of a second generic product does not accelerate substitution. *See, e.g.*, CD, Mar. 23, 2005 ("No correlation between brand erosion and the number of generic entrants."). In contrast, the expectation that brand sales are not eroded by AGs might conflict with the empirical findings of Table 3-8, which show lower expenditures on brand-name products with AG introduction. However, as previously suggested, the analysis that underlies that table cannot distinguish between an AG increasing brand erosion and brands having greater incentives to introduce AGs for products that would rapidly lose sales to generics regardless of whether an AG is introduced. *See supra*, Chapter 3, note 51. The documentary evidence points toward the latter explanation.

[169] *See supra* Chapter 3, Table 3-9 (showing statistical significance for models without controls but not for models with controls). Similarly, analysis of the post-exclusivity data shows a positive average effect on brand-name firm wholesale relative expenditures from marketing an AG. *See infra* Chapter 6, Table 6-6. Results for the latter period, however, were not statistically significant.

[170] Other than when AGs were introduced, brands cut price only 20% as much as the ANDA-generics during the 180-day exclusivity period (based on unweighted prices). Weighting showed brand price reductions that were 65% of those of ANDA-generics. *Compare supra* Chapter 3, Table 3-2 *with* Chapter 3, Table 3-5.

[171] *See* CD, undated (indicating that AGs are preferable to price equalization because AGs "allow for market segmentation," i.e., they "[m]aintain branded price for patients with low price sensitivity"); CD, undated (powerpoint prepared for June 2005 presentation listing as the first benefit of an AG strategy, "Segment the market"). The technique of selling both low- and high-priced versions of the same product is not unique to pharmaceutical drugs; price discrimination has long been recognized as a potential means for enhancing a firm's total revenues. *See, e.g.*, ROBERT S. PINDYCK & DANIEL L. RUBINFELD, MICROECONOMICS 381–82 (4th ed. 1997) (explaining that a company that sells the same product in different bottles at different prices to different segments of the market "does it because the practice is profitable"); DENNIS W. CARLTON & JEFFREY M. PERLOFF, MODERN INDUSTRIAL ORGANIZATION 293 (4th ed. 2005) (explaining that, under certain conditions, "[a] firm price discriminates to increase its profits").

[172] *See, e.g.*, Thomas Chen, Note, *Authorized Generics: A Prescription for Hatch-Waxman Reform*, 93 VA. L. REV. 459, 473–77 (2007), *available at* http://www.virginialawreview. org/content/pdfs/93/459.pdf (discussing physician prescription practices and consumer loyalties to brand-name drugs).

[173] *See* CD, undated; CD. Feb. 17, 2005.

[174] *See* CD, undated.

[175] In contrast, the brand may find it easier to take advantage of such developments when it need merely limit availability of an AG. *See* CD, Sept. 17, 2004 (noting that if the brand-name firm's AG subsidiary launches before a TRO decision is reached and the generic competitor is forced to pull back, "we would pull back also"); CD, Mar. 29, 2006 (discussing plans for transitioning to withdrawal of AG following anticipated withdrawal of ANDA-generic competition after reversal of a lower court's patent unenforceability ruling).

[176] *See* CD, undated (noting "[d]ifficulty in justifying price of follow-on compounds" if a discounted price serves as the reference).

[177] *Id.* at 0010; CD, undated (explaining that because generics must be priced lower than brand-name drugs in order to be eligible for substitution, a price equalization effort would just force the generics to reduce price further); *see also* Kent S. Bernard & Willard K. Tom, *Antitrust Treatment of Pharmaceutical Patent Settlements*, 15 FED. CIR. B.J. 617, 624 (2006) (citing a 2005 Novartis study finding mandatory generic-use policies applicable to nearly all Medicaid enrollees and a 97.1 percent generic substitution rate for Medicaid plans); Nicole Hubersfeld, *Clear Notice for Conditions on Spending, Unclear Implications for States in Federal Healthcare Programs*, 86 N.C. L. REV. 441, 479 (2008) (noting that "some states limit their [Medicaid] formularies to generic drugs").

[178] CD, undated.

[179] *See* CD, undated (discussing retail chains); CD, undated ("PBM's will substitute with a generic regardless of how much the branded price is discounted").

[180] The documents add insight regarding the implications of our finding that "first-filer generics make considerably less revenue when an AG enters the market," Chapter 3, Section IV, with the magnitude of the AG-entry effect during exclusivity ranging between -39.6% and -52.0%, depending on the model employed. *See supra* Chapter 3, Table 3-7; *cf.* CD, Oct. 6, 2005 (projecting that a first-filer generic's product would lose 29–32% of its net present value over roughly a five-year time frame if faced with AG competition).

[181] CD, June 7, 2003; *see also* CD, 2006 (denoted "DRAFT") ("AGs have had a significant impact on market pricing especially during the 180-day exclusivity period. . . . The increased competition has led to significant price erosion and reduced revenue for generic companies.").

[182] CD, Oct. 2005. The same document, however, lists above the quoted entry the point that AGs"[m]aximize profits for brands facing generic competitors." *Id.*

[183] CD, Apr. 25 (year unspecified).

[184] CD, Mar. 27, 2006.

[185] *See supra* Chapter 2, Section II.B.

[186] *See supra* Chapter 2, Figure 2-10.

[187] *See* CD, Nov. 2004 (AG's share is enhanced by launching before the brand loses exclusivity because "historically the first generic to market captures significant value during 'duopoly period' and gains a significant foothold in market share"); CD, undated ("[f]ive day pre-emptive launch would secure added retail share"); CD, Feb. 2, 2004 (concluding that AG marketing "make[s] the launch of subsequent generic product more difficult by establishing a strong early market share, and the product placed on appropriate formularies"); Chen, *supra* note 21, at 478–79 (arguing that pharmacies' tendency to stock only one generic confers a substantial advantage on first generic to enter).

[188] CD, Mar. 31, 2004 (considering whether the brand's AG subsidiary should adopt a strategy of early launch to deter patent challenges). However, another brand-name firm that considered launching an AG slightly before generic entry carefully evaluated effects on brand and AG revenue but did not include any disincentive effect in its calculus. *See, e.g.*, CD, Mar. 8–9, 2005.

[189] *See, e.g.*, CD, undated; Saami Zain, *Sword or Shield? An Overview and Competitive Analysis of the Marketing of "Authorized Generics,"* 62 FOOD & DRUG L.J. 739, 774 n.199 (2007) (noting that "the earlier the authorized generic enters the market, the more it cannibalizes the branded drugs' profits").

[190] *See* CD, Nov. 4, 2004 ("financial risk to brand [of early launch is] significant" because brand erosion cannot be "made up by benefit of 2 week early launch"; that risk is exacerbated if the first generic entrant is delayed for any reason, because the AG would cannibalize the brand during the delay); CD, Feb. 2, 2005 ("**Do not put Rx brand at risk** (i.e., do not launch in advance of a generic, but can have contracts in place and inventory at wholesalers")) (emphasis original); CD, Jan. 5, 2007 ("[generic subsidiary] and [brand-name company] agree it is not financially viable to launch an AG prior to launch of other AB rated generics in the US"); CD, Mar. 31, 2004 (disadvantages of launching the AG early include "Uncertainty over ultimate LOE date [that] could cause unnecessary brand erosion; Additional incentive for earlier 'at risk' launches by generics; Potential public relations issue; Legislative Risks").

[191] For example, some AG supply agreements require the AG marketer to compensate the brand for profits lost due to early launch of the AG. *See, e.g.,* Agreement, 2007; Agreement, 2003; Agreement, 2002, amended 2003. Alternatively, an agreement might require that the AG marketer pay the brand a high percentage of net revenues or profits from AG sales before third-party launch. *See, e.g.,* Agreement, 2005 (distributor must pay brand 100% of net profits on AG during the time when the AG is the only generic on the market).

[192] *See, e.g.,* CD, undated ("An authorized generic should NEVER be launched before a competitor in order to avoid eroding the brand prematurely."); CD, July 2004 ("Launch generic versions of [brand-name company] products that lose patent protection *in response* to generic competitive launch: Rule #1: First do no harm to the brand . . ."); CD, undated ("[AG Subsidiary] strategy is never to launch first. The strategy is to launch simultaneous (or as close as possible) to formidable generic competition (to protect brand profitability)."); *see also* Agreement, 2005 (launch date after entry by specified competitor); Agreement, 2005 (launch when "Third Party Generic . . . Product" is available, as verified by independent sources); Agreement, 2002, amended 2003 (launch when "third party delivers any Equivalent Product to any retail pharmacy").

[193] The figure does not include three instances where the brand settled with the first-filer and made the first-filer its exclusive AG marketer because, under those circumstances, there was no competition between the AG and the ANDA-generic during the 180-day exclusivity period. In the one instance where the figure identifies AG entry more than five days before the first-filer's entry, the AG entered on one strength of the product eleven months before ANDA-generic entry on that specific strength, but ten months after ANDA-generic entry on the other strengths.

[194] *See, e.g.,* Public Comment from the Prescription Access Litig. Project et al. to the Fed. Trade Comm'n 4 (June 5, 2006), http://www.ftc.gov/os/comments/genericdrugstudy3/060605pal. pdf ("[T]he fact that most authorized generics disappear from the market after the 180 days shows that they are neither intended to promote competition nor in fact do so.").

[195] For 2001–2007, discontinuation dates were based on company responses to the Special Orders. The 2010 Red Book, company websites, and other sources were used to determine whether AGs were marketed through the end of 2009.

[196] CD, July 26, 2004 ("working draft").

[197] *See, e.g.,* Agreement, 2006 ("Distributor shall have sole discretion over Distributor's price for the Product"); Agreement, 2004 (distributor "has sole authority and discretion to implement pricing changes"); Agreement, 2005 (distributor solely responsible for pricing).

[198] CD, Mar. 31, 2004 ("Potential [Company] Strateg[y]" of "Substantially Reduc[ing] Generic Price of All [Brand-Name Co.] LOEs During the 180-day Exclusive Period").

[199] As of 2003, the brand-name firm noted that its AG subsidiary "historically follows pricing down (never leads) . . . . Customers expect [AG subsidiary] to follow competitor price changes (both up and down) within 30 days." CD, Sept. 23, 2003. When the firm's AG subsidiary later considered "Refocus[ing] objective . . . From: Maximizing value capture for [the branded parent], To: Deterring patent challenges" by "aggressively pricing" its AGs, CD, Feb. 1, 2006, it described the "deterrence" option strategy as a potential change from the "[s]tatus quo." *Id.* A subsequent strategy document, which continues to describe the firm's strategy as "do not lead on price," CD, Oct. 19, 2006, indicates that the aggressive pricing option was not selected.

[200] *See, e.g.,* CD, undated ("An authorized generic should always be a price follower while letting the competition establish market value."); CD, undated ("As a 'price follower,' the authorized generic will never be the initiator of a price war leading to market price erosion."); CD, undated ("[AG subsidiary's] launch strategy is defensive in that the overall strategy id [sic] to protect the brand and delay the erosion of brand units and overall market price."); *cf.* CD, Feb. 8, 2002 ([Subsidiary's] plan was to be "a price follower to [the ANDA-generic], not a price leader" and to "offer a slightly higher contract price to the trade versus [ANDA-generic rival] to avoid price competition," but "with major customers the [subsidiary's] price will likely net down to an estimated 5% lower than [ANDA-generic competitor] . . . .").

[201] CD, Mar. 31, 2004 (listing as "Cons" of reducing price during exclusivity, "Loss of . . . high margin during 180 days; Negative financial reimbursement impact on retailers; Additional incentive for earlier 'at risk' launches by generics; Can accelerate brand erosion; Potential public relations issues; Lose some of the benefits of 'settlements' . . .").

[202] *See* CD, undated ("[AG Subsidiary] will share the 6-month exclusivity with first filer(s) and capture a 40% share of the generic market"); CD, undated ("An authorized generic should strive to achieve only a minority

share (40%) of the substitution market and not encourage price cuts."); CD, Feb. 8, 2002 ("[Subsidiary] will compete with [ANDA-generic] on select accounts and attempt to obtain between 40% and 60% of the generic market. Anything greater than a 60% share may incite severe pricing competition from [ANDA-generic] which is NOT a goal of [subsidiary].").

[203] *See supra* Chapter 3, Section III.A.3.

[204] CD, Dec. 12, 2005.

[205] *See* Agreement, 2006 ("Distributor shall not sell the Product as a loss leader"); Agreement, 2004 (similar); Agreement, 2005 (similar); *id.* (distributor shall not discount AG in a way not applied to the majority of distributor's other products).

[206] *See, e.g.,* Agreement, 2004 (profit split is 50% to the brand); Agreement, 2005 (profit split is 92% to brand if there is one ANDA-generic competitor); CD, Oct. 12, 2004 ("Historically, generic partners received 20–35% of the economics, but this has now been driven down to 10% or less"). In settlement contexts, by contrast, generics often pay less than 35 percent, and a number of agreements – involving both litigated and other products—have brand-name firm profit splits of ten percent or less. *See, e.g.,* Settlement Agreement (requiring generic to pay brand 10% of Net Sales of AG of litigated product); Settlement Agreement (requiring generic to pay brand 8% of Profits on sales of AG of non-litigated product); Settlement Agreement (requiring generic to pay brand 5% of Net Profit on sales of AG of litigated product); *cf.* Settlement Agreement (requiring generic to pay brand 1–25% of profits on AGs of litigated and non-litigated products, depending on the time after launch and the number of entrants).

[207] *See infra* Appendix E, ¶¶ 18–19, at E-4, E-5. Request 18 sought documents on the impact of AGs on ANDA-generic profitability and the decision of whether to file a Paragraph III or Paragraph IV ANDA. Request 19 focused on documents relating to the marketing of AGs by generic companies. Of the 57 generic companies that received the Order, 16 provided some documents in response to one or both specifications, although several of the submissions were minimal, and several of the largest generic companies produced no documents in response to either Request. Subsequently, one large generic company supplemented its production with company documents and a third-party, interpretive analysis.

[208] *See, e.g.,* Public Comment from the Generic Pharm. Ass'n ("GPhA") to the Fed. Trade Comm'n (June 27, 2006), http://www.ftc.gov/os/comments/genericdrugstudy3/062806gpha. pdf ("The sale of authorized generics during the generic exclusivity period reduces the value of the 180-day exclusivity and consequently reduces the incentive for generic drug companies to challenge questionable patents.").

[209] *See supra* Chapter 2, Section I.B.2.b.ii.

[210] Company Document ("CD"), July 15, 2004.

[211] *Id.* A later analysis submitted to the FTC asserted that the firm "typically forecasts that an AG will reduce its revenue during the [180-day] exclusivity period by roughly 70%" and that "[d]epending on the drug, upwards of 60% of total lifetime revenues and profits come during this exclusivity period." CD, Apr. 2011.

[212] CD, July 15, 2004.

[213] *Id.*

[214] *See, e.g.,* CD, Mar. 24, 2004 (providing Apotex Comment in Support of Mylan Citizen Petition, Food & Drug Admin. Docket No. 2004P-0075/EMC1 (Mar. 24, 2004), http:// www.fda.gov/ohrms/dockets/dailys/04/apr04/ 040204/04P-0075-emc00001.pdf).

[215] CD, undated.

[216] CD, undated.

[217] CD, Feb. 1, 2005; *see also* CD, Dec. 6, 2004 (Bear Stearns report noting that "[a generic company's] attorneys said that the company expected to earn $41 mil. during the exclusivity period, but that with Watson's generic on the market, the anticipated return was less than $9 mil.").

[218] *E.g.,* CD, Nov. 2, 2005; CD, Feb. 15, 2006; *cf.* CD, Feb. 8, 2006 ("Forecast . . . is based on [firm] having exclusivity. Substitution rate = 80% with [firm] generic market share being at 60% (exclusivity + Authorized Generic)"). Other documents from the same company note the company's failure to meet 2004 work plan projections in part because of AGs. CD, 2004 (stating that "[firm] continued to face with the Authorized Generics phenomena, gained share from the AG portion on few products," and noting that "77% of new products sales related to products with AG competition in comparison to 42% in Q3").

[219] Typically, the generic firm forecasts project lower prices when an AG is present. Although some forecasts predict greater discounts than found by the analysis in Chapter 3, others are consistent with our findings. The projections were too few, and in some cases too ambiguous, to permit compilation of meaningful results.

[220] *See, e.g.,* CD, Apr. 19, 2005 (e-mail and sales forecast noting, "[w]e would always assume an authorized generic."); CD, undated (noting, "AG impact assumed for every new generic product launch; [d]espite FTC review of AGs, studies show AG presence increases competition and reduces price and cost"); CD, Jan. 5, 2006 (new products launch summary, including forecasts for four products based on assumptions of 180-day exclusivity and the presence of an AG); CDs, Sept. 14, 2007 and May 8, 2008 (four new product forecasts by another generic firm assuming the presence of AG competition during the 180-day exclusivity period); *see also* CD, Feb. 1, 2005 ("We believe investors should assume that most new generic product launches will include an authorized generic player.").

[221] CD, May 23, 2005 (also noting as contributing to price erosion, "India disadvantage: increasing bulk availability and competition").

[222] CD, July 19, 2005.

[223] CD, Mar. 2005 (emphasis omitted); *see also* CD, Feb. 20, 2005 (noting change in projections for specific drugs marketed by Pfizer – "I have changed the competitive lay of the land and included Pfizer's authorized generic"). The concerns quoted in the text should be placed in context, however: AG competition was only the tenth of thirteen trends identified by the Business Plan, and the entire discussion was a single paragraph (with one follow-up sentence) in a 93-page report.

[224] CD, Nov. 2004.

[225] CD, July 14, 2005 (Powerpoint presentation citing as the other major focuses "[c]learing a path for approval of generic biopharmaceuticals" and "[k]eeping door firmly closed to imports and price controls").

[226] CD, Dec. 8, 2004.

[227] *See, e.g.*, CD, Mar. 3, 2005 ("For generic drug companies, authorized generics are only one of a number of factors that appear to have accelerated competition, which include shared exclusivities, expanded capabilities of existing companies, and new entrants into the U.S. market leading to price erosion."); CD, Feb. 1, 2005 (noting citizen petitions and AGs as "two important risk factors affecting the generic industry").

[228] *See supra* Chapter 2, Figure 2-6 and accompanying text.

[229] At one end of the spectrum, Prasco markets itself as "The Authorized Generics Company," and explains that it is "not structured to compete with brand companies," but rather focuses on "providing Pharma companies access into the generic marketplace." *See Our Business: Authorized Generics*, PRASCO, http://www.prasco.com/default.asp?contentid=12&img= ourbusiness.jpg.

[230] CD, July 14, 2005 (proposing to "[p]ursue PIV ANDAs; [p]ursue authorized generics . . . If you can't beat-em join-em"); *see also* CD, Dec. 8, 2004 (stating that "most major generic companies have participated in authorized generic opportunities").

[231] *See* CD, Mar. 26, 2004 (providing Leila Abboud, *"Authorized" Generics Are Under Fire*, WALL ST. J., March 25, 2004, at D4) (e-mail attaching Wall Street Journal article reporting that "[a]uthorizedgeneric deals are dividing the generic-drug industry. Some companies such as Watson Pharmaceuticals and Pharmaceutical Resources Inc.'s Par Pharmaceuticals unit think partnering with brands is a good strategy. But generic industry heavyweights Teva Pharmaceutical Industries Ltd., Mylan Laboratories and Barr Pharmaceuticals Inc. say authorized generics threaten the profitability and long-term health of the industry."); CD, undated (chart entitled "Generic Manufacturers Differ in Strategic Approach," showing Teva, Mylan and Barr "Against" AGs and Sandoz, Watson and Ivax "For").

[232] *See supra* notes 4-7 and accompanying text.

[233] *See, e.g.*, CD, Jan. 9, 2006 (noting "authorized generic/piggybacking" as one objective); CD, Dec. 8, 2004 (detailing five "near term authorized generic opportunities actively pursued"); CD, June 18, 2004 (e-mail from company CEO stating "I believe we should approach the innovators about authorized generics").

[234] *See, e.g.*, CD, Dec. 21, 2005 (e-mail asking brand-name companies to consider generic company as AG distributor).

[235] *See* CD, Dec. 8, 2004 (chart showing that AGs contribute significantly to the bottom lines of certain generic companies and explaining for two different firms that "authorized generic growth covers base business erosion" and "two authorized generics cover base business erosion").

[236] *See* CD, May 6, 2005 (describing options as "Stay the course . . . ; Limiting to High Barrier to Entry (HBE), including PIV exclusive opportunities . . . ; Limiting to HBE, not including PIV exclusive opportunities unless they are HBE post exclusivity; [and] Terminate AG activities").

[237] CD, Oct. 12, 2004; *see also* CD, Dec. 8, 2004 ("Authorized generics will be a continued focus as blockbusters reach the end of exclusivity;" while "[s]ingle product deals open the door to additional opportunities," "the deal value continues to shrink in the US.").

[238] *See supra* Section I.A.

[239] One document includes a one-sentence statement memorializing a decision to drop a generic project "[d]ue to launch of the authorized generic." CD, Aug. 9, 2005. The context, however, did not involve the issues of concern. The patent had expired years before, so there was no elimination of a patent challenge. The firm that decided against entering would have faced three established, ANDA-generic competitors in addition to the newly-launched AG.

[240] *See, e.g.,* CD, undated (describing company's "Limited Paragraph IV FTF pipeline" as a weakness and identifying as a "Market Objective[]" the need to "Focus on First-to-File (FTF) Paragraph IV opportunities"); CD, May 23, 2005 ("[f]ocus on FTF opportunities").

[241] CD, Sept. 20, 2005.

[242] For example, one investment report identified "the potential impact of multiple 180-day exclusivities as a crucial factor in [the company's] earnings outlook" and emphasized that "patent challenges are the key near-term drivers in the 2005 to 2008 time frame." CD, June 27, 2005.

[243] CD, Oct. 27, 2005. In particular, it noted that Paragraph III pricing had declined "from over 10% of brand to under 2% of brand" and that Paragraph IV pricing had declined "from ~60% of brand to ~40% of brand." *Id.*

[244] *Id.*
[245] *See id.* (noting that one AG deal alone "[c]ould add $6M[million]–$24M margin potential inFY06–07").
[246] CD, Jan. 12, 2005.
[247] CD, undated (noting that the "loophole [that] allows the brand manufacturer's 'authorized generic' to immediately compete with the generic manufacturer's product that was granted 180 day exclusivity . . . is significant because the company that was granted market exclusivity must lower its price to compete with the authorized generic, resulting in decreased profits. Over time, this strategy will lower funding available to generic manufacturers for legal challenges of brand patents.").
[248] CD, June 27, 2005. *But cf. infra* text accompanying note 60 (explaining that the report ultimately concludes that the exclusivity opportunities studied would be profitable even with AG competition).
[249] CD, undated.
[250] *Id.*
[251] CDs, Sept. 14, 2007 & May 8, 2008 (new product forecasts).
[252] CD, Apr. 2011.
[253] *Id.*
[254] *Id.* The firm's quantitative analysis, however, shows that a generic version of a third drug (with annual sales of $36 million) would have been profitable with or without an AG competitor and finds generic entry for a fourth drug (with annual sales of $20 million) unprofitable under both circumstances. *Id.*
[255] CD, Apr. 9, 2004 (exclamation marks in original); *see also* CD, July 9, 2005 (deciding to launch an ANDA-generic despite anticipated presence of AG).
[256] CD, Mar. 26, 2004.
[257] CD, Dec. 8, 2004. In support of AGs, the document cites "Increased competition; Decreased prices; Pro-consumer; Additional tool for generic companies to fill 'holes' in their pipeline or to enter new treatment areas; Respects innovator marketing rights; Support generic industry reputation of access to lower cost pharmaceuticals." The points cited in opposition are: "Potential disincentive to file Paragraph IV's; Long term financial impact on generic industry; Arguably not in 'spirit' of Hatch-Waxman; Reduced value of 180-day exclusivity to those who have it."
[258] *Id.* ("Brand companies may choose to launch an authorized generic via a generic partner to: Settle patent litigation; Maximize profits by participating in the generic market once generic competition starts; Solve a manufacturing capacity issue." "Generic companies may choose to launch an authorized generic to: Settle litigation; Compete in a market they otherwise could not have entered; Quickly add additional products to portfolio; Add new source of business.").
[259] *Id.*
[260] *Id.*
[261] *Id.*; *see also id.* (finding "[f]ewer opportunities to earn an exclusivity [–] NCE-1 products now have shared exclusivity in most cases" and noting that "[f]orfeiture events could cause a loss of exclusivity").
[262] *Id.* ("Authorized generic products have effectively ended the sole exclusivity product launch for all high-value innovator products. All launches face price competition."); *id.* (AG marketing "[h]as become a common industry practice diluting value of 180-day exclusivity; [r]educes value of all competing generic products").
[263] *Id.* (concluding, in an example showing nearly $200 million of annual profit on a drug with $1 billion of annual sales, "[v]alue of generic product is reduced during the 6 month exclusivity period; [h]owever, considerable value is still generated when competing with an authorized generic"); *see also id.* (chart showing an average $42 million pre-manufacturing profit (after legal expenses and other costs of bringing the product to market) for six Paragraph IV entrants facing AG competition during 180-day exclusivity). Similarly, other firms provided projections showing ANDA-generics operating profitably in competition with AGs. *See, e.g.,* CD, Aug. 2, 2005 (projecting, over the first ten months following launch, a gross profit margin of $170 million for a drug strength with almost $500 million in annual brand sales and a $240 million margin for a drug strength with approximately $700 million in annual brand sales, despite AG competition).
[264] CD, Dec. 8, 2004.
[265] CD, June 27, 2005.
[266] *Id.*
[267] CD, Mar. 3, 2005. Similarly, a study, commissioned and reported publicly by a generic firm that often has partnered with brand-name companies to market AGs, observes that "[t]he literature contains no empirical evidence that the prospect of competition from authorized generics has reduced either patent challenges by other generic manufacturers or the development of new generic products." CD, Apr. 2007 (providing Kevin A. Hassett & Robert J. Shapiro, The Impact of Authorized Generic Pharmaceuticals on the Introduction of Other Generic Pharmaceuticals (2007), http://www.authorizedgenerics.com/downloads/ ImpactofAuthorizedGeneric Pharmaceuticals.pdf (written for Prasco)). With respect to the latter point, the authors present their own quantitative analysis, concluding that "competition from authorized generics does not reduce R&D by generic manufacturers, and therefore should not reduce or delay the introduction of future generic products." *Id.*

[268] IMS CONSULTING, IMS HEALTH, ASSESSMENT OF AUTHORIZED GENERICS IN THE U.S. 11 ("IMS Study") (2006) (written for the Pharm. Research and Mfrs. of Am. ("PhRMA")), http://replay.web.archive.org/20061009134405/http://www.phrma.org/files/IMS%20 Authorized%20Generics%20Report_6-22-06.pdf.

[269] *Id.* at 14–15.

[270] Ernst R. Berndt et al., *Authorized Generic Drugs, Price Competition and Consumers' Welfare*, 26 HEALTH AFF. 790 (2007).

[271] *Id.* at 792–93. The study did not distinguish AGs from other generic competitors.

[272] Ernst R. Berndt, Richard Mortimer & Andrew Parece, *Do Authorized Generic Drugs Deter Paragraph IV Certifications? Recent Evidence* (2007) (working paper written for PhRMA), http://www.analysisgroup.com/uploadedFiles/Publishing/Articles/PhRMA_Authorized_ Generic_Entry.pdf.

[273] *Id.* at 4.

[274] *Id.* at 4. Chapter 7, *infra*, presents findings based on our own analysis of Paragraph IV certifications.

[275] MARC GOODMAN, GARY NACHMAN & LOUISE CHEN, MORGAN STANLEY, QUANTIFYING THE IMPACT FROM AUTHORIZED GENERICS (2004).

[276] *Id.* at 8–9.

[277] David Reiffen & Michael R. Ward, *Branded Generics as a Strategy to Limit Cannibalization of Pharmaceutical Markets*, 28 MAN. & DEC. ECON. 251, 263 (2007).

[278] As in Chapter 3, the data analyzed in this chapter consist of monthly observations of market outcomes for "products," which are defined as a full specification of active ingredient(s), dosage form, and strength. Each product accounts for a number of observations equal to the number of months the product is observed in the data, so the results reported may differ substantially from a listing that combined all observations for the same drug. For instance, suppose 600mg Gabapentin tablets account for an observation in the three-manufacturer row of Table 6-1 in a particular month. Then if another manufacturer enters, that product accounts for one of the observations in the four-manufacturer row for the next month. If the number of manufacturers stays at four for several months, each of those months counts as another observation in the four-manufacturer row. In some of those months, there are also four manufacturers selling 800mg Gabapentin tablets, which also would be counted in the four-manufacturer row.

[279] This decline does not necessarily indicate that firms exited the market; it is in part due to some of the products with a relatively high number of competitors experiencing first generic entry with less than 30 months left in our data window, so that we do not observe the 30th month of generic competition for these products.

[280] Some of the steps leading up to generic entry often occur years in advance of actual entry. Therefore, some of the costs associated with entry will have been sunk long before the entry actually occurs. Potential entrants presumably use their expectations about the competitive environment before sinking these costs for a particular product, but they may not know with certainty whether an AG will enter when making some of these decisions.

[281] In technical terms, the problem is that both the decision to issue an AG and the entry decisions of ANDA-generic manufacturers are endogenous, i.e., they have causal links with other variables in the model. An instrumental variables regression analysis utilizing market size and brand-name firm identity as instruments to control for this endogeneity was investigated. The results suggested that these instruments did not control well for the endogeneity of the number of ANDA-generic manufacturers, so the results are not reported here.

[282] For concreteness, the effect of an AG during exclusivity typically was characterized as the impact of going from just one ANDA-generic competitor to an ANDA-generic plus an AG. Outside of exclusivity, the analysis will estimate the impact of switching from five ANDA-generic competitors, for example, to four ANDA-generics plus an AG. One piece of evidence supporting this approach is provided by an examination of market shares of generic competitors in the first several months following generic entry in "No Exclusivity" markets that experienced AG entry. ("No Exclusivity" markets are considered because no competitor enjoys a first-mover advantage from an FDA-granted exclusivity period in them, so generic competitors can enter on equal ground.) The average market share of AGs in these situations is similar in magnitude to the average market share of individual ANDA-generic competitors, and the difference is not statistically significant. This is consistent with treating an AG as equivalent to a typical generic competitor. Further support for this assumption comes from analyzing data on the number of generics present in markets two years after first generic entry to determine whether the eventual number of generic competitors differed in AG markets. Controlling for pre-entry brand sales, the number of generic competitors present in the market after two years, including the AG, was not statistically different between markets with an AG and those without.

[283] A second model was estimated in which the effect of the AG also was allowed to vary flexibly across the observed number of manufacturers. The estimated effects from this model are difficult to interpret, not robust across specifications, and hard to identify because products facing a large number of manufacturers are rarely observed without an AG. Although the results of this model were somewhat erratic, the overall inferences about the impact of an AG did not differ from those produced by the basic model reported here.

[284] *See* Company Document ("CD"), undated ("historically the first generic to market . . . gains a significant foothold in market share"); *cf. supra* Chapter 4, note 36 and accompanying text (discussing potential first-mover advantages in connection with AG launch timing).

285 Because these are shares of current-month expenditures, and as shown in Figure 6-1, the generic price is declining, these are shares of a pie that typically is shrinking over time.

286 The sample is limited to first-filer firms. A firm is identified in the data as a first-filer for a product if it is an ANDA-generic firm and had positive sales during exclusivity. The sample of products is therefore implicitly limited to products with an exclusivity period. In the uncommon case in which the product has multiple first-filers, expenditures on the products produced by these firms are aggregated. Revenues of known re-packagers are excluded.

287 *See supra* Chapter 3, Table 3-9.

288 This rough calculation assumes that drug prices increase at a rate consistent with the rate at which the brand-name company discounts future revenue streams.

289 *See* GOODMAN ET AL., *supra* note 8.

290 *See infra* Appendix E, ¶ 17, at E-4.

291 The Morgan Stanley analysis assumed that pre-entry brand profit margins were 90%, which is to say that the brand's marginal cost is equal to 10% of its price, and that generics had the same marginal cost as the brand. This is consistent with our use of the generic price following extensive generic entry as an estimate of marginal costs.

292 To see this, start with the initial expression for annual profits, and perform the following steps:

$$(p_g - c_g)q_g = (p_g - 0.1p_b)q_g = \frac{(p_g - 0.1p_b)}{p_b}q_gp_b = (\hat{p}_g - 0.1)q_gp_b = (\hat{p}_g - 0.1)\frac{q_gp_g}{q_bp_b}\frac{p_b}{p_g}q_bp_b = (\hat{p}_g - 0.1)\hat{r}_g\frac{1}{\hat{p}_g}r_b$$

This must be divided by two in order to account for the exclusivity period lasting only half a year.

293 Because it was not possible to reliably estimate effects more than three years after first generic entry, analysis is truncated at the three-year mark. This almost certainly causes some understatement of the profits associated with generic entry. However, the bulk of the AG effect likely is recognized during the exclusivity period and the few years that follow, so ignoring the impact past three years probably is not a significant source of error. Furthermore, future profits are not discounted: assuming that the inflation rate in a given drug market will roughly equal the discount rate of market participants, the use of current dollars in the analysis is appropriate.

294 HOWREY LLP, THE SHORT-TERM AND LONG-TERM COMPETITIVE IMPACT OF AUTHORIZED GENERICS 22–23 (2009) (written for PhRMA), http://www.ftc.gov/os/comments/ genericdrugstudy3/091028pharmresearch.pdf. Also, Morgan Stanley used an estimate of $10 million per challenge, which includes $1–2 million in costs associated with the ANDA approval process. *See* GOODMAN ET AL., *supra* note 8, at 8. That is within the range of expenditures observed in the data, and, given the relatively low rate of usable responses, the evidence does not suggest that Morgan Stanley's estimated $8–$9 million of challenge expenses was inaccurate. However, there is no apparent reason to believe that any accounting idiosyncrasies that may have affected responses to the Special Orders produced a biased sample, so the $5 million estimate of typical expenditures on a Paragraph IV challenge will be used as the baseline here.

295 Because this analysis is meant to apply to small drugs as well as large drugs, it relies on estimates from unweighted regressions from Chapter 3 and earlier in this chapter.

296 The lower break-even market sizes reported here are consistent with evidence presented in Chapter 7, that drugs with market sizes smaller than $50 million do attract Paragraph IV challenges.

297 The market sizes reported here are aggregated over strength and dosage form. In other words, market size is calculated for all strengths and forms of a particular combination of active ingredients.

298 Some drugs, with very small market sizes, may not have drawn Paragraph IV challenges even if there had been no prospect of AG competition.

299 Again, the calculation of market size aggregates all strengths and dosage forms associated with a particular combination of active ingredients. *See supra* note 30.

300 To the degree a generic company is overly optimistic about its challenge, however, AG competition would deter challenges when the generic's actual chance of winning was even lower than four to ten percent. Conversely, if the generic were overly pessimistic about its chances, AG competition would deter challenges when the real chance of success was higher than the subjective assessments shown in Figure 6-6.

301 In this analysis, future profits are not discounted. Firms do not typically use the same discount rates when making entry decisions, and therefore the choice of any specific discount rate is admittedly arbitrary. The effects of a higher discount rate would likely shift the profiles of the break-even drugs towards larger drugs. However, changing the discount rate by any reasonable amount would not drastically alter the basic conclusions of the analysis: an AG would affect the profitability of a paragraph IV filing only where the brand sales are small.

302 Unlike Chapter 3 and Chapter 6, where analysis examined different "products," *see supra* Chapter 3, note 16 and Chapter 6, note 11, this chapter focuses on "drugs," which include all strengths covered by an NDA. This unit of observation is most appropriate for an analysis of patent challenge data because Paragraph IV challenges typically target all strengths of a drug. In addition, ANDA records in the relevant FDA database were organized by application number, and usually included all strengths of a drug in a single application. The chief consequence is that different strengths, which had been treated as separate observations in Chapters 3 and 6, here are treated together as a single observation.

[303] *See supra* Chapter 6, Section V.

[304] *See, e.g.*, David Reiffen & Michael R. Ward, *Branded Generics as a Strategy to Limit Cannibalization of Pharmaceutical Markets*, 28 MAN. & DEC. ECON. 251, 263 (2007) (concluding that the introduction of AGs is "least problematic . . . in relatively large markets").

[305] The dates of the first Paragraph IV certifications made in ANDAs for a particular drug (i.e., for a particular dosage form and NDA) were obtained from the U.S. Food and Drug Administration's ("FDA") Paragraph IV Patent Certifications website. *See Paragraph IV Patent Certifications*, FDA, http://www.fda.gov/Drugs/DevelopmentApprovalProcess/HowDrugsareDevelopedandApproved/ApprovalApplications/AbbreviatedNewDrugApplicationANDAGenerics/ucm047676.htm (last updated May 11, 2011) (reporting the dates of first challenges after March 2, 2004). When Paragraph IV certifications for different strengths were made on different dates, the earliest date was used. For more details, *see infra* Appendix H.

[306] The table shows the number of drugs subject to first patent challenges, not the number of challenges per drug. Because certain dosage forms, such as injectables, are sold primarily outside the retail channels included in National Prescription Audit sales data from IMS Health, the table is limited to tablet and capsule forms.

[307] *See* Howrey LLP, THE SHORT-TERM AND LONG-TERM COMPETITIVE IMPACT OF AUTHORIZED GENERICS 26 (2009) (written for Pharm. Research and Mfrs. of Am. ("PhRMA")), http://www.ftc.gov/os/comments/genericdrugstudy3/091028pharmresearch.pdf (finding break-even points of $50.2 million without an AG and $110 million with an AG); MARC GOODMAN, GARY NACHMAN, & LOUISE CHEN, MORGAN STANLEY, QUANTIFYING THE IMPACT FROM AUTHORIZED GENERICS 6–9 (2004) (break-even point of $48 million without an AG and $110 million with an AG); *see also* Pfizer, Do Authorized Generics Benefit Consumers? (2005) (presentation slides showing break-even points of $48 million without an AG and $89 million with an AG). The analysis in Chapter 6 suggests that for a drug with $50 million in pre-entry brand-name sales, a generic firm that does not expect AG competition would expect that a patent challenge would be profitable if it anticipated a 12% probability of winning; however, if the firm expected to face an AG, it would require at least a 26% probability of winning to expect profitability. *See supra*, Chapter 6, Figure 6-6.

[308] *See supra* Chapter 6, Figure 6-6. For higher probabilities of winning, the break-even level is even lower, e.g., $6.8–$14.9 million when the generic believes it has a 100% probability of winning, depending on whether or not it anticipates AG competition.

[309] *See supra* Chapter 2, Figure 2-9 and accompanying text. Between April 2003 and December 2008, there were six exclusivity periods on products with sales below $50 million; in none of those situations did the brand launch an authorized generic during the exclusivity period. *But cf. supra* Chapter 5, note 14 and accompanying text (noting that some generic companies produced documents indicating that the firms always assume AG competition).

[310] Even assuming companies are less likely to challenge patents on low-sales drugs, similar numbers of low- and high-sales drugs subject to a first patent challenge could arise if there are more low-sales drugs available for first challenge than high-sales drugs.

[311] *See infra* Appendix I, Figure I-1 (frequency of Paragraph IV challenges increases as pre-entry brand sales increase).

[312] The data are based on sales at the time of certification rather than at generic entry. (Because the length of time between certification and generic entry is often many years, generic entry has not yet occurred for many of the drugs with first patent challenges in 2003–2008.) It is possible that a company might have challenged a patent on a low-sales drug because it anticipated an increase in sales by the time of generic entry. If so, a low sales level at certification might not represent the company's view of the financial incentive underlying its challenge.

[313] For example, patent challenges for a new formulation of a blockbuster drug (sales greater than $2 billion) began less than a year after approval of the new formulation, when annualized sales were about $14 million. Five years later, the year before generic entry, sales of the new formulation had risen to about $90 million. *See infra* Appendix H, Section IX, regarding annualization of sales.

[314] This might have contributed to two companies' patent challenges regarding three contraceptives; the companies offer a number of estrogen hormone-related drugs.

[315] The most dramatic example of such a strategy concerned a company's challenge to patents on a drug with sales under $1 million, which could be explained by its simultaneous challenge to the same patents listed for an older dosage form of the drug with sales of nearly $2 billion. The low-sales drug was a line extension of the high-sales drug, i.e., it contained the same active ingredient, and was part of the same "franchise" as the high-sales drug. Five other low-sales drugs involved challenges to patents that covered other drugs with substantially higher sales.

[316] The declines were statistically significant for comparisons of 2003 sales with 2007 and 2008 (5% statistical significance level, using a two-tailed t-test, variances not assumed equal). Other pair-wise comparisons were not statistically significant. The observed declines in the mean and median sales levels of drugs subject to a first patent challenge could be explained by an increase in challenges to small-market drugs or by a decrease in the market size of drugs available for challenge; the data do not distinguish between the possibilities.

[317] These graphs are based on the patent certifications entered in ANDA records maintained in the FDA's application database. Although patent certifications must be made with respect to every patent listed in the Orange Book, the FDA application database lists only the highest certification made. Thus, if an ANDA contains a Paragraph IV certification for any patent, the database shows a Paragraph IV certification even if the applicant also made Paragraph II (the patent is expired) or Paragraph III certifications for other patents. Changes in the FDA's application database precluded compiling the ANDA information through 2008.

[318] *See, e.g.*, FTC, PHARMACY BENEFIT MANAGERS: OWNERSHIP OF MAIL-ORDER PHARMACIES 15 (2005), http://www.ftc.gov/reports/pharmbenefit05/050906pharmbenefitrpt.pdf (discussing increased utilization of prescription drugs).

[319] *See* PhRMA, 2007 ANNUAL REPORT 20 (2007), http://web.archive.org/web/20080329043525/ http://www.phrma.org/files/2007%20Annual%20Report. pdf; *see also* GENERIC PHARM. ASS'N ("GPhA"), 2009 ANNUAL REPORT 28 (2009), http://www.gphaonline.org/sites/ default/files/gpha-low-res.pdf (also citing IMS Health data). The increase from the years 2000 to 2007 in ANDA filings, including those with patent challenges, does not appear to arise from an increase in NDAs. The number of NDA approvals varied from year to year but did not exhibit an upward trend in this period and the years preceding it. *See* U.S. GOV'T ACCOUNTABILITY OFFICE, NEW DRUG DEVELOPMENT: SCIENCE, BUSINESS, REGULATORY, AND INTELLECTUAL PROPERTY ISSUES CITED AS HAMPERING DRUG DEVELOPMENT EFFORTS 24 (2006), http://www.gao.gov/new.items/d0749.pdf; CTR. FOR DRUG EVAL. AND RESEARCH ("CDER"), FDA, 2007 UPDATE: IMPROVING PUBLIC HEALTH THROUGH HUMAN DRUGS 12–15 (2007), http://www.fda.gov/downloads/ AboutFDA/CentersOffices/CDER/WhatWeDo/UCM121704.pdf.

[320] *See* 21 C.F.R. § 314.94(a)(12) (2010).

[321] Because a drug may draw multiple ANDA filings, the relative numbers of PIII and PIV ANDA filings (shown above in Figure 7-2) do not necessarily reflect the relative numbers of drugs for which PIII and PIV certifications were made.

[322] There is a limitation on this data. If companies wait longer to file Paragraph III ANDAs than Paragraph IV ANDAs, it could be that there are products for which a generic would have filed a Paragraph IV ANDA if it did not expect an authorized generic but has not yet filed its Paragraph III ANDA. Nonetheless, this analysis is still helpful and is consistent with the other evidence examined in this chapter.

[323] Data on yearly patent challenges were obtained from the FDA's Paragraph IV website, *see supra* note 4. A previous study that examined the numbers of drugs facing a first Paragraph IV certification observed little change from 2004 through May 2006. *See* Ernst R. Berndt et al., *Authorized Generic Drugs, Price Competition, and Consumers' Welfare*, 26 HEALTH AFF. 790, 794 (2007).

[324] Staff examined the FDA's application database to determine whether a particular ANDA contained the first PIII certification for a given drug (i.e., for a particular dosage form and NDA), and whether any previous or subsequent ANDAs for the same drug contained a PIV certification. This allowed staff to identify PIII drugs, for which no ANDAs with PIV certifications were filed, either before or after the first PIII certification. Because complete PIII ANDA filing information for 2008 was unavailable, staff limited the analysis to 2003–07.

[325] Of the 286 ANDAs with PIII certifications filed in 2006 and 2007, only four were first PIII certifications; rather, the bulk of the ANDAs with PIII certifications were either filed after a first PIII certification in a previous year, or were filed with regard to a drug for which another applicant made a PIV certification.

[326] This percentage could fall if a "first PIII filer" amends its certification to PIV, or if a subsequent ANDA makes a PIV certification for any of the four drugs.

[327] These findings are consistent with a recent industry study that concluded that "the vast majority of products enter[] the market via paragraph IV challenges (92%)." AARON GAL & NIKHIL R. CHARI, BERNSTEIN RESEARCH, THE LONG VIEW: U.S. GENERIC PHARMACEUTICALS -A BOTTOM-UP MODEL OF THE U.S. COMMODITY GENERICS MARKET IN 2009–2013, at 3 (2009); *see also id.* at 7, 14 (by dollar or prescription volume, Paragraph IV drugs comprise the bulk of generic market entry).

[328] The difference between the mean sales of PIII drugs ($136,245,673) and PIV drugs ($541,720,294) was statistically significant at the 1% level, using a two-tailed t-test, variances not assumed equal.

[329] In contrast, many PIV drugs had sales above $500 million, while no PIII drugs exceeded that amount.

[330] In addition to an increased likelihood of sharing exclusivity with another generic competitor in the NCE context, there is also the possibility of an authorized generic, further reducing the expected profits from a successful Paragraph IV certification.

[331] *See* 21 C.F.R. § 314.108 (2010). The percentage was calculated from New Molecular Entity (NME) and NDA approvals from 2000–07, as reported by the FDA. *See Summary of NDA Approvals & Receipts, 1938 to the present*, FDA, http://www.fda.gov/AboutFDA/WhatWeDo/History/ProductRegulation/SummaryofNDA ApprovalsRe ceipts1938tothepresent/default.htm (last updated Feb 16, 2011); *NME Drug and New Biologic Approvals*, FDA, http://www.fda.gov/Drugs/DevelopmentApprovalProcess/How DrugsareDevelopedand Approved/DrugandBiologicApprovalReports/ucm121136.htm (last updated Feb 23, 2011); CDER, *supra* note 18, at 11.

[332] *See* JOHN THOMAS, PHARMACEUTICAL PATENT LAW 432-35 (2d ed. 2010). ANDAs with PIV certifications cannot be filed until four years and six months have elapsed if the FDA has granted pediatric exclusivity.

[333] *See id.*; CDER & CTR. FOR BIOLOGICS EVAL. AND RESEARCH ("CBER"), FDA, GUIDANCE FOR INDUSTRY: QUALIFYING FOR PEDIATRIC EXCLUSIVITY UNDER SECTION 505A OF THE FEDERAL FOOD, DRUG, AND COSMETIC ACT 13 (1999), http://www.fda.gov/downloads/Drugs/GuidanceComplianceRegulatory Information/Guidances/UCM080558.pdf (explaining that pediatric exclusivity attaches to NCE exclusivity).

[334] *See* CDER, FDA, GUIDANCE FOR INDUSTRY: 180-DAY EXCLUSIVITY WHEN MULTIPLE ANDAS ARE SUBMITTED ON THE SAME DAY 4 (2003), http://www.fda.gov/downloads/ Drugs/GuidanceCompliance RegulatoryInformation/Guidances/ucm07 2851.pdf.

[335] This practice began in July 2003, when the FDA issued its guidance on sharing 180-day exclusivity among multiple ANDAs submitted on the first day. *See id.* at 6. Subsequently, the Medicare Prescription Drug, Improvement, and Modernization Act of 2003 ("MMA"), Pub. L. No. 108-173, 117 Stat. 2066 (codified in scattered sections), defined "first applicant" in such a way that all applicants who submit a substantially complete application containing a Paragraph IV certification on the first day the FDA receives such an application may be granted 180-day exclusivity. *See* 21 U.S.C. § 355(j)(5)(B)(iv)(I)–(II)(bb) (2010) (awarding 180-day exclusivity to a "first applicant" as defined). The law also called for granting exclusivity on a product basis rather than a patent-by-patent basis, which likely enhances a generic firm's incentive to file an ANDA with at least one PIV certification on the first day. *See* SHASHANK UPADHYE, GENERIC PHARMACEUTICAL PATENT AND FDA LAW § 13:16 (2010 ed. 2010) (observing that it may be "fruitful to file the ANDA with at least one Paragraph IV certification to reserve [the] right to convert any Paragraph III certifications to Paragraph IV later on").

[336] An advantage of studying decision-making for challenges of patents covering NCEs is that because the challenges leading to shared exclusivity generally occur at a consistent time after NDA approval, comparisons of sales levels and other factors that may reflect the attractiveness of a drug for a patent challenge are standardized with respect to the stage of a brand's life cycle.

[337] The increase in first-day challenges may reflect the added certainty, with shared exclusivity, that any given first-day filer will be permitted to participate in the exclusivity period. The gradual nature of the increase likely reflects the time required for generic companies to take advantage of the broadened opportunity for sharing exclusivity by developing and filing ANDAs for NCE drugs for which first-day filing opportunities were approaching.

[338] The number of first-day ANDAs with a PIV certification is based on the number of apparent first-day ANDAs in the FDA's application databases. Because the FDA may not deem all such filings as "substantially complete" or approvable, these numbers should be considered estimates of the number of companies that will compete during exclusivity. *See infra* Appendix H, Section X.

[339] The companies likely anticipated that they would share 180-day exclusivity with several other first-day filers. Although ANDA filings are confidential, firms would be aware of the prospect of sharing exclusivity, both because of such sharing for a few NCEs for which generic entry already has occurred (e.g., Protonix), and because of court documents and other sources that indicate that many companies undertake first-day challenges. *See, e.g.*, Company Document ("CD"), Dec. 8, 2004 ("NCE-1 products now have shared exclusivity in most cases"); Sara Stefanini, *The Best and Worst Patents for Generics To Fight,* IP Law360, at 1, 4, May 6, 2008 ("People are going to be filing on that four-year date, and everybody knows that everybody is going to file . . . .").

[340] *See, e.g.*, CONG. BUDGET OFFICE, HOW INCREASED COMPETITION FROM GENERIC DRUGS HASAFFECTED PRICES AND RETURNS IN THE PHARMACEUTICAL INDUSTRY 31 (1998), http://www.cbo.gov/ftpdocs/ 6xx/doc655/pharm.pdf.

[341] In some cases, the brand appoints the generic to distribute the brand's AG during the 180-day period of marketing exclusivity. In such circumstances, there is still no competition between an ANDA-generic's product and a brand's AG.

[342] In this chapter, when used in the context of categorization of an agreement, a "first-filer" is defined as a generic entitled to 180 days of marketing exclusivity at the time of the settlement agreement. Under some circumstances, there can be competition from other first-filers during the 180-day exclusivity period. *See* 21 U.S.C. § 355(j)(5)(B)(iv)(II)(bb) (2010) (providing that exclusivity may be shared by applicants filing on the same day).

[343] Pursuant to settlement, a generic company may pay a royalty to the brand to gain an earlier entry date than it would get by compromising on the date alone, while an exclusion payment – a payment from the brand to the generic – buys a later entry date. *See* Alden F. Abbott & Suzanne T. Michel, *The Right Balance of Competition Policy and Intellectual Property Law: A Perspective on Settlements of Pharmaceutical Patent Litigation*, 46 IDEA 1, 14 (2005).

[344] H.R. Rep. No. 98-857(I), at 14, 28 (1984), *reprinted in* 1984 U.S.C.C.A.N. 2647, 2647, 2661. Although initial judicial reactions reflected concern with such arrangements, *see In re* Cardizem CD Antitrust Litig., 332 F.3d 896, 908 (6th Cir. 2003), subsequent appellate rulings adopted a far more permissive position. *See* Ark. Carpenters Health & Welfare Fund v. Bayer AG (*In re* Ciprofloxacin Hydrochloride Antitrust Litig.), 544 F.3d

1323, 1336 (Fed. Cir. 2008), *cert. denied*, 129 S.Ct. 2828 (2009); Ark. Carpenters Health & Welfare Fund v. Bayer AG, 604 F.3d 98 (2d Cir. 2010), *cert. denied,* 131 S.Ct. 1606 (2011); Joblove v. Barr Labs., Inc. (*In re* Tamoxifen Citrate Antitrust Litig.), 429 F.3d 370 (2d Cir. 2005), *amended by*, 466 F.3d 187 (2d Cir. 2006); Schering Plough Corp. v. FTC, 402 F.3d 1056 (11th Cir. 2005). Other cases remain in litigation. *See* King Drug Co. of Florence v. Cephalon, Inc., 702 F. Supp. 2d 514 (E.D. Pa. 2010) (denial of motion to dismiss); FTC v. Watson Pharms., Inc., No. 10-12729-DD (11th Cir. first notice of appeal of dismissal filed June 10, 2010); *In re* K-Dur Antitrust Litig., Nos. 10-2077, -2078, -2079, -4571 (3d Cir. first notice of appeal filed Apr. 30, 2010).

[345] In FY 2010 there were 31 final settlements filed under the MMA that involved compensation to the generic patent challenger and an agreement by the generic firm to refrain from launching its product for some period of time. BUREAU OF COMPETITION, FED. TRADE COMM'N, AGREEMENTS FILED WITH THE FEDERAL TRADE COMMISSION UNDER THE MEDICARE PRESCRIPTION DRUG, IMPROVEMENT, AND MODERNIZATION ACT OF 2003: OVERVIEW OF AGREEMENTS FILED IN FY 2010 (2011), http://www.ftc.gov/os/2011/05/1105mmaagreements.pdf. These agreements involved 22 different brand-name drugs with combined annual U.S. sales of $9.3 billion. *Id.*

[346] This reflects the fact that competition typically dissipates total profits accruing to suppliers so that the sum of duopoly profits is less than monopoly profits. *See, e.g.*, Mark A. Lemley & Carl Shapiro, *Probabilistic Patents*, J. ECON. PERSPECTIVES, Spring 2005, at 75, 91 n.15.

[347] *See* CD, Oct. 6, 2005 (comparing forecasted net present values for early and late launches, with and without an AG).

[348] This Report cites all agreements arising from settlements or patent litigation, including settlements, licenses, and supply and distribution agreements as "Settlement Agreements."

[349] Agreements were counted based on the number of New Drug Applications involved in the litigation. For instance, if a spray formulation and a tablet formulation of a pharmaceutical involved two NDAs and both were subject to the litigation, the settlement arrangements were considered two agreements. In one agreement included in the total, the brand and a first-filing generic settled their patent dispute without litigation, with the brand-name firm promising not to offer AG competition for a period of time.

[350] Examples of the types of agreements omitted from this total include agreements that precluded launch of an AG by a third party but allowed the brand to launch an AG and agreements that specified that the generic could accelerate its entry upon launch of an AG but had no other provisions regarding AGs.

[351] A brand can compete with an AG either by launching it on its own or by authorizing another firm to market the AG. *See supra* Chapter 2, Sec. I.B.2. An explicit commitment not to compete can take different forms, for example, the brand company's granting the first-filer an exclusive license to a generic version of the brand. In these settlements, the brand agreed not to launch or sponsor its AG in competition with the first-filer's generic product for some period of time.

[352] Hatch-Waxman rewards the first-filer to challenge a brand-name drug patent with 180 days of market exclusivity, and bars the FDA from approving any later applicants until the period has expired or been forfeited. Thus, an agreement with a first-filer that defers entry may create a "bottleneck," blocking the approval of subsequently filed ANDAs. *See* FED. TRADE COMM'N, GENERIC DRUG ENTRY PRIOR TO PATENT EXPIRATION ch. 5 (2002), www.ftc.gov/os/2002/07/genericdrugstudy.pdf. Congress amended Hatch-Waxman in 2003 to provide that first-filers forfeit their exclusivity under certain circumstances, but even with the amendments, settlement agreements still have significant potential to create bottlenecks that block subsequent applicants. *See Protecting Consumer Access to Generic Drugs Act of 2009: Hearing on H.R. 1706 Before the Subcomm. on Commerce, Trade, and Consumer Protection of the H. Comm. on Energy and Commerce*, 111th Cong. (2009), http://www.ftc. gov/os/2009/03/P859910payfordelay.pdf (prepared statement of the FTC) (forfeiture provisions of the MMA do not relieve bottleneck when a first generic applicant enters a settlement agreement with the brand-name company and there is no court decision of invalidity or non-infringement); *see also* Letter from Gary J. Buehler, Dir., Office of Generic Drugs, U.S. Food and Drug Admin., to Marc A. Goshko, Executive Dir., Teva Parenteral Medicines, regarding Docket No. 2007N-0389, at 5 n.6 (Jan. 17, 2008), http://www.fda.gov/ohrms/dockets/DOCKETS/07n0389/07n0389-let0003.pdf (noting that when a first-filer enters a settlement agreement without a final judgment of invalidity or non-infringement, the "inability to force a forfeiture of 180-day exclusivity could result in delays in the approval of otherwise approvable ANDAs").

[353] *See infra* note 16 (discussing why restrictions on AG marketing usually do not exceed 180 days).

[354] All sales figures are for the full calendar year prior to the settlement agreement or for the last full year prior to generic entry. The annual sales data are from IMS Health, IMS National Prescription Audit Plus 7™, Years 2003 to 2008, Data Extracted January 2009; and from Top 200 Drugs for 2009 by Sales, http://www.drugs.com/top200.html (last visited June 2, 2011). In one instance, when IMS data for the product at issue were unavailable, information was drawn from Top 200 Drugs for 2005 by Sales, http://www.drugs.com/ top200_2005.html (last visited June 19, 2009). In another instance, sales information was obtained from a press release. Sales information could not be obtained for one drug with an agreement in

FY 2010. Accordingly, total, average, and median market size were calculated on the basis of 38 drugs (14 for 2010).

355 In large markets, a restriction on AG marketing of more than 180 days likely provides little benefit to either of the settling parties; longer restrictions keep the brand from selling its AG in a valuable market, but probably provide little compensation to a first-filer because many ANDA-generic competitors are likely to enter upon the expiration of exclusivity.

356 Under four such settlements, the agreed-upon entry date gave the brand the entire length or nearly the entire length of a composition of matter patent covering the drug. Another provided for entry six months before expiration of the only listed patent, which had claims to a method of use. Another settlement barred entry until 6–8 months before expiration of late-issued patents confined to a single form of the drug's active ingredient.

357 *See, e.g.,* Settlement Agreement, 2005 (entry on low-sales product, about 2 months after settlement; on blockbuster product, more than 3 years); Settlement Agreement, 2005 (entry on low-sales product, about 7 months after agreement; on blockbuster product, nearly 5 years); Settlement Agreement, 2008 (products with similar sales, one with entry about one week after execution of the agreement, the other about 3 years). For these agreements, both products contain the same active ingredient, i.e., one is a line extension of the other, and the generic was the first-filer for both products.

358 To avoid double counting, four agreements with declining royalties after expiration of an explicit "No AG" provision are not included in the eleven Type (2) agreements.

359 One ANDA was ineligible for 180-day exclusivity because the applicant made a "Section viii" statement explaining that it did not seek approval for a patented use. *See* 21 U.S.C. § 355(j)(2)(A)(viii); Purepac Pharma. Co. v. Thompson, 354 F.3d 877, 880 (D.C. Cir. 2004) ("a section viii does not entitle a successful applicant to the 180-day period of exclusivity bestowed on paragraph IV applicants."). Another application was an NDA approved under Section 505(b)(2) of the Federal Food, Drug, and Cosmetic Act, 21 U.S.C. § 355(b)(2), which does not provide for 180-day exclusivity.

360 The eight Type (3) agreements include only those that provide for the marketing or possible marketing by a subsequent filer of an AG during the first-filer's 180-day exclusivity period. Nine other agreements provided for the marketing of an AG by a subsequent filer, but only after the expiration of 180-day exclusivity.

361 Under the original provisions of the Hatch-Waxman Act, a victory by a subsequent filer triggered the first-filer's exclusivity, allowing the FDA to approve the subsequent filer's ANDA 180 days later. 21 U.S.C. § 355(j)(5)(B)(iv)(II) (2000). This court-judgment trigger has been eliminated and does not apply to ANDAs filed after December 8, 2003.

362 Pursuant to amendments contained in the MMA, a final court decision is a forfeiture event: if the first-filer does not launch its product within 75 days of a court decision, it forfeits its exclusivity, and the FDA is permitted to approve subsequent filers. *See* 21 U.S.C. § 355(j)(5)(D); Caraco Pharm. Labs. v. Forest Labs., 527 F.3d 1278, 1284–88 (Fed. Cir. 2008).

363 *Caraco*, 527 F.3d at 1284.

364 Under these agreements, the brand retains the ability to offer a "No AG" promise to the first-filer, which could act as an incentive for the first-filer to settle and defer entry.

365 Absent a settlement between the first-filer and the brand, the agreement allows the subsequent filer to launch the AG on the day the first-filer launches its ANDA-generic product following a final court decision of patent invalidity, unenforceability, or non-infringement. *See* Settlement Agreement, 2006.

366 *See* Settlement Agreement, 2006 (appointing the first-filer the exclusive AG distributor for 180-days but requiring the brand to supply the AG only if the first-filer was unable to obtain final FDA approval of its ANDA).

367 *See infra* note 30 and accompanying text.

368 For most of these agreements, the other product is a different drug (NDA), but for three agreements, the other products are dosage strengths of the litigated drug that were not at issue in the litigation. For two other agreements, the other products are future dosage strengths of the litigated drugs for which the brand had requested FDA approval. In addition to the twelve Type (4) agreements appointing the generic as the AG for another product, four Type (1) agreements and one Type (3) also contained such provisions.

369 *See* Settlement Agreement, 2008 (allowing launch during 180-day exclusivity if the first-filer launches at risk, but not if the first-filer defers entry until after a decision by a court of appeals). This agreement was made publicly available in the brand-name firm's 8-K filing with the Securities and Exchange Commission. For further discussion of these issues, *see* FED. TRADE COMM'N, AUTHORIZED GENERICS: AN INTERIM REPORT ch. 2, sec. III.B (2009), http://www.ftc.gov/os/2009/06/P062105authorizedgenericsreport.pdf.

370 FTC, "Generic Drug Entry Prior to Patent Expiration: An FTC Study," Chapter 2, July 2002.

371 Id.

372 Under the Paperwork Reduction Act, as amended, an agency may not conduct or sponsor, and a person is not required to respond to, a collection of information unless it displays a currently valid OMB control number.

373 Section 6003 of the Deficit Reduction Act of 2005, P.L. 109-171, which became effective on Jan. 1, 2007, amends Section 1927(b)(3)(A) of the Social Security Act (42 U.S.C. § 1396r-B8(b)(3)(A)) to include all drugs approved pursuant to 21 U.S.C. § 355(c), including AGs, in Medicaid best price calculations.

[374] *See* FDA, APPROVED DRUG PRODUCTS WITH THERAPEUTIC EQUIVALENCE EVALUATIONS v, 2-2 (27th ed. 2007) [hereinafter Orange Book].

[375] Generally, AGs are marketed under a different product code, labeler code, trade name, trademark, and/or packaging (other than repackaging the listed drug for use in institutions) than the listed drug. *See* Medicaid Program; Prescription Drugs, 71 Fed. Reg. 77,174, 77,183-84, 77,198 (Dec. 22, 2006). Typically, the name of an AG is the nonproprietary established name of its active ingredients, but in some cases a trade name different from the brand-name of the listed drug is used. Also, AGs are usually marketed by a subsidiary or division of the brand-name manufacturer or a third party in a manner equivalent to the marketing practices of holders of an approved ANDA for a drug. *See* Letter from William K. Hubbard, FDA, to Stuart A. Williams, Mylan Pharmaceuticals, Inc., and James N. Czaban, Heller Ehrman White & McAuliffe 2 n.2 (July 2, 2004) (responding to the citizen petitions of Mylan and Teva regarding AG drugs and 180-day exclusivity).

[376] *See* http://www.usp.org/pdf/EN/mmg/modelGuidelinesV2.0-2006-02-06.pdf. *See also* Drug List Table, at http://www.usp.org/pdf/EN/mmg/drugListingV2.0-2006-02-06.pdf.

[377] *See* P.L. 108-173, tit. XI, Subtit. B, § 1112, 117 Stat. 2066, 2461-2 (2003).

[378] Under the Paperwork Reduction Act, as amended, an agency may not conduct or sponsor, and a person is not required to respond to, a collection of information unless it displays a currently valid OMB control number.

[379] *See* FDA, APPROVED DRUG PRODUCTS WITH THERAPEUTIC EQUIVALENCE EVALUATIONS v, 2-2 (27th ed. 2007) [hereinafter Orange Book].

[380] Generally, AGs are marketed under a different product code, labeler code, trade name, trademark, and/or packaging (other than repackaging the listed drug for use in institutions) than the listed drug. *See* Medicaid Program; Prescription Drugs, 71 Fed. Reg. 77,174, 77,183-84, 77,198 (Dec. 22, 2006). Typically, the name of an AG is the nonproprietary established name of its active ingredients, but in some cases a trade name different from the brand-name of the listed drug is used. Also, AGs are usually marketed by a subsidiary or division of the brand-name manufacturer or a third party in a manner equivalent to the marketing practices of holders of an approved ANDA for a drug. *See* Letter from William K. Hubbard, FDA, to Stuart A. Williams, Mylan Pharmaceuticals, Inc., and James N. Czaban, Heller Ehrman White & McAuliffe 2 n.2 (July 2, 2004) (responding to the citizen petitions of Mylan and Teva regarding AG drugs and 180-day exclusivity).

[381] *See* P.L. 108-173, tit. XI, Subtit. B, § 1112, 117 Stat. 2066, 2461-2 (2003).

[382] Under the Paperwork Reduction Act, as amended, an agency may not conduct or sponsor, and a person is not required to respond to, a collection of information unless it displays a currently valid OMB control number.

[383] Section 6003 of the Deficit Reduction Act of 2005, P.L. 109-171, which became effective on Jan. 1, 2007, amends Section 1927(b)(3)(A) of the Social Security Act (42 U.S.C. § 1396r-8(b)(3)(A)) to include all drugs approved pursuant to 21 U.S.C. § 355(c), including AGs, in Medicaid best price calculations.

[384] *See* FDA, APPROVED DRUG PRODUCTS WITH THERAPEUTIC EQUIVALENCE EVALUATIONS v, 2-2 (27th ed. 2007) [hereinafter Orange Book].

[385] Generally, AGs are marketed under a different product code, labeler code, trade name, trademark, and/or packaging (other than repackaging the listed drug for use in institutions) than the listed drug. *See* Medicaid Program; Prescription Drugs, 71 Fed. Reg. 77,174, 77,183-84, 77,198 (Dec. 22, 2006). Typically, the name of an AG is the nonproprietary established name of its active ingredients, but in some cases a trade name different from the brand-name of the listed drug is used. Also, AGs are usually marketed by a subsidiary or division of the brand-name manufacturer or a third party in a manner equivalent to the marketing practices of holders of an approved ANDA for a drug. *See* Letter from William K. Hubbard, FDA, to Stuart A. Williams, Mylan Pharmaceuticals, Inc., and James N. Czaban, Heller Ehrman White & McAuliffe 2 n.2 (July 2, 2004) (responding to the citizen petitions of Mylan and Teva regarding AG drugs and 180-day exclusivity).

[386] This definition, which was used in the Special Orders, is very similar to the definitions of authorized generic drug in the Federal Food, Drug and Cosmetic Act, 21 U.S.C. § 355(t)(3), and in Centers for Medicare and Medicaid regulations, 42 C.F.R. § 447.506.

[387] *See* 21 C.F.R. § 299.4 ("Established names for drugs.").

[388] Generally, drugs that have AGs have them for all multisource strengths. Exceptions may involve settlement agreements in which the generic markets its ANDA-generic product for some strengths and AGs for others. Similarly, most ANDAs filed during the period covered by the study include all strengths of a drug. *See* CTR. FOR DRUG EVAL. AND RESEARCH, U.S. FOOD AND DRUG ADMIN., GUIDANCE FOR INDUSTRY: VARIATIONS IN DRUG PRODUCTS THAT MAY BE INCLUDED IN A SINGLE ANDA 1 (Dec. 28, 1998), http://www. fda.gov/downloads/Drugs/GuidanceComplianceRegulatoryInformation/Guidances/ucm07 2892.pdf.

[389] OFFICE OF GENERIC DRUGS, U.S. FOOD AND DRUG ADMIN., APPROVED DRUG PRODUCTS WITH THERAPEUTIC EQUIVALENCE EVALUATIONS ("Orange Book") (31st ed. 2011), http:// www.accessdata.fda.gov/ scripts/cder/ob/eclink.cfm. "Capsule" includes capsule; capsule, delayed release; capsule, delayed release pellets; and capsule, extended release. "Tablet" includes tablet; tablet, chewable; tablet, coated particles; tablet, delayed release; tablet, delayed release, orally disintegrating; tablet, extended release; tablet, orally disintegrating. *See id.* at App. C (Uniform Terms – Dosage Forms).

[390] IMS Health, IMS National Prescription Audit Plus 7™, Years 2003 to 2008, Data Extracted January 2009.

[391] The monthly Producer Price Index (PPI) for finished goods, seasonally adjusted (WPSSOP3000), over the period of our data (January 2003 through December 2008) is obtained from the Bureau of Labor Statistics. *See Producer Price Indexes*, BUREAU OF LABOR STATISTICS, http://www.bls.gov/ppi/data.htm (last updated June 14, 2011).

[392] The cumulative NDC database, provided by the FDA, contains all NDC records available when it was compiled, whereas the online NDC Directory contains current but not discontinued NDC records. *National Drug Code Directory*, U.S. FOOD AND DRUG ADMIN., http://www.fda.gov/Drugs/InformationOnDrugs/ucm142438.htm (last updated June 15, 2011).

[393] The nature of the "labeler" also helped identify AGs; NDA products with active ingredient names and labeler codes for generic companies (including generic subsidiaries of brand-name parent companies) or authorized generic companies were usually AGs.

[394] *See FDA Listing of Authorized Generics*, U.S. FOOD AND DRUG ADMIN., http://www.fda.gov/AboutFDA/CentersOffices/CDER/ucm126391.htm (last updated Mar. 25, 2011). This list became available on June 27, 2008. Because the list is based on annual reports provided by companies to the FDA, it may not identify all recent AGs.

[395] THOMPSON HEALTHCARE, RED BOOK (2010 ed. 2010).

[396] Also, one AG launched before 2001 was included in the study because a new strength was launched after 2001.

[397] One such AG was included because of competitive implications – it had been distributed by a generic company pursuant to settlement, but not long before generic entry (including the settling generic's ANDA-generic) the brand-name company became the AG distributor.

[398] *See* ILL. DEPT. OF PUBLIC HEALTH, ILLINOIS FORMULARY FOR THE DRUG PRODUCT SELECTION PROGRAM x–xii (21st ed. 2003), http://www.idph.state.il.us/about/fdd/ Formulary21st_edition.pdf. The 21st edition was the last edition of the Illinois Formulary. Since the list of AGs in the Illinois Formulary is cumulative, editions 14–20 (1994–2002, provided by the Division of Food, Drugs and Dairies, Illinois Department of Public Health) were used to determine the likely year of launch.

[399] *See supra* Appendix C for a list of companies included in the study. Because predecessors and subsidiaries were also considered, more companies were actually studied than Appendix C suggests. *See infra* Section IV.B.

[400] Predecessor and subsidiary relationships were determined from the Directory of Corporate Affiliations (2007), company websites, and other sources.

[401] *See* Agency Information Collection Activities; Comment Request, 72 Fed. Reg. 25,304, 25,306 (May 4, 2007) (discussing drugs included in the study).

[402] In addition, the FTC relied on a cumulative Orange Book database provided by the FDA. Identification of licensees is discussed *infra* at Section III.A.4.

[403] For a description of the drugs covered by each type of Order, *see* Appendix D, at D-11, D-12 (Brand-Name Drug Company Special Order, *Instructions for Specific Items,* ¶¶ 4-6); Appendix E, at E-9, E-10 (Generic Drug Company Special Order, *Instructions for Specific Items,* ¶¶ 4, 5 and 7); and Appendix F, at F-8 (Authorized Generic Drug Company Special Order, *Instructions for Specific Items,* ¶¶ 4 and 5).

[404] Generic companies were also asked to provide information on any AGs that they distributed, but companies were categorized as generic companies on the basis of their ANDAs, not AGs.

[405] For example, licensee relationships include situations in which one company develops a drug and holds the NDA or ANDA, and another, contractually-related company, sells or promotes the brand-name or ANDA-generic drug. Assignments involve the sale of the NDA or ANDA from one company to another. Although AGs often are distributed via licenses or assignments (e.g., an external generic company enters into a license with the NDA holder to distribute an AG, or distributes an AG pursuant to a mature NDA purchased from an innovator company), the licenses and assignments discussed in this section refer to arrangements for the distribution and sale of brand-name and ANDA-generic drugs by a company other than the original developer, not arrangements for distribution of an AG.

[406] The RED BOOK'S "manufacturers" are actually "labelers" – a term that includes both manufacturers and distributors of drugs. *See, e.g.,* THOMPSON HEALTHCARE, *supra* note 10, at 186 (2008) (noting that RED BOOK'S manufacturers include distributors and labelers other than the holder of the NDA or ANDA listed in the Orange Book); *National Drug Code Directory*, *supra* note 7 ("A labeler is any firm that manufactures . . . or distributes (under its own name) the drug.").

[407] The FDA's List of Authorized Generic Drugs, the Orange Book, the NDC database, and the FDA's application databases, often list original NDA-holders that merged with, or were acquired by, other companies; many such original NDA-holders no longer exist. Thus, the NDA-holding companies as set forth in this study often differ from those in these sources.

[408] There were few instances in which a brand-name successor company's AG counts included AGs launched by a company that it acquired. The most notable example is Pfizer, for which six of the 19 AGs counted in Figure 2-2 were launched by Pharmacia's subsidiary, Greenstone, *before* Pharmacia and Greenstone were acquired by Pfizer in 2003. Otherwise, inclusion of a predecessor's AGs in a successor company's count had little effect on companies' counts.

[409] Assignees of NDAs are often generic companies that may market both brand-name and AG versions of a drug.

[410] Information about other companies that merged later, near the end or after the period covered by the study (e.g., Barr and Teva, which merged Dec. 23, 2008), is also presented separately.

[411] For example, Figure 2-2 shows that Biovail had one AG pursuant to its NDA. Biovail, however, does not appear in either Figures 2-3 or 2-4 because the brand-name drug under its NDA is distributed by Forest, and the AG is distributed "in house" by Forest's subsidiary, Inwood.

[412] For example, in Figure 2-6, 7 of Teva's 26 exclusivities are for drugs for which other companies also earned exclusivity.

[413] Medicare Prescription Drug, Improvement, and Modernization Act of 2003 ("MMA"), Pub. L. No. 108-173, 117 Stat. 2066 (codified in scattered sections).

[414] Rarely, the first strength with generic entry via exclusivity lacks an AG, but AGs of all strengths are launched later, and are marketed during a subsequent exclusivity.

[415] End dates for 180-day exclusivities for different strengths of a drug are usually the same, except when different generic companies have exclusivity with respect to different strengths. The calculated start date is generally very close (within days) to the launch date of the ANDA-generic drug(s). In the unusual case when ANDA-generic launch was so late that it missed exclusivity altogether (e.g., when exclusivity was triggered by court decision and the generic was not ready to launch), the "exclusivity period" was excluded from the results.

[416] Also, in one instance the first-filer marketed, and discontinued, an AG before its 180-day exclusivity period began.

[417] Rarely, the first strength of an AG is launched at the time of generic entry without exclusivity, but subsequently AGs for other strengths enter during exclusivity periods.

[418] Wholesale data are from IMS Health, IMS National Sales Perspectives™, January 2003 to December 2008, Retail and Non-Retail Channels, Data Extracted February 2009.

[419] *See infra,* note 35 and accompanying text. For each NDA, we determined the highest patent certification as of the date the database was compiled, May 13, 2008.

[420] COMIS was used by the FDA "to track information about the receipt and review status of investigational new drug applications (INDs), new drug applications (NDAs), and abbreviated new drug applications (ANDAs)." *See Drugs@FDA Frequently Asked Questions*, U.S. FOOD AND DRUG ADMIN., http://www.fda.gov/Drugs/InformationOn Drugs/ucm075234.htm. The FDA provided information from the database to the FTC in 2008, including applications filed by May 13, 2008. Beginning in 2009, the FDA tracked applications in its Document Archiving, Reporting, and Regulatory Tracking System (DARRTS). Because of difficulties in working with 2008 information that arose from two different systems, we were unable to extend most of our analyses based on application data past the end of 2007.

[421] *Paragraph IV Patent Certifications*, U.S. FOOD AND DRUG ADMIN., http://www.fda.gov/ Drugs/DevelopmentApprovalProcess/HowDrugsareDevelopedandApproved/ApprovalApplications/AbbreviatedNewDrugApplicationANDAGenerics/ucm047676.htm (last updated June 10, 2011) (reporting the dates of first PIV certifications after March 2, 2004).

[422] Although expressly limited to first PIV certifications after March 2, 2004, the FDA's Paragraph IV Patent Certification website includes two first PIV certifications between January 1, 2004, and March 2, 2004, with dates generally consistent with those we estimated from the FDA's application database.

[423] Analysis by drug also avoids counting repeated "first PIVs" in anomalous situations such as when the brand adds a new strength many years after initial NDA approval, or a generic company files an ANDA with a PIV certification for a strength not approved under an NDA.

[424] Drugs *not* subject to a PIII or PIV may lack patent protection or may be covered by regulatory exclusivities that extend beyond the drug's patent protection or prohibit a challenge.

[425] Unlike PIV patent certifications, no website reports PIII patent certifications.

[426] The first PIV certifications for these drugs occurred 2–11 months after NDA approval, and the length of time from NDA approval to the end of the year ranged from 6.5–11.3 months.

[427] *See* 21 C.F.R. § 314.108.

[428] For the few instances in which more than one dosage form of the same active ingredient had NCE exclusivity, the figure includes only the first dosage form (NDA) that was approved, for which ANDAs with PIV certifications cannot be filed for four years after NDA approval. The figure does not include later-approved dosage forms of the same active ingredient because NCE exclusivity for all dosage forms of the same active ingredient because NCE exclusivity for all dosage forms of the same active ingredient ends on the same date, and the period for which ANDAs with PIV certifications cannot be filed is less than four years for the later approved dosages forms. *See* Abbreviated New Drug Application Regulations, 54 Fed. Reg. 28,872, 28,897 (July 10, 1989) (NCE exclusivity applies to active moiety, not specific drug product).

[429] Lists of NCEs with approval dates from 1998–2004 (first PIV dates from 2002–2008) were obtained from the FDA website and from the cumulative Orange Book database obtained from the FDA. *NME Drug and New Biologic Approvals*, U.S. FOOD AND DRUG ADMIN., http://www.fda.gov/Drugs/DevelopmentApprovalProcess/HowDrugsareDevelopedandApproved/Drug andBiologicApprovalReports/ucm121136.htm. The set of NCEs with NDAs approved from 1998–2004 included all NCEs for which the first possible day for a challenge occurred from 2002 through 2008: No NCE with an NDA approved during the last six months of

1997 had pediatric exclusivity that made the first possible day for a patent challenge occur in the first half of 2002 instead of the last half of 2001. Similarly, no NCE with an NDA approved during the last six months of 2004 had pediatric exclusivity that extended the first possible day for a challenge from the last half of 2008 to the first half of 2009.

[430] For ANDAs filed Jan. 1, 2002–May 13, 2008, we used the COMIS database, while the DARRTS database was used for ANDAs filed May 14, 2008–Dec. 31, 2008. *See supra* note 35. ANDA filings determined with the DARRTS database were cross-checked against publicly available litigation filings and other documents.

[431] The Federal Trade Commission received prescription sales information from over 100 drug firms representing product-level sales information over the period 1/1/2000–3/31/2007. Unfortunately, much of the firm data proved intractable due in part to inconsistencies across firms, and sometimes across products within a firm. For example, the firms often applied discounts, charge-backs, returns, drug expirations and other product flow information as periodic accounting adjustments. These adjustments were made on irregular bases over time and could differ in timing across dollar and quantity sales of the same product. As a consequence, the sales adjustments frequently led to negative sales dollars and quantities, which made calculation of meaningful prices problematic. These issues led us to purchase sales information from a data vendor.

[432] Certain discounts may not be accounted for in this data. IMS CONSULTING, IMS HEALTH, ASSESSMENT OF AUTHORIZED GENERICS IN THE U.S. 19 (2006) (written for the Pharm. Research and Mfrs. of Am. ("PhRMA")), http://replay.web.archive.org/20061009134405/http://www.phrma.org/files/IMS%20 Authorized %20Generics%20Report_6-22-06.pdf ("[P]rompt-payment cash discounts and bottom-line invoice discounts are not reflected in the dollar purchase amounts. Also, it should be noted that volume purchase estimates may not always reflect drop shipment activity.") As long as these omitted discounts do not vary systematically between authorized and ANDA-generic products, the absence of information on these discounts should not bias the analysis.

[433] Most molecules were assigned to the most prevalently observed therapeutic class observed in the data. However, the molecule, Bupropion, represents an important exception. The molecule Bupropion must be distinguished by whether it is used to treat smoking addiction or depression. Nitrofurantoin was excluded from the analysis because it is associated with several molecular names in the FDA data.

[434] Dosage forms were defined using the "three-lettered" code defined by IMS. The mapping of this variable into dosage forms used in the analysis is provided in Table I-4. This mapping was necessary in order to match the IMS and FDA data.

[435] Several market outcomes, such as prices, have been normalized based on the market conditions that existed prior to generic entry. Consequently, even though data for the first three months of 2003 were available, that information was used only to calculate pre-generic entry market characteristics for products that experienced generic entry early in 2003.

[436] This process dropped Clopidogrel 75mg tablets, Ondansetron 24mg tablets, Fenofibrate 160mg tablets, Fenofibrate 54mg tablets, Trimethobenzamide 300mg capsules, and Amantadine 100mg tablets.

[437] On occasion, positive but small sales figures were observed for a generic firm earlier than other reliable information suggests it could be on the market. Therefore, generic sales that occurred prior to the FDA-defined exclusivity period and that represented less than 0.5% of pre-entry brand sales were excluded.

[438] The six-month limitation on the length of the exclusivity period affects only products in "AG Only" markets. The three-year window considered outside exclusivity is a maximum length. The analysis considers drugs with shorter time horizons. The three-year mark was chosen because less than half of the drugs in the sample were observed for more than three years.

[439] The IMS data do not always differentiate between manufacturers and repackagers. Although repackagers were not included in the count of manufacturers, the sales associated with them were used to construct price and sales figures. A list of companies treated as repackagers is provided in Table I-5. Incorrect identification of the repackagers could cause over- or under-statement of the number of active generic manufacturers of a product.

[440] *See* FED. TRADE COMM'N, PHARMACY BENEFIT MANAGERS: OWNERSHIP OF MAIL-ORDER PHARMACIES ch. VI (2005), http://www.ftc.gov/reports/pharmbenefit05/050906pharm benefitrpt.pdf (providing additional information on repackagers).

[441] *See, e.g., FDA Listing of Authorized Generics*, U.S. FOOD AND DRUG ADMIN., http://www. fda.gov/AboutFDA/CentersOffices/CDER/ucm126391.htm (last updated Mar. 25, 2011).

[442] *See Paragraph IV Patent Certifications*, U.S. FOOD AND DRUG ADMIN., http://www.fda.gov/Drugs/DevelopmentApprovalProcess/HowDrugsareDevelopedandApproved/Approval Applications/AbbreviatedNewDrugApplicationANDAGenerics/ucm047676.htm (last updated June 10, 2011) (list updated twice a month).

[443] For example, if the exclusivity period as identified by the FDA ended on June 15, 2005, then the exclusivity would include the months December 2004 through May 2005 but would exclude June. However, if the end date of the exclusivity was June 29th, then the month of June would also be included in the exclusivity period.

[444] *See Producer Price Indexes*, BUREAU OF LABOR STATISTICS, http://www.bls.gov/ppi/data. htm.

[445] Another way to group products would be by chemical properties of the active ingredients, but the condition treated by the product is, arguably, the single most important characteristic relating the products in a category.

For example, the molecule Bupropion is used to treat two conditions, smoking addiction and clinical depression. Bupropion is categorized into two therapeutic codes that represent the treatment of these conditions, despite being the exact same molecule and thus having identical chemical properties.

[446] Even without considering dollars sold, some therapeutic classes may represent a large fraction of total products sold in the market, but represent a small number of products beginning to face generic competition during the time window of this analysis.

[447] The market-size metric is the ratio between the average market size of the therapeutic class against the average overall market size. For example, a value of 3 indicates that the therapeutic class has a market size that is three times larger than the average product.

[448] For example, some of the products in the sample are ineligible to face a Paragraph IV challenge.

[449] *See* Omnibus Budget Reconciliation Act of 1990, Pub. L. No. 101-508, Title IV, § 4401 (a)(3), 104 Stat. 1388-143 (codified at 42 U.S.C. § 1396r-8 (2010)).

[450] The program is administered by the Centers for Medicare & Medicaid Services ("CMS") in the Department of Health and Human Services.

[451] *See, e.g.*, Company Document ("CD"), undated (contending that "the failure of the Department of Health and Human Services (HHS) to enforce the inclusion of authorized generics in the Medicaid rebate calculation for the brand product is . . . depriving state Medicaid programs of hundreds of millions of dollars in rebates").

[452] Deficit Reduction Act of 2005 ("DRA"), Pub. L. No. 109-171, 120 Stat. 4 (codified at 42 U.S.C. § 1396r (2010)).

[453] *See id.* §§ 1396r-8 (b)(3)(A), (c)(1)(C)(i)(ii).

[454] *See* Medicaid Program; Prescription Drugs, 71 Fed. Reg. 77,174 (Dec. 22, 2006).

[455] *Id.* at 77,183–84, 77,198.

[456] *See* Medicaid Program; Prescription Drugs, 72 Fed. Reg. 39,142, 39,151, 39,199 (July 17, 2007).

[457] *See id.* at 39,199–200; *id.* at 39,243 (final rule § 447.506).

[458] *See, e.g.*, CD, July 13, 2007.

[459] *See* Public Comment from Ronald W. Davis, Attorney, to the Fed. Trade Comm'n 3 ("Davis Comment") (June 4, 2006), http://www.ftc.gov/os/comments/genericdrugstudy3/060604 davis.pdf (submitted on behalf of an undisclosed client) ("Among other things, the new provision, effective in 2007, amends the definition of 'best price,' for purposes of calculating the Medicaid rebate, to include prices charged for authorized generics sold by an affiliate or other licensee of the NDA holder. The purpose, and the likely effect, of this amendment is to fundamentally reduce the incentives of branded firms to introduce authorized generics."); Public Comment from the Pharm. Research and Mfrs. of Am. ("PhRMA") to the Fed. Trade Comm'n 10 n.17 (June 5, 2006), http://www.ftc.gov/os/ comments/genericdrugstudy3/060605pharma.pdf (cautioning that the inclusion of AGs in the calculation of best price "could impact . . . the incentives for brand drug companies to introduce authorized generics").

[460] *See* CD, Oct. 5, 2006 (DRA a "[b]ig win for generic lobbyists . . . ; [c]ould cost [Brand Co.] approximately $25–50 million a year in additional Medicaid rebates"); CD, Feb. 5, 2007 (DRA provisions are "intended to discourage AG's by increasing the Medicaid rebate liability of the brand drugs"; "AG provisions may discourage some brand companies on some products from entering into AG agreements due to increased Medicaid rebates on their brand sales and increased complexity of AMP/BP price reporting requirements for AG's."); CD, Mar. 3, 2006 (law firm analysis predicting that the "new [DRA] provision may significantly complicate the ability of manufacturers to enter the generic market by use of an authorized generic"); *see also* CD, Sept. 28, 2006 (DRA "designed to discourage authorized generic introduction during the Hatch Waxman 180 day generic exclusivity period, also penalizes innovators launching authorized generics during the first quarter of generic sales").

[461] Davis Comment, *supra* note 11, at 3 ("[T]he purported 'problem' that gave rise to the proposed study will likely disappear, or be substantially reduced, without any further regulatory or legislative action. And the regulatory environment will be materially altered, so that the information sought will be of little practical utility to any possible Commission action or change in statutory law.").

[462] The DRA became effective on January 1, 2007. As reported in Chapter 2, twelve AGs were launched that year, and fifteen were launched in 2008. *See supra* Chapter 2, Section I.A.

[463] *See supra* Appendix D, ¶ 30, at D-7 (Brand-Name Drug Company Special Order); *see supra* Appendix F, ¶ 12, at F-3 to -4 (Authorized Generic Drug Company Special Order).

[464] The DRA changes were signed into law in February 2006, and had an effective date of January 1, 2007. The proposed rule was issued on December 22, 2006, but the final rule was not issued until July 17, 2007. The document request applied to documents dated January 1, 2006 to April 29, 2007. Accordingly, most of the financial and analytical documents that the companies produced were based on the proposed rule rather than the final rule, which, as noted above, likely imposed significantly higher Medicaid rebates than the proposed rule.

[465] Eighteen brand companies and one specialized AG firm that received the Special Orders provided some documents in response to the DRA document request.

466 *See, e.g.*, CD, Sept. 28, 2006 (noting that DRA provisions would take effect on January 1, 2007 and that "detailed financial analysis is required on a product by product basis to determine the most effective strategy for [company] to implement upon loss of patent or market exclusivity").

467 *See, e.g.*, *id.* ("[t]he % of Medicaid [p]articipation is key to the financial impact of [the] Authorized Generic on [the brand company]").

468 *See, e.g.*, *id.* ("Since the Medicaid rebate is calculated on a quarterly basis, the timing of generic launch in the quarter is also a critical factor . . . ."); CD, Oct. 5, 2006 ("launch at the end of a quarter will cost more than at the beginning"); CD, Mar. 2, 2007 ("The amount it costs us will vary from product to product depending on when the generic is launched in the quarter.").

469 In one of the few post-final rule documents produced, a brand company with a substantial AG program estimated that under the final rule, the DRA would increase its rebates for the fourth quarter of 2007 by approximately $18 million, to a total of roughly $113 million; in contrast, the firm projected that under the proposed rule its rebates would have increased by only $1 million. CD, Sept. 21, 2007; *see also,* CD, Aug. 1, 2007 (retrospective analysis of rebates using data for the first and second quarters of 2007, again finding a much greater increase under the final rule).

470 The Part D Medicare program provides expanded Medicare coverage for prescription drugs. As part of this program, "dual eligibles" (those who qualified for prescription coverage under both Medicaid and Medicare) were transferred to Medicare. *See, e.g.*, CD, Apr. 25, 2006 (noting shift of Medicaid patients to Medicare coverage with respect to osteoporosis drugs); CD, Feb. 12, 2007 (noting "[n]egligible Medicaid rebate impact" on osteoporosis drug since "[m]ost patients covered by Medicare"). Accordingly, some drugs previously provided through the Medicaid program to the elderly are now provided under Medicare, to which the DRA provisions do not apply. *See* CD, undated (noting that "[t]otal payments for Medicaid rebates in 2006 fell dramatically as a result of the conversion of Medicaid/Medicare dual eligibles to Medicare effective January 1, 2006. Approximately 60% of total Medicaid business converted to Medicare in 2006.").

471 Under the 340B Program pharmaceutical companies provide prescription drugs to various types of government-operated or assisted health care facilities at heavily discounted prices based on a formula that takes into account the amount of the Medicaid rebate. *See* 42 U.S.C. § 256b (2010).

472 In fact, application of the formula can result in a negative price for some drugs, triggering the so-called "penny pricing" policy for those drugs. *See, e.g.*, CD, Oct. 2007. Under the penny pricing policy, drug manufacturers are told to submit a 340B ceiling price of $0.01 whenever the ceiling price would otherwise be negative. *See, e.g.*, *Authorized Generic Law Resulting In Growing Number of Penny Priced Drugs*, FED. DRUG DISCOUNT & COMPLIANCE MONITOR, July 2008, at 1, 8 (quoting a representative of Schering-Plough as saying that "340B pricing for the drug [Desogen] has been, and in all likelihood will continue to be, dramatically affected by the new CMS rule regarding the calculation of AMP and best price for brand-name products that have authorized generic versions" and predicting that "penny pricing would have a 'substantial' impact on the marketplace").

473 *See* CD, Feb. 12, 2007.

474 CD, Nov. 28, 2006, Jan. 5, 2007.

475 *See* CD, undated.

476 *See* CD, Sept. 25, 2007 (agreeing to "suspend" their AG contract "as a result of [the DRA] final rule").

477 *See, e.g.*, CD, undated; CD, Jan. 9, 2006; CD, Mar. 2007; *see also,* CD, Jan. 5, 2007 (deciding to launch two AGs shortly before issuance of the final rule when AG revenues were expected to offset increased rebates).

478 *See* CD, Jan. 5, 2007 ("Consider strategic implications in addition to financials (customer expectations, inventory and production capacity utilization)").

479 Entry by 180-day exclusivity could occur following a successful patent challenge with a court determination of invalidity, non-infringement, or unenforceability or when a brand fails to sue the generic or the parties enter a settlement.

480 The count of generic manufacturers in the market includes the AG and was constructed, separately, for wholesale and retail data. Manufacturers were considered to have exited if they experienced three consecutive months of zero sales. Discrepancies in manufacturer counts between the NSP and NPA data were allowed to remain.

481 Pre-entry sales of the brand-name product refer to the sum total of brand-name product sales three months prior to generic entry.

482 For the analysis reported in Table 3-1, this price, p, is the average retail price of all generic versions of the product, including the AG. Table 3-2 is based on the same model; the only difference is that p is the average wholesale price of all generic versions of the product. In Table 3-3, the average ANDA price and the AG price in a given month are treated as two separate observations instead of being combined in a weighted average, and the AG indicator is turned on when the observation is an AG price. Tables 3-4 and 3-5 report analysis very similar to that in Tables 3-1 and 3-2, except that p is the price of the brand-name product in the month as opposed to an average generic price.

483 Although the indicator variable for month 0 was excluded, data from month 0 were not excluded. When estimating a regression model that has a constant, such as α in this model, it is necessary to have indicator

variables for all but one of the possible categories. The effect of the omitted category is picked up by the constant.

484 The results of this prediction are not very sensitive to specification or to the point of evaluation. For example, estimation of a model with a log-linear specification that imposes a constant AG effect at any point in the data produces effects of similar magnitudes.

485 The mdft subscripts have been suppressed for the sake of exposition.

486 The pre-entry brand revenue, R_0, is constructed to be the total expenditures on the brand-name product for the three months immediately prior to generic entry, divided by three.

487 Once again, the results of this analysis displayed some robustness with respect to an alternate log-linear model specification.

488 The effect of the AG may depend on the number of manufacturers in the market. Interacting the AG indicator with the number of manufacturers captures these differential effects. Because some markets involve many manufacturers, the number of interaction terms in this model is large, producing many estimates of the impact of an AG (one for each interaction). The effects from this model are difficult to interpret, unstable across specifications, and difficult to estimate because products facing large numbers of manufacturers are rarely observed without an AG. Moreover, the results do not provide enough evidence to contradict or significantly buttress the conclusions reached from the simpler analysis reported in the text. For all these reasons, the analysis is omitted.

489 Determining the actual number of products displaced by the AG outside exclusivity is beyond the scope of this Report. As described in the text, in markets where no generic firm ever had an exclusivity period, the AG takes a market share that is very close to the average market share of the ANDA-generics that enter in the first several months of generic competition. Consequently, the AG appears to behave similarly to ANDA-generic manufacturers in these markets, suggesting that it is reasonable to assume that an AG displaces one, and only one, ANDA-generic manufacturer.

In: Authorized Generic Drugs
Editors: Edward R. Nelson and Jerry G. Wright
ISBN: 978-1-62257-075-1

Chapter II

AUTHORIZED GENERIC PHARMACEUTICALS: EFFECTS ON INNOVATION*

John R. Thomas

SUMMARY

The practice of "authorized generics" has recently been the subject of considerable attention by the pharmaceutical industry, regulators, and members of Congress alike. An "authorized generic" (sometimes termed a "branded," "flanking," or "pseudo" generic) is a pharmaceutical that is marketed by or on behalf of a brand-name drug company, but is sold under a generic name. Although the availability of an additional competitor in the generic drug market would appear to be favorable to consumers, authorized generics have nonetheless proven controversial. Some observers believe that authorized generics potentially discourage independent generic firms both from challenging drug patents and from selling their own products.

These perceived disincentives result from the provisions of the Drug Price Competition and Patent Term Restoration Act of 1984. Better known as the Hatch-Waxman Act, this legislation provides independent generic firms with a reward for challenging patents held by brand-name firms. That "bounty" consists of a 180-day generic drug exclusivity period awarded to the first patent challenger. During the 180-day period, the brand-name company and the first generic applicant are the only firms that receive authorization to sell that pharmaceutical. At the close of this period, other independent generic competitors may obtain marketing approval and enter the market, ordinarily resulting in lower prices for generic medicines.

Some commentators view the 180-day exclusivity period as a crucial incentive for generic firms to challenge patents held by brand-name firms. Under this view, the launch of an authorized generic during the 180-day exclusivity period makes the recovery of litigation

* This is an edited, reformatted and augmented version of the Congressional Research Service Publication, CRS Report for Congress RL33605, dated January 27, 2012.

expenses more difficult. In turn, the possibility that a brand-name firm will sell an authorized generic during the 180-day exclusivity period may decrease the incentives of generic firms to challenge patents in the first instance.

Other observers believe that authorized generics benefit consumers by increasing competition in the generic market. Because the authorized generic is manufactured by the brand-name firm and identical to its own product, consumers may be encouraged to switch to the lower-cost authorized generic alternative. Authorized generics may also facilitate the settlement of patent litigation between brand-name and independent generic firms. As an historical matter, certain of these settlement agreements have allowed authorized generics to enter the market, and therefore promoted competition, prior to the expiration of the relevant patent term.

Recent judicial opinions have upheld FDA practices allowing authorized generics. If authorized generic practice is deemed appropriate, then no action need be taken. The approach taken by legislation introduced in the 112th Congress, H.R. 741 and S. 373, presents another option. Under these bills, authorized generics may not be sold during the term of the 180-day generic exclusivity. This legislation was not yet been enacted.

Rising health care costs have for many years focused congressional attention upon the development and availability of prescription drugs. Recently, the presence of "authorized generic" pharmaceuticals in the drug marketplace has been the subject of congressional concern.[1] An "authorized generic" is a pharmaceutical that is marketed by or on behalf of a brand-named drug company, but is sold under a generic name. The brand-name firm may distribute the drug under its own auspices or via a license to a generic drug company. The price of this "authorized copy" is ordinarily lower than that of the brand-name drug.[2] Some sources refer to authorized generics as "branded," "flanking," or "pseudo" generics."[3]

Authorized generics may be pro-consumer in that they potentially increase competition and lower prices, particularly in the short-term. They have nonetheless proven controversial. Authorized generics ordinarily enter the market at about the time the brand-name drug company's patents are set to expire.[4] Some observers argue that such products may possibly discourage independent generic firms both from challenging drug patents and from selling their own generic products.[5] The potential diminution in independent generic incentives may in turn lead to less desire on the part of brand-name firms to market authorized generics themselves.

Legal challenges to authorized generics practice have thus far been unsuccessful in the courts. Legislation has been introduced regarding authorized generic practice, however. Legislation introduced but not yet enacted in the 112th Congress, H.R. 741 and S. 373, proposes to prevent pharmaceutical firms from selling authorized generics.

This report presents an analysis of the innovation and public health issues relating to authorized generic drugs. The report begins with a review of the procedures through which independent generic drug companies receive government permission to market their products and resolve patent disputes with brand-name firms. It then provides detailed background information pertaining to the concept of authorized generics and assesses their potential impact upon patent challenges and consumer welfare. The report closes with a summary of congressional issues and possible alternatives.

MARKETING APPROVAL AND PATENT ISSUES FOR GENERIC DRUGS

The practice of authorized generics has arisen within a complex statutory framework established by the Drug Price Competition and Patent Term Restoration Act of 1984,[6] legislation more commonly known as the Hatch-Waxman Act.[7] Under parameters established by that statute, a manufacturer that wishes to sell a generic drug must both obtain marketing approval from the Food and Drug Administration (FDA) and account for any patent rights that pertain to that product. This report first addresses FDA marketing approval procedures for generic drugs, and then turns to possible patent implications.

FDA Approval Procedures

The FDA regulates the marketing of pharmaceuticals in the interest of public health.[8] Under this regime, the developer of a new drug must demonstrate that the product is safe and effective before it can be distributed to the public. This showing typically requires the drug's sponsor to conduct both preclinical and clinical investigations.[9] In deciding whether to issue marketing approval or not, the FDA evaluates the test data that the sponsor submits in a so-called New Drug Application (NDA).

Prior to the enactment of the Hatch-Waxman Act, the federal food and drug law contained no separate provisions addressing marketing approval for independent generic versions of drugs that had previously been approved by the FDA.[10] The result was that a would-be independent generic drug manufacturer had to file its own NDA in order to sell its product.[11] Some independent generic manufacturers could rely on published scientific literature demonstrating the safety and efficacy of the drug by submitting a so-called paper NDA. Because these sorts of studies were not available for all drugs, however, not all independent generic firms could file a paper NDA.[12] Further, at times the FDA requested additional studies to address safety and efficacy questions that arose from experience with the drug following its initial approval.[13] The result was that some independent generic manufacturers were forced to prove once more that a particular drug was safe and effective, even though their products were chemically identical to those of previously approved pharmaceuticals.

Some commentators believed that the approval of an independent generic drug was a needlessly costly, duplicative, and time-consuming process.[14] These observers noted that although patents on important drugs had expired, manufacturers were not moving to introduce independent generic equivalents for these products due to the level of resource expenditure required to obtain FDA marketing approval.[15]

In response to these concerns, Congress enacted the Hatch-Waxman Act, a statute that has been described as a "complex and multifaceted compromise between innovative and generic pharmaceutical companies."[16] Its provisions included the creation of two statutory pathways that expedited the marketing approval process for independent generic drugs. The first of these consist of Abbreviated New Drug Applications, or ANDAs. An ANDA allows an independent generic applicant to obtain marketing approval by demonstrating that the proposed product is bioequivalent to an approved pioneer drug, without providing evidence of safety and effectiveness from clinical data or from the scientific literature. The second are so-called § 505(b)(2) applications, which are sometimes still referred to as "paper NDAs." Like an NDA, a § 505(b)(2) application contains a full report of investigations of safety and effectiveness of the proposed product. In contrast to an NDA, however, a § 505(b)(2) application typically relies at least in part upon published literature providing pre-clinical or clinical data.

The availability of ANDAs and § 505(b)(2) applications often allow an independent generic manufacturer to avoid the costs and delays associated with filing a full-fledged NDA. They may also allow an independent generic manufacturer, in many cases, to place its FDA-approved bioequivalent drug on the market as soon as any relevant patents expire.[17]

As part of the balance struck between brand-name and independent generic firms, Congress also provided patent proprietors with a means for restoring a portion of the patent term that had been lost while awaiting FDA approval. The maximum extension period is capped at a five-year extension period, or a total effective patent term after the extension of not more than 14 years.[18] The scope of rights during the period of extension is generally limited to the use approved for the product that subjected it to regulatory delay.[19] This period of patent term extension is intended to compensate brand-name firms for the generic drug industry's reliance upon the proprietary pre-clinical and clinical data they have generated, most often at considerable expense to themselves.[20]

Resolution of Patent Disputes

In addition to being the holder of an FDA-approved NDA, the brand-name pharmaceutical firm may own one or more patents directed towards that drug product.[21] The product described by an independent generic firm's ANDA or § 505(b)(2) application may possibly infringe those patents should that product be approved by the FDA and sold in the marketplace. The Hatch-Waxman Act therefore establishes special procedures for resolving patent disputes in connection with applications for marketing generic drugs.

In particular, the Hatch-Waxman Act requires each holder of an approved NDA to identify patents it believes would be infringed if a generic drug were marketed before the expiration of these patents.[22] The FDA then lists these patents in a publication titled *Approved Drug Products with Therapeutic Equivalence Evaluations*, which is more commonly known as the "Orange Book."[23] Would-be manufacturers of independent generic drugs must then engage in a specialized certification procedure with respect to Orange Book-listed patents. An ANDA or § 505(b)(2) applicant must state its views with respect to each Orange Book-listed patent associated with the drug it seeks to market. Four possibilities exist:

(1) that the brand-name firm has not filed any patent information with respect to that drug;
(2) that the patent has already expired;
(3) that the generic company agrees not to market until the date on which the patent will expire; or
(4) that the patent is invalid or will not be infringed by the manufacture, use or sale of the drug for which the ANDA is submitted.[24]

These certifications are respectively termed paragraph I, II, III, and IV certifications.[25] An ANDA or § 505(b)(2) application certified under paragraphs I or II is approved immediately after meeting all applicable regulatory and scientific requirements.[26] An independent generic firm that files an ANDA or § 505(b)(2) application including a paragraph III certification must, even after meeting pertinent regulatory and scientific requirements, wait for approval until the drug's listed patent expires.[27]

The filing of an ANDA or § 505(b)(2) application with a paragraph IV certification constitutes a "somewhat artificial" act of patent infringement under the Hatch-Waxman Act.[28] The act requires the independent generic applicant to notify the proprietor of the patents that are the subject of a paragraph IV certification.[29] The patent owner may then commence patent infringement litigation against that applicant.

If the NDA holder demonstrates that the independent generic firm's proposed product would violate its patents, then the court will ordinarily issue an injunction that prevents the generic drug company from marketing that product. That injunction will expire on the same date as the NDA holder's patents. Independent generic drug companies commonly amend their ANDAs or § 505(b)(2) applications in this event, replacing their paragraph IV certifications with paragraph III certifications.[30]

On the other hand, the courts may decide in favor of the independent generic firm. The court may conclude that the generic firm's proposed product does not infringe the asserted patents, or that the asserted patents are invalid or unenforceable.[31] In this circumstance, the independent generic firm may launch its product once the FDA has approved its ANDA or § 505(b)(2) application. In addition, the independent generic firm may benefit from a 180-day period of marketing exclusivity, a concept this report describes next.

Generic Marketing Exclusivity

The Hatch-Waxman Act provides prospective manufacturers of independent generic pharmaceuticals with a reward for challenging the patent associated with an approved pharmaceutical. The reward consists of a 180-day generic drug exclusivity period awarded to the first ANDA applicant to file a paragraph IV certification. During this 180-day period, the FDA may not approve another ANDA containing a paragraph IV certification with respect to the same drug.[32] Notably, the 180-day generic drug exclusivity applies only to ANDA applicants, and not to those filing § 505(b)(2) applications.[33]

Commentators have long referred to this provision as creating "generic exclusivity" or "180-day exclusivity."[34] As originally enacted, the Hatch-Waxman Act allowed the brand-name firm and the first independent generic applicant to share the market for the first 180 days of generic competition. At the close of this period, other independent generic competitors could receive FDA marketing approval. Because market prices often drop considerably following the entry of additional generic competition, the first independent generic applicant could potentially obtain more handsome profits than subsequent market entrants.[35]

Congressional enactment of the Medicare Modernization and Improvement Act of 2003[36] clarified that more than one patent challenger can enjoy "generic exclusivity," provided that certain conditions are met. Following the 2003 statute, all "first applicants" are potentially entitled to the 180-day generic exclusivity.[37] The statute defines the term "first applicant" to mean all applicants who, on the first day on which a substantially complete generic application with paragraph IV certification is filed, did themselves file a substantially complete generic application with a paragraph IV certification.[38] The statute therefore makes clear that multiple first applicants—that is to say, more than one generic that filed a paragraph IV generic application on the same day—may each enjoy "shared exclusivity."

The 180-day generic exclusivity period is intended to ameliorate collective action problems that may arise with regard to pharmaceutical patent challenges.[39] Stated less technically, an independent generic firm that challenges a patent must bear the expensive, up-front cost of litigation. If the independent generic firm is successful, however, the challenged patent is declared invalid with regard to the entire pharmaceutical industry. Any firm—not just the one who challenged the patent—could then introduce a competing product to the marketplace. Understandably, this forced sharing may undermine the incentives any one independent generic firm would possess to challenge a brand-name firm's patent. The award of 180 days of generic exclusivity is therefore intended to allow a successful patent challenger to capture an individual benefit for its effort, in turn encouraging such challenges in the first instance.[40]

The Concept of Authorized Generics

Authorized Generics Practice

As noted previously, an "authorized generic" is a pharmaceutical that is marketed by or on behalf of a brand-name drug company, but is sold under a generic name.[41] Authorized generics are thus similar to "private label" products, which are manufactured by one firm but sold under the brand of another. Although private label products are commonplace in food, cosmetic, and other markets, they have only recently attracted attention in the pharmaceutical industry.[42]

Current interest in authorized generics is largely due to a shift in corporate strategies that has been traced to the early 1990s. Until that time, many entrants in the pharmaceutical industry engaged exclusively either in selling brand-name, innovative drugs, or in selling generic drugs. Several other brand-name firms began to market authorized generics shortly before patents on their products were due to expire. Among such products were Nolvadex® (tamoxifen), authorized by the Stewart Pharmaceutical Division of ICI Americas (now AstraZeneca) and sold by Barr Laboratories; Dyazide® (triamterene/hydrochlorothiazide), marketed by SmithKline Beecham Pharmaceuticals (now GlaxoSmithKline); and Ventolin® (albuterol), authorized by GlaxoSmithKline and sold by Dey LP.[43]

Many brand-name firms did not continue to sell authorized generics at that time, however, reportedly due to a lack of profitability.[44] One reason for the "resurgence" of authorized generics in the early 2000's is that physicians, pharmacists and patients more rapidly switch to generic drugs upon their introduction to the marketplace than a decade ago.[45] Because the rate of generic adoption is much greater now, brand-name firms reportedly are more willing to "genericize" their own brands in order to capture a share of that market.[46] The expanding generic adoption rate has also reportedly led to an industry trend where brand-name houses acquire generic firms.[47] This development too may encourage authorized generics practice in the future.

In line with current trends, a number of successful paragraph IV ANDA applicants have faced competition from authorized generics during the 180-day generic exclusivity period. These independent generic firms include Barr, for the product Allegra® (fexofenadine);[48] Eon, for the product Wellbutrin SR® (bupropion SR);[49] and Teva, for the product Glucophage®.[50] Some industry analysts believe that authorized generics will form an increasingly prominent feature of the U.S. pharmaceutical market in the future.[51] Other commentators believe that this time has already arrived: According to one account, since 2004 "authorized generic versions have appeared for nearly all drugs with expiring U.S. patents."[52]

Authorized Generics within the Hatch-Waxman Framework

Authorized generics practice has proven controversial due to the Hatch-Waxman Act's architecture and incentive structures. Some commentators have voiced concerns that the introduction of authorized generics, particularly during the 180-day market exclusivity granted to the independent generic firm that brought a paragraph IV challenge, thwarts the policy goal of encouraging the introduction of generic pharmaceuticals.[53] In particular, critics argue that the use of authorized generics may discourage firms from filing paragraph IV patent challenges if their litigation expenses cannot be recouped through the 180-day market exclusivity period.[54] As antitrust attorney David A. Balto explains:

> The bounty from challenging a patent is very important. Pharmaceutical patent litigation is a multimillion-dollar proposition. But for the potential reward of six-month exclusivity that represents the vast majority of potential profits from generic entry, many firms might forgo challenging patents.[55]

For example, the FDA ruled that the generic manufacturer Apotex was entitled to 180-day exclusivity for its version of the anti-depressant drug Paxil® in 2003. The brand-name drug company, GlaxoSmithKline, introduced an authorized generic version of Paxil®. Although Apotex anticipated sales of up to $575 million during the 180-day generic exclusivity period, its sales were reported to be between $150 million and $200 million.[56] In a 2004 filing with the FDA, attorneys for Apotex asserted "that the authorized generic crippled Apotex's 180-day exclusivity—it reduced Apotex's entitlement to about two-thirds—to the tune of approximately $400 million."[57]

In addition, brand-name firms commonly introduce authorized generics on the eve of generic competition. Without an independent generic patent challenger in the first instance, brand-name firms may themselves make diminished, or delayed, use of the authorized generic strategy. As a result, the pro-competitive benefits of authorized generics may be postponed, or not realized at all, should independent generic rivals become less willing to challenge patents held by brand-name firms.[58]

On the other hand, authorized generics potentially offer several benefits both to drug companies and to consumers. Authorized generics are commonly less expensive than the brand-name drug. The introduction of an authorized generic therefore allows a lower-cost product to be made available to the consumer.[59] As the FDA opined in a statement issued in July 2004:

> Marketing of authorized generics increases competition, promoting lower prices for pharmaceuticals, particularly during the 180-day exclusivity period in which the prices for generic drugs are often substantially higher than after other generic products are able to enter the market.[60]

More particularly, a June 2009 study conducted by the Federal Trade Commission (FTC) found that retail prices decreased by an average of 4.2% and wholesale prices decreased by an average of 6.5% when an authorized generic competed with an ANDA generic. This level of competition led to an estimated average decline of 50% of the generic firm's revenue.[61]

In addition, once a generic version of a drug becomes available following patent expiration, brand-name firms may lose considerable market share. Indeed, many health management organizations and insurance companies reportedly promote the use of generic substitutes for brand-name medications once they become available.[62] Absent participation in the generic market, brand-name firms may not be able to take advantage of investments they previously made with respect to their manufacturing facilities. Authorized generics therefore allow brand-name firms to continue to employ their manufacturing facilities at or near peak capacity even following patent expiration.[63]

Authorized generics may also support the research and development efforts of brand-name firms by providing them with additional revenue. Authorized generics may supply the brand-name firm with an additional income source, such as a royalty on sales made by its generic subsidiary or contracting partner.[64] These funds, or some portion of them, can potentially be employed in support of pharmaceutical innovation.

Authorized generics may also facilitate settlement of patent infringement suits between brand-name and independent generic firms. A judicial holding of patent invalidity may have a severe impact upon a brand-name firm in terms of its lost revenue. Many observers also believe that patent litigation is an uncertain venture.[65] By settling patent litigation, and allowing an ANDA applicant to produce an authorized generic, brand-name firms may potentially better manage risk. Such a technique provides a more stable revenue stream, both in support of the brand-name firm's research and development activities and for its investors. The generic company making an authorized generic can also benefit by not having to expend funds on litigation with an uncertain outcome or pursue an ANDA at the FDA, while expanding its product line, acquiring manufacturing experience, and gaining the first-mover advantage in the generic market.[66]

The use of authorized generics as a litigation settlement mechanism also impacts consumers, but in a manner that is both less certain and likely varies on a case-by-case basis. On one hand, particular settlement agreements may provide for the sale of authorized generics years before the disputed patent is set to expire. As a result, consumers may gain early access to a lower-cost alternative to the brand-name drug. On the other hand, had the generic firm refused to settle and ultimately prevailed in the litigation, then the market would have been open to full competition even earlier. The impact upon competition of a litigation settlement likely depends upon a number of complex factors, including the strength of the patent, the number of potential generic competitors, and the precise terms of the litigation settlement agreement.

A Federal Trade Commission Report issued on August 31, 2011, addressed the topic of authorized generics and may contribute to policy debate over the impact of these products. Titled *Authorized Generic Drugs—Short-Term Effects and Long-Term Impact*, makes four primary findings:

- Competition from authorized generics during the 180-day marketing exclusivity period has led to lower retail and wholesale drug prices. During this time, competition by an authorized generic is associated with retail prices that are 4%to 8% lower, and wholesale prices that are 7% to 14% lower, than those without an authorized generic.
- Authorized generics have a substantial effect on the revenues of competing generic firms. During the 180-day exclusivity period, the presence of an authorized generic competitor on average reduces the first-filing generic's revenues by 40% to 52%. In addition, revenues of the first-filing generic are between 53% and 62% lower during the first 30 months after the exclusivity period ends, if it is facing authorized generic competition. Introduction of an authorized generic can mean hundreds of millions of dollars in lost revenue for the first generic competitor to enter the market.
- Lower expected profits could affect a generic company's decision to challenge patents on products with low sales. However, the reduced revenues resulting from authorized generic competition during the 180-day exclusivity period have not substantially reduced the number of challenges to branded drug patents by generic firms. Despite the presence of authorized generic competition, generic companies have continued to challenge patents, even on brand-name drugs in small markets.
- There is strong evidence that agreements not to compete using authorized generics have become a way that some branded firms compensate generic firms for delaying entry to the market.[67]

Legality of Authorized Generics

The policy debate concerning authorized generics has been accompanied by legal challenges before the FDA and the courts concerning this practice. Opponents of authorized generics have contended that the Hatch-Waxman Act's generic exclusivity provisions should be understood as excluding authorized generics from the marketplace for the 180-day period.[68] The FDA has taken the opposite view, however, reasoning that the Hatch-Waxman Act does not require a brand-name pharmaceutical company to file any sort of application in order to market the drug as an authorized generic.[69] In turn, the 180-day period of generic exclusivity provided by the Hatch-Waxman Act only applies to ANDA or § 505(b)(2) applications with paragraph IV certifications. As a result, the 180-day generic exclusivity period does not bar authorized generics from entering the market.

Two notable judicial opinions have upheld the FDA's position favoring authorized generics. In the first of these opinions, *Teva Pharmaceutical Industries, Ltd. v. Crawford*,[70] the Court of Appeals for the D.C. Circuit found no reasonable reading of the Hatch-Waxman Act that would allow authorized generics to be barred by the 180-day generic exclusivity period. In that case, independent generic manufacturer Teva had previously entered into an arrangement with Purepac Pharmaceutical Co., the first paragraph IV ANDA applicant with respect to the drug gabapentin. Teva and Purepac had agreed to share the 180-day generic exclusivity period. During that period, however, Pfizer sold its own authorized generic version of gabapentin, which was priced substantially below the price of its brand-name drug.[71]

Teva responded by petitioning the FDA to prohibit the marketing of authorized generic versions of gabapentin during the 180-day generic exclusivity period. Alternatively, Teva asserted that Pfizer should be required to file a supplemental NDA before selling an authorized generic.[72] According to Teva, the impact of the latter proposed ruling would lead to the same outcome as the first: Pfizer would be compelled to respect the 180-day generic exclusivity period established by the Hatch-Waxman Act.

The FDA denied the petition, resulting in a Teva lawsuit against the FDA. The district court confirmed the FDA's views, concluding that "[n]othing in the statute provides any support for the argument that the FDA can prohibit NDA holders from entering the market with [an authorized] generic drug during the exclusivity period."[73] Teva then appealed to the Court of Appeals for the D.C. Circuit, which affirmed.

Chief Judge Ginsburg began his opinion by observing that the Hatch-Waxman Act did not stipulate the manner in which the holder of an approved NDA must market its drug. Further, prior to the enactment of the Hatch-Waxman Act, nothing in the Food, Drug, and Cosmetic Act prevented the NDA holder from marketing an authorized generic. The D.C. Circuit thus saw the issue as whether it should "declare that a previously lawful practice became unlawful when the Congress passed a statute that said nothing about that practice."[74]

The Court of Appeals further rejected Teva's "functional" interpretation of the Hatch-Waxman Act. According to Teva, the practice of authorized generics had "developed only recently as a routine brand-name business strategy" and therefore had not been anticipated by Congress. Further, authorized generics practice severely diminished generic incentives to challenge pharmaceutical patents. According to Teva, then, "adhering to the 'literal' terms of the statute would lead to an absurd result, namely, that [the Hatch-Waxman Act] grants only a 'meaningless' exclusivity against subsequent ANDA filers rather than a 'commercially effective' exclusivity that runs against the NDA holder as well."[75]

The D.C. Circuit responded by reasoning that the balance between innovation and competition struck by the Hatch-Waxman Act was "quintessentially a matter for legislative judgment," such that "the court must attend closely to the terms in which the Congress expressed that judgment."[76] Here, Chief Judge Ginsburg reasoned, the statute was unambiguous. Although the Hatch-Waxman Act barred the approval of subsequent ANDAs for 180 days, the statutory language simply did not speak to marketing arrangements made by the holder of the approved NDA. The court of appeals further observed that, even in the event that an NDA holder authorized a generic, the 180-day exclusivity period continued to bar other firms from marketing a generic version of the drug. As a result, authorized generic practice hardly rendered the Hatch-Waxman Act's generic exclusivity provisions "meaningless."[77] In conclusion, because the Hatch-Waxman Act "clearly does not prohibit the holder of an approved NDA from marketing, during the 180-day exclusivity period, its own 'brand-generic' version of its drug," FDA practices concerning authorized generics were affirmed.[78]

A second judicial opinion, *Mylan Pharmaceuticals, Inc. v. U.S. Food and Drug Administration*,[79] also concluded that the Hatch-Waxman Act "does not grant the FDA the power to prohibit the marketing of authorized generics during the 180-day exclusivity period.... "[80] That case involved the pharmaceutical nitrofurantoin, which is used to treat urinary tract infections. When the FDA approved a paragraph IV ANDA filed by Mylan Pharmaceuticals, Inc, to sell nitrofurantoin, NDA holder Proctor & Gamble Pharmaceuticals, Inc., licensed a third party generic firm to sell an authorized generic version of the drug. Mylan reportedly lost sales of "tens of millions" of dollars due to this arrangement.[81]

Mylan challenged the FDA approval of authorized generics practice before the U.S. District Court for the Northern District of West Virginia. Mylan appealed the district court's dismissal of its case to the Court of Appeals for the Fourth Circuit, which affirmed. Citing the D.C. Circuit's decision in *Teva v. Crawford* with approval, the Fourth Circuit similarly concluded that the statute clearly defined the 180-day exclusivity period only with respect to other paragraph IV ANDAs, not to authorized generics.[82] The Fourth Circuit therefore concluded that "[a]lthough the introduction of an authorized generic may reduce the economic benefit of the 180 days of exclusivity awarded to the first paragraph IV ANDA applicant, § 355(j)(5)(B)(iv) gives no legal basis for the FDA to prohibit the encroachment of authorized generics on that exclusivity."[83] As a result, the district court's judgment was affirmed.

It is possible to criticize the statutory construction of both *Teva v. Crawford* and *Mylan v. FDA*. In particular, neither court of appeals stressed that the Hatch-Waxman Act describes the 180-day time frame as an "exclusivity period."[84] The term "exclusivity" might be viewed as a curious drafting choice in view of the ruling that generic firms must potentially compete alongside authorized generics during the 180-day period.

On the other hand, the notion of "shared exclusivity" that arose following the Medicare Modernization Act amendments may be viewed as codifying congressional intent that multiple generic applicants may enter the market during the 180-day marketing exclusivity period.[85] In addition, many prescription drugs are available in a number of different dosage forms and strengths. Under current Hatch-Waxman Act practice, each strength and dosage form is considered a separate drug product for which a distinct generic applicant can qualify for 180-day exclusivity.[86] As a result, the term "exclusivity" may be considered to have a particular meaning in the Hatch-Waxman Act—one that does not necessarily mean that independent generic firms will not face competition during the 180-day period even in the absence of authorized generics. Of course, these provisions may also impact the incentives that independent generic firms possess to challenge pharmaceutical patents.

In any event, *Teva v. Crawford* and *Mylan v. FDA* currently represent the law of the land. Absent further judicial developments or congressional activity, authorized generics will be judged as legitimate means for NDA holders to market their products under the Hatch-Waxman Act.[87]

Concluding Observations

Although Congress made significant amendments to the Hatch-Waxman Act as recently as 2003,[88] authorized generics were not subject to discussion at that time. The rise of this practice, as well as the vigor of the debate surrounding it, suggests both the pace of change within the industry and the prominence of the pharmaceutical industry within the national public health system.

As discussion of authorized generics continues, Congress may wish to have a sense of its legislative options. Should Congress conclude that authorized generics are appropriate, then it may simply take no action. The opinions of the D.C. and Fourth Circuits suggest that, as currently drafted, the Hatch-Waxman Act does not allow the FDA to restrict the ability of brand-name firms to sell or approve of authorized generics.[89] Absent legislative input, the FDA may be unlikely to alter its interpretation of the Hatch-Waxman Act in this respect in the future.

Alternatively, Congress could simply disallow authorized generics practice. In the 112th Congress, H.R. 741 and S. 373 would prohibit NDA holders from manufacturing, marketing, selling, or distributing an authorized generic drug. The term "authorized generic drug" was defined as "any version of a listed drug ... that the holder of new drug application ... seeks to commence marketing, selling, or distributing, directly or indirectly, after receipt of a notice" that an ANDA has been filed.[90] Drugs marketed by firms eligible for the 180-day generic exclusivity, or that were sold by anyone after that exclusivity has expired, were not considered to be authorized generic drugs. This legislation has not yet been enacted.

Another option is to require brand-name firms to file a supplemental NDA, or a similar application, with the FDA when they market authorized generics.[91] This filing would then place the brand-name firm in the same category as generic applicants who did not qualify as the first to file. In turn, the 180-day generic exclusivity period would then apply against the authorized generic.

Notably, whether the 180-day generic exclusivity period strikes an appropriate balance between encouraging patent challenges and ensuring prompt access to generic medications is itself a contested proposition within the pharmaceutical industry.[92] Discussion of the authorized generics issue may also prompt further reflection on the basic structure of incentives within the Hatch-Waxman Act.

Current interest in authorized generics reflects long-standing congressional concern for the appropriate balance between innovation and competition within the pharmaceutical industry. Although academic inquiry into authorized generics practice remains in its early phases, it is notable that knowledgeable commentators have reached disparate views of the benefits or detriments of this practice. Some observers stress that authorized generics benefit consumers by providing enhanced access to lower-cost alternatives to branded drugs, while others express concerns that authorized generics will defeat the incentives that independent generic firms possess to challenge pharmaceutical patents. Future studies may shed additional light on the impact of authorized generics upon consumer welfare.

End Notes

[1] See Thomas Chen, "Authorized Generics: A Prescription for Hatch-Waxman Reform," 93 *Virginia Law Review* (2007), 459; Saami Zain, "Sword or Shield? An Overview and Competitive Analysis of the Marketing of 'Authorized Generics'," 62 *Food & Drug Law Journal* (2007), 739.

[2] See Leila Abboud, "'Authorized Generics' Duel Grows," *Wall Street Journal* (March 25, 2004); Leila Abboud, "Drug Makers Use New Tactic to Ding Generic-Drug Firms," *Wall Street Journal* (January 27, 2004).

[3] See "Blockbuster Drugs with Expiring Patents Gain New Hope: Generic Drugs," *Drug Week* 352 (April 15, 2005).

[4] Stephen Barlas, "'Authorized' Generics May Pose Unauthorized Problems: Government Worries About Potential Brand-Name Blocking Technique," 30 *Pharmacy and Therapeutics* no.8 (2005), 435.

[5] See Michelle L. Kirsche, "Despite Challenges, Generics Dispensing is on the Rise," 27 *Drug Store News* no. 4 at20 (March 21, 2005).

[6] P.L. 84-417, 98 Stat. 1585 (1984).

[7] See, e.g., Laura J. Robinson, "Analysis of Recent Proposals to Reconfigure Hatch-Waxman," 11 *Journal of Intellectual Property Law* (2003), 47.

[8] CRS Report RS22946, *Food and Drug Administration (FDA): Overview and Issues*, by Erin D. Williams.

[9] See G. Lee Skillington and Eric M. Solovy, "The Protection of Test and Other Data Required by Article 39.3 of the TRIPS Agreement," 24 *Northwestern Journal of International Law and Business* (2003), 1.

[10] See Alfred B. Engelberg, "Special Patent Provisions for Pharmaceuticals: Have They Outlived Their Usefulness?," 39 *IDEA: Journal of Law and Technology* (1999), 389.

[11] See James J. Wheaton, "Generic Competition and Pharmaceutical Innovation: The Drug Price Competition and Patent Term Restoration Act of 1984," 34 *Catholic University Law Review* (1986), 433.

[12] See Kristin E. Behrendt, "The Hatch-Waxman Act: Balancing Competing Interest or Survival of the Fittest?," 57*Food and Drug Law Journal* (2002), 247.

[13] *Id.*

[14] See, e.g., Justina A. Molzon, "The Generic Drug Approval Process," 5 *Journal of Pharmacy and Law* (1996), 275 ("The Act streamlined the approval process by eliminating the need for [generic drug] sponsors to repeat duplicative, unnecessary, expensive and ethically questionable clinical and animal research to demonstrate the safety and efficacy of the drug product.").

[15] See Jonathan M. Lave, "Responding to Patent Litigation Settlements: Does the FTC Have It Right Yet?," 64 *University of Pittsburgh Law Review* (2002), 201 ("Hatch-Waxman has also increased the generic drug share of prescription drug volume by almost 130% since its enactment in 1984. Indeed, nearly 100% of the top selling drugs with expired patents have generic versions available today versus only 35% in 1983.").

[16] Natalie M. Derzko, "A Local and Comparative Analysis of the Experimental Use Exception—Is Harmonization Appropriate?," 44 *IDEA: Journal of Law and Technology* (2003), 1.

[17] See, e.g., Sarah E. Eurek, "Hatch-Waxman Reform and Accelerated Entry of Generic Drugs: Is Faster Necessarily Better?," 2003 *Duke Law and Technology Review* (August 13, 2003), 18.

[18] 35 U.S.C. § 156(b) (2004).

[19] 35 U.S.C. § 156(b)(1) (2004).

[20] CRS Report RL32377, *The Hatch-Waxman Act: Legislative Changes Affecting Pharmaceutical Patents*, by Wendy H. Schacht and John R. Thomas.

[21] Patents, which are administered by the United States Patent and Trademark Office (USPTO), provide their owner with the ability to exclude others from making, using, selling, offering to sell or importing into the United States the patented invention. 35 U.S.C. § 271(a) (2004). The term of the patent is ordinarily set at twenty years from the date the patent application was filed, 35 U.S.C. § 154 (2004), although pharmaceutical patents may be extended in order to compensate for a portion of the patent term that was lost during FDA marketing approval procedures. 35 U.S.C. § 156 (2004). Patent proprietors are permitted to file a civil suit in federal court in order to enjoin infringers and obtain monetary damages. 35 U.S.C. § 281 (2004). Although issued patents enjoy a presumption of validity, accused infringers may assert that the patent is invalid or unenforceable on a number of grounds. 35 U.S.C. § 282 (2004).

[22] 21 U.S.C. § 355(c)(2) (2004).

[23] See, e.g., Jacob S. Wharton, "'Orange Book' Listing of Patents Under the Hatch-Waxman Act," 47 *St. Louis University Law Journal* (2003), 1027.

[24] 21 U.S.C. § 355(j)(2)(A)(vii) (2004).

[25] See Douglas A. Robinson, "Recent Administrative Reforms of the Hatch-Waxman Act: Lower Prices Now In Exchange for Less Pharmaceutical Innovation Later?," 81 *Washington University Law Quarterly* (2003), 829.

[26] 21 U.S.C. § 355(j)(5)(B)(i) (2004).

[27] 21 U.S.C. § 355(j)(5)(B)(ii) (2004).

[28] Eli Lilly and Co. v. Medtronic, Inc., 496 U.S. 1047, 15 USPQ2d 1121 (1990).

[29] 21 U.S.C. § 355(j)(2)(B)(i) (2004).

[30] 21 C.F.R. § 314.94(a)(12)(viii)(C)(1)(i) (2006).

[31] Although patents enjoy a presumption of validity, 35 U.S.C. § 282 (2004), that presumption is not uncontestable. Accused infringers may demonstrate that the patent does not meet the standards established by the Patent Act, and as a result should not have been issued by the U.S. Patent and Trademark Office. *Id.* In addition, an accused infringer may demonstrate that the patent is unenforceable on a number of grounds, among that its owner has engaged in "misuse" of the patent. *Id.*

[32] 21 U.S.C. §355(j)(5)(B)(iv) (2004).

[33] U.S. Dept. of Health and Human Services., Food and Drug Admin., Center for Drug Evaluation and Research, *Guidance of Industry, Listed Drugs, 30-Month Stays, and Approval of ANDAs and 505(b)(2) Applications Under Hatch-Waxman, As Modified by the Medicare Prescription Drug, Improvement, and Modernization Act of 2003*, at 5 n.14 (October 2004).

[34] See, e.g., Valerie Junod, "Drug Marketing Exclusivity Under United States and European Union Law," 59 *Food and Drug Law Journal* (2004), 479; Gerry J. Elman, "FDA Approval of Generic Drugs: Instituting a First Successful Defense Requirement for Generic Exclusivity," 22 *Biotechnology Law Reporter* 97 (April 2003);

Frederick Tong, "Widening the Bottleneck of Pharmaceutical Patent Exclusivity," 24 *Whittier Law Review* (2003), 775.

[35] See Michael Bobelian, "1984 Act Led to a Boom in Prescription Drug Litigation," 231 *New York Law Journal* 1, col.3 (May 24, 2004).

[36] P.L. 108-173, 117 Stat. 2066 (2003).

[37] 21 U.S.C. §355(j)(5)(B)(iv)(I) (2004).

[38] 21 U.S.C. §355(j)(5)(B)(iv)(II)(bb) (2004).

[39] Mova Pharm. Corp. v. Shalala, 140 F.3d 1060, 1064 (D.C. Cir. 1998).

[40] See generally Joseph Scott Miller, "Building a Better Bounty: Litigation-Stage Rewards for Defeating Patents," 19 *Berkeley Technology Law Journal* (2004), 667.

[41] See Leila Abboud, "'Authorized Generics' Duel Grows," *Wall Street Journal* (March 25, 2004); Leila Abboud, "Drug Makers Use New Tactic to Ding Generic-Drug Firms," *Wall Street Journal* (January 27, 2004).

[42] See John Schmeltzer, "Upscale Generics Make Gains: 'Private Label' Items Battling Brand Names," *Montgomery County Herald* (May 19, 2006).

[43] "As brand-generic alliances grow, opponents cry foul," *Drug Store News* (August 23, 2004).

[44] Sanda Levy, "Why authorized generics are making a comeback," *Drug Topics: The Online Newspaper for Pharmacists*, available at http://www.drugtopics.com/drugtopics/article/ articleDetail.jsp?id=111159.

[45] *Id.*

[46] *Id.*

[47] See Andrew Humphries and Nick D'Amore, "Generic Deluge: As U.S. Regulators Receive a Record Number of Generic Drug Applications, Pharmaceutical Companies Continue to Align With or Combat Generic Competition," 24 *Med Ad News* no. 11 (November 1, 2005), 1.

[48] See Beth Understahl, "Authorized Generics: Careful Balance Undone," 16 *Fordham Intellectual Property, Media, and Entertainment Law Journal* (Autumn 2005), 355.

[49] *Id.*

[50] See Tara Croft, "Building Teva," *Daily Deal* (October 25, 2004).

[51] See James Richie, "Prasco's market share Rx: authorized generic drugs: Firm helps pharmaceutical companies retain profits," *Cincinnati Business Courier* (February 6, 2006).

[52] Tony Pugh, "Drug companies battle generics with their own copies," *Duluth News-Tribune* (April 30, 2006).

[53] See Understahl, *supra* note 48.

[54] Tony Pugh, "Loophole may dampen generic-drug boom," *San Jose Mercury News* (May 3, 2006), A1.

[55] David A. Balto, "We'll Sell Generics Too: Innovator drug makers are gaming the regulatory system and harming competition," 39 *Legal Times* no. 12 (March 20, 2006).

[56] See Jenna Greene, "The Drug Industry Has Figured Out a Way to Best Generic Competition, and Pharmaceutical Patent Litigation Could Free-Fall," 183 *New Jersey Law Journal* (January 23, 2006), 217.

[57] See Pugh, *supra* note 54.

[58] See Narinder Banait, "Authorized Generics: Antitrust Issues and the Hatch-Waxman Act," Mondaq (November 4, 2005).

[59] Morton I. Kamien and Israel Zang, "Virtual Patent Extension by Cannibalization," *Southern Economic Journal*, July1999.

[60] U.S. Food and Drug Administration, *FDA Supports Broader Access to Lower Priced Drugs*, FDA Talk Paper, July 2, 2004. A study prepared by IMS Consulting for the Pharmaceutical Research and Manufacturers of America reached a similar conclusion, determining that the average price discount to brand-name drugs during the 180-day exclusivity period is greater when an authorized generic has been marketed than when one has not. IMS Consulting, *Assessment of Authorized Generics in the U.S.* (Spring 2006), available at http://www. phrma.org/files/IMS%20Authorized%20Generics%20Report_6-22-06.pdf.

[61] Federal Trade Commission, *Authorized Generics: An Interim Report* (June 2009).

[62] Kathleen Kerr, "Prescription Hurdles: Need Brand-Name Drug? Generic May Come First," *Newsday* (March 16, 2006), B13.

[63] Jon Hess and Elio Evangelista, *Authorized Generics: Lifecycle Management's Compromise in the Patent Wars* (Cutting Edge Information, August 23, 2005), 4.

[64] *Id.*

[65] See James Bessen and Michael J. Meurer, "Lessons for Patent Policy from Empirical Research on Patent Litigation," 9 *Lewis and Clark Law Review* 1 (2005).

[66] Christopher Worrell, *Authorized Generics*, presentation given at The 5th Generic Drugs Summit, September 27-29,2004, and David Reiffen and Michael R. Ward, *"Branded Generics" as a Strategy to Limit Cannibalization of Pharmaceutical Markets*, May 2005, 2-4 available at http://www.uta.edu/faculty/mikeward/branded generics.pdf.

[67] See Federal Trade Commission, *FTC Report Examines How Authorized Generics Affect the Pharmaceutical Market* (Aug. 31, 2011), available at http://www.ftc.gov/opa/2011/08/ genericdrugs.shtm).

[68] See Generic Pharmaceutical Association, *Comment in Support of Citizen Petition Docket No. 2004P-0075/CP1* (May 21, 2004), available at http://www.fda.gov/ohrms/dockets/dailys/04/ June04/060404/04p-0075-c00003-vol1.pdf.

[69] See M. Howard Morse and Richard E. Coe, "Authorized Generics Are Good for You: Competition from drug pioneers shouldn't trouble the FTC," 29 *Legal Times* no. 15 (April 10, 2006).

[70] 410 F.3d 51 (D.C. Cir. 2005).

[71] *Id.* at 52.

[72] *Id.* at 52-53.

[73] Teva Pharm. Indus. v. FDA, 355 F.Supp.2d 111, 117 (D.D.C. 2004).

[74] 410 F.3d at 53.

[75] *Id.* at 54.

[76] *Id.*

[77] *Id.*

[78] *Id.* at 55.

[79] 454 F.3d 270 (4th Cir. 2006).

[80] *Id.* at 271.

[81] *Id.* at 273.

[82] *Id.* at 275.

[83] *Id.* at 276

[84] 21 U.S.C. § 355(j)(5)(B)(iv) (2004).

[85] See *supra* notes 36-38 and accompanying text.

[86] See Apotex, Inc. v. FDA, 414 F. Supp. 2d 61, 64 (D.D.C. 2006).

[87] See generally Thomas P. Noud and Paul T. Meiklejohn, "The Developing Law of Pharmaceutical Patent Enforcement," 87 *Journal of the Patent and Trademark Office Society* (2005), 921.

[88] Medicare Modernization and Improvement Act, P.L. 108-173, 117 Stat. 2066 (2003).

[89] See *supra* notes 68-81 and accompanying text.

[90] H.R. 573, § 1.

[91] This option is essentially the same as the one that Teva unsuccessfully argued before the Court of Appeals for the District of Columbia Circuit in the *Teva v. Crawford* case. See *supra* note 70 and accompanying text.

[92] Letter of Robert A. Armitage, Eli Lilly and Company, Re: Authorized Generic Study (June 5, 2006), available at http://www.ftc.gov/os/comments/genericdrugstudy3/060605lilly.pdf.

INDEX

M

N

O

P

Q

R

S